THE COMPLETE
HOMEOPATHIC RESOURCE
FOR COMMON ILLNESSES

THE
COMPLETE
HOMEOPATHIC
RESOURCE
—for—
COMMON
ILLNESSES

Dennis K. Chernin, M.D., M.P.H.

North Atlantic Books
Berkeley, California

Homeopathic Educational Services
Berkeley, California

Published by   and
North Atlantic Books   Homeopathic Educational Services
P.O. Box 12327   2124 Kittredge Street
Berkeley, California 94712   Berkeley, California 94704

Cover and book design © Ayelet Maida, A/M Studios
Printed in the United States of America

The Complete Homeopathic Resource for Common Illnesses is sponsored by the Society for the Study of Native Arts and Sciences, a nonprofit educational corporation whose goals are to develop an educational and cross-cultural perspective linking various scientific, social, and artistic fields; to nurture a holistic view of arts, sciences, humanities, and healing; and to publish and distribute literature on the relationship of mind, body, and nature.

North Atlantic Books' publications are available through most bookstores. For further information, call 800-337-2665 or visit our website at www.northatlanticbooks.com.

Substantial discounts on bulk quantities are available to corporations, professional associations, and other organizations. For details and discount information, contact our special sales department.

Library of Congress Cataloging-in-Publication Data
Chernin, Dennis, 1949–
The complete homeopathic resource for common illnesses / by Dennis Chernin.
   p. cm.
Includes bibliographical references.
ISBN-13: 978-1-55643-608-6 (trade paper)
ISBN-10: 1-55643-608-4 (trade paper)
1. Homeopathy—Materia medica and therapeutics I. Title.
RX601.C44 2006
615.5'32—dc22
                                        2006009464
1 2 3 4 5 6 7 8 9 UNITED 12 11 10 09 08 07 06

Contents

Preface

Looking back at my medical school experience at the University of Michigan, I remember hearing the word *homeopathic* only once. I believe it was when one of my internal medicine professors talked about the small amount of replacement thyroid hormone needed for someone whose thyroid had been irradiated (and destroyed) as a treatment for Graves' disease, a form of hyperthyroidism. He referred to this minute amount as a "homeopathic dosage." Despite using this term, I'm virtually certain he had no idea what homeopathy really was. At the time, I wondered what he meant, but quickly moved on as I was trying to absorb the volumes of information coming my way. Little did I know that I would later spend so much of my life studying, contemplating, absorbing, and practicing this absolutely fascinating, therapeutic system of medicine.

My first exposure to homeopathy came in 1975, when I was studying meditation and yoga with an American trained psychologist and meditation teacher, Swami Ajaya. I was doing a residency in psychiatry at the University of Wisconsin and he introduced me to the work of his teacher, Swami Rama, and to one of his fellow students, Rudolph Ballentine, M.D. They were living and practicing holistic medicine in the Chicago area, incorporating conventional medicine with the complementary approaches of nutrition, yogic therapies, meditation, psychotherapy, Ayurveda (traditional medicine in India), and homeopathy. Their work was brilliant, unique, and inspiring.

Swami Rama invited my wife, Jan, and me to study with him at the Himalayan Institute and to work in Dr. Ballentine's medical clinic, the Center for Holistic Medicine. Our one-year commitment turned into a four-year stay that included the birth of two of our four children, two years of supervised training in homeopathy, and two years of helping teach many other young physicians the art and science of homeopathy. In the mid-'70s, there were only a few living homeopaths in the U.S. and these people were bridges to the great physicians of homeopathy's golden years. We were fortunate to study and learn from these elder statesmen, including Drs. Rood, Panos, Sutherland, White, Williams, and Rodgers.

During this period, the doctors and staff would have weekly clinics to discuss difficult cases with Swami Rama, himself an experienced Indian trained homeopath (and accomplished yogi), seeing many patients in a short time. We would all share huge Indian lunches, teach classes, and meditate in the evening together. We were a community brought together with a common goal of healing, study, and meditation. This was a time of tremendous growth and learning, challenging and fun.

Moving with my family to Ann Arbor, Michigan in 1981, I set up a solo medical practice, using and refining the modalities I had studied at the Himalayan Institute. In 1987, we bought two beautiful Victorian homes and moved these buildings three miles from downtown Ann Arbor, restoring and connecting them together. In this setting, we created a truly complementary and holistic medical center. I continue to treat patients there and to teach interested doctors, health care practitioners, medical students, and laypeople about homeopathy.

In 1996, an engineer from Minneapolis, Kurt Swanson, asked me to write the information for a software program on homeopathy. Because I had already co-written one book about homeopathy *(Homeopathic Remedies for Health Professionals and Laypeople)* and another on holistic medicine that included a chapter on homeopathy *(Health: A Holistic Approach),* I thought creating a CD on homeopathy would present an interesting new challenge. After a year of hard work, we finished the program and won an award as the best new software program of 1997.

Many patients, colleagues, and friends, especially those with Apple computers and others who don't especially like using computers, have suggested over the past few years that I write a book containing the same information in the CD. This book is in response to these suggestions.

Acknowledgments

I would like to thank several people who have helped and studied with me on my thirty-year homeopathic odyssey. Swami Rama, who died in 1996, initiated me into this science and for this I am extremely grateful. Rudolph Ballentine, M.D., helped me get started and encouraged me to be precise and at the same time to think creatively. Several fellow homeopathic physician colleagues who studied with me in those early years still remain good friends and confidants: Greg Manteuffel, Rick Frires, Jerry Gore, Dale Buegel, and Barb Bova. Kurt and Carla Swanson were instrumental in helping to compile and edit the original information on homeopathy for the CD.

I also want to thank Dana Ullman, M.P.H., for his encouragement and help in editing and revising this book. He also allowed me to use several of his writings and references in Chapter 4 on scientific research as well as in the Resources section at the end of the book. And I really appreciate Homeopathic Educational Services for co-publishing this book and CD with North Atlantic Books.

Finally, I want to thank my family whom I love dearly and who make my life so complete. My wife, Jan, still amazes me when out of the blue she'll suggest a specific remedy (and one that is usually right on target) for an ailing friend or colleague. My children Abe, Ethan, and Ari are wonderful people whose great senses of humor about their slightly alternative father constantly bring a smile and a laugh to all of us.

Introduction

Disease generally falls into three categories—acute, acute exacerbations of chronic illness, and chronic illness. While homeopathic remedies can be used to treat all categories, or levels, of disease, this book and accompanying CD are generally oriented toward the former two. Treatment of chronic illness with homeopathy is somewhat more complex because the practitioner needs to take into account factors such as family history including genetic predispositions (what homeopaths call "miasms"), old accidents, suppressed illnesses, and the long-term effects of medication. While I touch upon some of the remedies used in chronic problems, it is really beyond the scope of this book to delve deeply into this complex area of disease treatment.

This book and CD teach the principles and concepts of homeopathy in great detail. Using the book, or CD, or both, readers can select a remedy for their family's health concern. Physicians and health care practitioners will find this book quite helpful as well, especially those who are beginning a homeopathic practice. It should be remembered, however, that this is not a substitute for professional advice—laypeople should always consult their health care provider for problems that are serious or persistent.

This book is divided into chapters: (1) the basics of homeopathy, introducing homeopathic theory and definitions; (2) the Clinical Repertory portion, covering common illnesses and their homeopathic treatments; (3) an overview of the different modules of the CD, corresponding to the content of the book, and how to use the CD; and (4) a summary of scientific study about homeopathy. The CD, from which this book was taken, includes a materia medica and a repertory. The Materia Medica (in Latin, "materials of medicine") module covers the various homeopathic medicines and their symptom pictures and applications. If included in this book, it would be a massive section of many hundreds of pages; I believe readers can more easily review the remedies by studying the CD. The Repertory module, essentially an index to the Materia Medica, containing a listing of symptoms and homeopathic remedies that can be used to treat the symptoms, also is not included in this book because it is designed as an interactive resource on the CD; it simply does not translate into usable book form.

In Chapter 1, we explore the definition and history of homeopathy, the basic laws of homeopathy, homeopathic and allopathic views of health and disease, the concept of the vital force, and susceptibility to disease. Basic facts are detailed as well as home prescribing approaches, how to prepare the remedies, and a comparison to standard medicines. Readers also learn how to choose the correct remedy, its dosage (potency), and when to repeat or change the remedy selection.

Chapter 2, Common Illnesses and Their Homeopathic Treatment, is the Clinical Repertory listing of many illnesses or conditions with the remedies that can be used to help each one. For each remedy, there is a description of associated symptoms. From the remedy options, a home prescriber may be able to choose which remedy best matches the person's illness. Using some thirty years of experience in practicing homeopathy, I created the Clinical Repertory in this book and CD. The conditions covered in the Clinical Repertory were determined by the conditions I have successfully treated with homeopathy in the past and by the types of problems encountered most frequently in my practice.

Chapter 3 covers in some depth the definitions and practical applications of the Clinical Repertory, as well as the other modules on the CD (the Materia Medica and the Repertory). This chapter helps readers understand how to use the CD most effectively.

In the fourth chapter, readers can find summary descriptions of the scientific research that supports the modern interest in homeopathy. We look at early research, meta-analysis studies, double-blind and placebo-controlled clinical studies, clinical outcomes studies, and laboratory studies.

Finally, in the Resources section, the last "chapter" in the book, are helpful lists of books on homeopathy, research, organizations involved with homeopathy, and Internet sites for further inquiry.

Homeopathy is a wonderful, effective, and fascinating system of medical care. This book and CD are great tools and offer clear and concise guidance on your journey toward improved health and well-being. This book will teach you how to treat many common acute ailments so that you do not have to resort to conventional drugs, which may be effective in eliminating your symptoms, but which do so by suppressing your body's immune and defense system. You and your family deserve safe treatments that help heal both your body and mind.

CHAPTER 1

What Is Homeopathy?

DEFINITION AND HISTORY

Homeopathy is a system for prescribing medicinal substances according to the *law of similars*. This law states that the appropriate medicine for a sick individual is a substance that would create a similar set of symptoms if administered to a healthy person. In other words, substances that could produce symptoms when given to a healthy person can, with proper preparation, be used to treat sick people with those same symptoms. The word *homeopathy* is derived from the Greek roots *homoios,* which means "similar or like treatment," and *pathos,* which means "of disease." Thus, the word means "like treatment of disease."

The roots of the law of similars are ancient, having been described in the treatises of Hippocrates in Greece and by the Ayurvedic physicians in ancient India. Paracelsus, a fifteenth-century European physician, referred to the principle underlying the law of similars in his discussion of the doctrine of signatures when he stated: "You bring together the same anatomy of the herbs and the same anatomy of the illness into one order. This simile gives you understanding of the way in which you shall heal."[1]

Practiced throughout the world for almost 200 years, homeopathy was rediscovered in the early 1800s by the great German physician, Samuel Hahnemann (1755–1843). Today homeopathy is widely practiced in North America, India, Mexico, South America, Germany, France, Great Britain, Russia, and other European countries. Homeopathy was first introduced in the United States in 1825, and the American Institute of Homeopathy, the first national medical association, was founded in 1844. (The second major medical association was the American Medical Association, founded in 1847.) In the late 1800s and early 1900s, many homeopathic hospitals and twenty-two homeopathic medical schools existed in this country, including the University of Michigan in Ann Arbor and four medical schools in Chicago.

Presently, there are no homeopathic medical schools in the United States. Instead, people attend one of the many homeopathic schools and training programs, most of which offer two- to four-year courses and some of which provide distance learning education (see pages 422–427 for a list of some of the educational opportunities in the U.S. and Canada).

There are many homeopathic medical schools in the world, including those in India and Mexico. In France, homeopathy is taught in several medical and pharmacy schools such as those in Bordeaux, Marseilles, Paris-Nord, and Lyon. Almost all pharmacies in France carry homeopathic remedies and 30 to 40 percent of the French population use homeopathy. In the United States, an increasing number of pharmacies now carry remedies.

LAW OF SIMILARS

Samuel Hahnemann, a practicing physician, became disillusioned by the dangers of existing therapies, such as the use of toxic doses of mercury for many ailments and the practices of bloodletting and blood leeching. He turned to studying the pharmacology and healing principles of ancient and indigenous medical systems. In his studies, Hahnemann became interested in the curative effect that quinine had in the treatment of malaria. He experimented with quinine by ingesting small amounts over a period of time and eventually developed many of the symptoms of malaria. His conclusion was that quinine could cure malaria because it could create the typical symptoms of this particular disease when given to a healthy person. Thus, Hahnemann rediscovered the law of similars.

In light of this discovery, Hahnemann began a systematic study of many commonly known medicinal substances. He administered very small amounts of these substances to himself and other healthy volunteers over an extended period of time, and carefully noted the symptoms that developed. This process of verifying the medicinal properties of these various substances is called "proving the medicine" and is derived from the German word *prüfung,* meaning "test." Through this work, a vast amount of knowledge was collected regarding the symptoms that these medicinal substances could produce in healthy people. According to the law of similars, one of these medicines could thus be administered and result in a curative effect in a sick person with a similar set of symptoms.

Conventional allopathic medicine, which uses drugs to treat sick people and is the dominant system practiced in the United States, also has treatments based on the law of similars. Immunizations use very small amounts of viruses, bacteria, or toxins to stimulate an individual's immune system. This produces antibodies that protect the person from the same infection normally caused by the injected substance.

Another standard practice in modern drug therapy that follows the homeopathic law of similars is allergy treatment. Giving people very small amounts of an allergen (dust, pollen, dander, and so on) often helps to desensitize them to the same substance. When these people come in contact with the allergen, their allergic reaction to it may then be lessened or eliminated.

HOMEOPATHIC VIEW OF DISEASE

An understanding of the concepts of health and disease from a homeopathic perspective is fundamental to comprehending the law of similars. The relationship of health versus disease can best be understood by examining the interaction of people and their environment. The nervous system, endocrine system, and immune system initiate and control the body's response to environmental pressures. These pressures may include internal or external factors such as inherited genetic weakness, emotional stress, mental or physical strain, injuries, environmental pollutants, bacteria and viruses, or nutritional deficiencies. If a person's adaptive powers are strong enough to withstand the disruptive effect of these influences, health prevails. On the other hand, disease results if pressures stress the individual's adaptive powers beyond his or her ability to cope.

Whether successful or not in the attempt to adapt, the body always strives for health. Consequently, a sick person's symptoms represent an attempt to overcome internal and external stresses and stimuli in an effort to re-establish health. The symptoms are not the result of these stimuli, but rather an expression of the body and mind's reaction to the stimuli.

Though people vary tremendously in their ability to adapt to stress in the environment, the homeopathic prescriber is concerned with all factors associated with the onset of a person's health problems. Characteristics such as oversensitivity, insecurity, lack of self-confidence, or laziness are important in understanding a person's illness and in choosing the correct remedy. Illnesses often date back to events that resulted in grief, worry, disappointment in love, or childhood feelings of neglect or abandonment.

Homeopathic philosophy contends that from birth until death the individual is reacting to his or her environment in the most intelligent way possible. A vital healing force is always moving in the direction of greater overall balance for the whole person, and this healing force is clearly expressed in every mental, emotional, and physical symptom. The symptoms of an illness clearly express this intelligence at work attempting to re-establish a state of health. In this context, a fever or nasal discharge represents the body's attempt to fight infection, and giving a medicinal substance that encourages the immune reaction should generally help this immune response. This is precisely what the homeopathic remedy does, working to stimulate the body in a similar way and in the same direction as the person's own response to illness.

The homeopathic prescriber obtains information about the cause of disease by studying the body's reaction to it. This reaction is depicted by symptoms such as fever, cough, diarrhea, or pain. Based on the law of similars, a remedy is chosen to reinforce the symptoms that are representative of the mind and body attempting to heal itself.

Not only can homeopathic remedies treat disease; they can also prevent it. Even if there is no specific diagnosis of the group of symptoms and all diagnostic study results are within the normal range, homeopathic treatment is possible. This is because the symptom complex accurately expresses the forces of the disease process. Signals or sensations of illness may appear long before actual tissue damage takes place. By administering the appropriate homeopathic remedy, a disease process may be halted before it progresses to pathological changes. In this respect, homeopathy can be a *preventive* medical system.

For example, conventional allopathic doctors generally disregard the liver as being the source of illness unless liver enzymes are elevated. Only when these blood-test changes occur, or when X-ray, ultrasonic scan, or biopsy prove pathological destruction, will medicine be given. Even then, few drugs are considered effective in such liver diseases as hepatitis or cirrhosis. The homeopath, on the other hand, recognizes that certain changes in mind and body are signs of underlying liver dysfunction. Even if the liver enzymes are normal, symptoms such as a heavily coated tongue, vague abdominal pain in the upper right side, sluggishness in the morning, and a melancholy mood or hypochondriasis all suggest liver dysfunction. The homeopathic physician prescribes a remedy based upon the totality of these symptoms so that liver function can return to normal. In this way, symptoms are eliminated and potential diseases are prevented. Similarly, other vague or poorly treated illnesses, such as viral infections or allergies, respond well to homeopathy, using the symptoms produced by the mind and body as a guide to prescribing.

It is fundamental in homeopathy to view the symptoms of an illness as a curative response by the entire organism. This means that, despite the presence of symptoms in various parts of the body such as the skin, lungs, or joints, there is nevertheless only one illness present. Each symptom is related to another, forming a single condition. In homeopathic treatment, the one medicine that can produce the entire constellation of symptoms in a healthy person is administered to cure the ailing person.

HOMEOPATHIC VIEW OF HEALTH

Homeopathic philosophy views health as a dynamic ongoing process in which a person constantly meets challenges in a positive way. Health is not simply the absence of disease, but represents the person's constant adaptation to internal and external stresses. From this perspective, a person with a chronic illness such as arthritis, who continually strives to have a positive attitude and takes responsibility for doing appropriate joint loosening exercises, may be healthier than a person who is pain free but is stubborn, constantly angry, or hypercritical.

Emotional health is characterized by a person who feels and experiences the full gamut of human feelings—love, anger, jealousy, compassion, and sadness. The emotionally healthy individual does not become overwhelmed by these feelings, does not feel enslaved by emotions, and does not dwell or brood on negative thoughts. Mental health is characterized by calmness, courage, patience, clarity of thinking, and creativity. Even after disappointment or loss of a loved one, emotionally healthy people are able to adjust to new life circumstances with reserves of strength.

LAW OF PROVING

The *law of proving* is the systematic verification of the law of similars. During the proving of a substance, healthy people take a remedy over a certain period of time and report any symptoms or sensations that represent a change from their normal state of health. When the symptoms are found to be common to a specified proportion of experimenters, they are considered the "proving" of that remedy. Hahnemann stated:

> There is . . . no other possible way in which the peculiar effects of medicines on the health of individuals can be accurately ascertained—there is no sure, no more natural way of accomplishing this object, than to administer the . . . medicine experimentally, in moderate doses, to healthy persons, in order to ascertain which changes, symptoms, and signs of their influence each individually produces on the health of the body and of the mind.[2]

Approximately 1,500 different remedies have been proven over the years. Plants, minerals, and extracts from animals, such as snake or bee venom, are among the many agents used in the preparation of homeopathic remedies.

Proving a remedy involves the observation of the mental,

emotional, and physical symptoms peculiar to each medicinal substance. Food cravings and aversions, mood fluctuations, memory and concentration, sleep quality, and sensitivity to external stimuli such as weather—these are all carefully recorded, along with the areas of bodily discomfort and any factors that increase or decrease the discomfort. In the proving of a remedy, mental and emotional symptoms are often reflected in physical signs and symptoms. For example, the remedy *Sulphur* is associated with a personality that tends to be easily angered, argues about philosophical matters, and is quite irritable and disorganized. Physical symptoms correspond with those of the mental sphere; hence, the person's emotional volatility is shown in a red, flushed, "hot" appearance, with profuse sweat and skin eruptions. He or she is often haggard looking, disheveled, and dirty—qualities that correspond to mental disorganization.

The specific mind and body symptoms that each medicine is capable of producing during the proving have been collected and compiled in books called *materia medica*. Other books called *repertories,* which are compendiums of symptoms, listing the substances that cause each physical and psychological symptom in the provings, complement the materia medica.

This detailed knowledge of the symptoms caused by each medicinal substance provides for a high degree of specificity in prescribing for each individual. The importance of sharp selectivity in prescribing medicinal substances has been emphasized by the Nobel Prize–winning microbiologist René Dubos:

> It is obvious that the sharper the selectivity of a biologically active substance, the greater the probability that it will be innocuous for cells and functions other than the one for which it has been designed. In other words, a substance is more likely to be therapeutically useful if it acts almost uniquely against a structure or an activity peculiar to the organism or function to be affected.[3]

Two children who suffer with middle ear infection (otitis media) might provide an example of specificity in homeopathic prescribing. One child may appear extremely irritable and oversensitive and may be sweaty, thirsty, and susceptible to drafts, wishing to be well covered with blankets. The pain in the ear may be worse with cold applications and better from warmth. Homeopathically prepared *Hepar sulph* (calcium sulphide) produces these symptoms in a healthy person and would act curatively in this particular case. The other child may display a mild and weepy disposition, wanting to be held and comforted. Lack of perspiration, thirstlessness, and wanting to be uncovered and outside in the open air may be apparent. The ear pain may improve with cold packs and become worse from the application of heat. *Pulsatilla* (windflower) would be needed to cure this child while *Hepar sulph* would probably not help at all. The reaction of the vitality as expressed through perspiration pattern, thirst, and reaction to weather and temperature are totally opposite in these two children. The selection of the remedy that is most similar to the symptoms will lead to a rapid and lasting cure of the illness.

LAW OF POTENTIZATION

When Hahnemann first began treating people according to the law of similars, many of the medicines he used were potentially toxic substances such as mercury and arsenic. To prevent toxic reaction to these substances, they were sequentially diluted before being administered. Though toxicity was reduced by dilution, there was also a decrease in therapeutic effect. As a result of his extensive knowledge of ancient medicinal systems and practices, Hahnemann was aware of a method of increasing the activity of a medicinal solution by vigorously shaking it in its container, so he methodically shook his medicines after each dilution. He found that as the toxic properties were steadily reduced with each dilution, the therapeutic efficacy increased with the shaking—a seemingly paradoxical effect. This method of increasing therapeutic effect with each sequential dilution by shaking is known as *potentization.* The resulting product of potentization is referred to as a *microdilution* or *potency.* The potency of small amounts of medicinal substances is not novel, as is demonstrated in the case of thyroid hormone: free thyroid hormone in the human is one part per 10,000 million parts of blood plasma. Potentization also provides a means for releasing medicinal qualities from supposedly inert substances such as common table salt *(Natrum mur).*

In the actual preparation of the potentized medicine, one part of the medicine is either diluted with ninety-nine parts of alcohol and water solution or ground with ninety-nine parts of milk sugar (lactose). This mixture undergoes vigorous shaking (succussion) or grinding (trituration) to produce what is called a 1c potency. One part of this mixture is added to another ninety-nine parts of alcohol and water solution or lactose, and the shaking or grinding is repeated, resulting in a 2c potency. Potencies may range from 1c to 100,000c. If the dilutions are one part remedy to nine parts of either alcohol and water or lactose, this is called an "x" (decimal) potency rather than a "c" (centesimal) potency.

Potentization is controversial because, according to the laws of chemistry, by the time the 12c or 24x potency is reached, there are few if any molecules of the substance left in the solution. However, potencies such as 200x, 200c, or 1,000c are effective over a longer period of time, and thus require fewer doses than the 3x, 6x, or 6c preparations. Homeopaths speculate that the process of potentization liberates the energetic essence of the substance and that the solvent (alcohol and water solution or lactose) acts as a template or vehicle in which the energy of the medicine is imprinted and preserved. This concept of a template can be better understood in light of the effects that pressure has on ice crystallization of freezing water. The late Harvard physics department chairman, P. W. Bridgman, reported different crystallization patterns for water freezing at higher altitude than for water freezing at lower altitude. When the ice from the higher altitude was melted and refrozen at lower altitude, the crystallization pattern of the higher-altitude ice was maintained.[4] The effect of pressure on crystallization was demonstrable and indelible. Perhaps the homeopathic remedy exerts a similar effect on its solute.

Critics of homeopathy suggest that homeopathic medicines could only exert a placebo effect because the high dilutions do not contain measurable amounts of the medicinal substance. However, provings of homeopathic medicines using dilutions greater than 12c or 24x are a strong argument against this suggestion. It is unlikely that many different people would experience the same set of symptoms from a given medicine if the medicine were simply a placebo.[5]

VITAL FORCE

The concept of the *vital force* is integral to understanding homeo-pathic medicine. This concept helps explain the dynamics of how the potentized remedy interacts with the sick person to effect a cure. Vital force is not a biochemical entity. Rather, it is a bio-electrical energy that affects a human's mental and physical functioning. It is that quality which animates living organisms and constantly seeks homeostasis and health in an inherently intelligent way.

All aspects of nature, whether mineral, vegetable, or animal, also have underlying energy patterns. Homeopathic remedies are derived from these three kingdoms. The energy pattern or vital force of these remedies is enhanced by potentization and, when matched with the vital force of people, promotes a healing response.

Homeopathy maintains that the vital force permeates all levels of human existence—body, mind, and spirit—and is similar to the energy stimulated by acupuncture needles. People are viewed as a dynamic whole, with the vital force acting as the integrating factor. Healthy people have a particular quality or pattern to their vital force, but when they become sick this subtle energy is distorted. Even during illness, however, this healing force reacts in the most self-preserving manner, and its plan is clearly articulated through the symptom complex.

In homeopathy, energy qualities of the remedy (as revealed by the proving of the remedy) are matched with the unhealthy person's energy qualities (as revealed by physical, mental, and emotional symptoms). Through the law of similars, unhealthy people can be cured. Perhaps the similar vibratory qualities of the remedy and the sick person produce a harmonic resonance that helps to balance the person's vital force.[6]

Western medical science describes the defense mechanisms of the human organism as physiochemical phenomena. Antibodies, lym-phocytes, gamma globulin, and interferon are thought to somehow interact to protect and rid the body of internal or external disease agents. The factors that underlie their functioning, however, remain elusive. Homeopathic theory states that the vital force underlies these defense mechanisms. If the vital force is aligned, then the defenses maintain homeostasis; if the life force is disturbed, illness results.

Allopathic medicine acknowledges that disease can result from the defective functioning of "physiologic energy," which generates heat, enhances metabolism, and, along with enzymes, maintains important physiochemical reactions in the body. These latter energy reactions are responsible for transmission of nerve impulses and production of ATP or cellular energy from oxygen and glucose. However, allopathic medicine does not recognize that disease and disharmony can manifest on a subtler energy level. As a consequence, no treatment is directed toward eliminating illness that reflects these energy imbalances.

The energy referred to in homeopathy is more fundamental and subtle; it underlies the physiologic energy of the body. Without this deep energy, the biochemical reactions could not occur. Technology has not been developed to a sufficient degree to analyze this vital energy. We cannot assume, however, that the energy is not real. Two hundred years ago people would have scoffed at the idea of electrical energy, and not long ago the concept of nuclear energy seemed preposterous. As technology advanced, these energies were isolated, channeled, and reproduced with amazing rapidity and skill. Eastern medical traditions and a few branches of Western medicine have discovered that the underlying subtle energy is not only real, but is fundamental to health and disease. In time it may be recognized in traditional allopathic medicine. Perhaps the modern technologies of nuclear magnetic resonance (MRI), PET scanners, or electron spectrometry will someday be able to detect the energy described by homeopathy.

SUSCEPTIBILITY TO DISEASE

Homeopathic philosophy has long understood the importance of susceptibility to disease. Individuals are continuously exposed to bacteria and viruses but do not always get sick. People actually have potentially deadly bacteria growing in their bodies. This includes meningococcus in the naso-pharynx, which can cause severe meningitis, and pneumococcus in the bronchial tubes, which can cause pneumonia. What keeps people from getting these diseases is their underlying susceptibility and the ability of their immune system to maintain health.

This susceptibility or predisposition to illnesses can also help explain why certain people respond to loss of a loved one or a job with anger or extreme depression, while others feel sad yet continue to lead productive lives.

Homeopathic practitioners recognize that the underlying susceptibility to disease is based on such complex factors as hereditary predisposition, childhood experiences, emotional traumas, accidents, life habits, and psychological attitudes. All of these factors affect and interact with a person's immune and nervous systems to lower or increase susceptibility to disease. Homeopaths believe this interaction is coordinated in an intelligent, coherent way by the person's vital force. It is this underlying energy on which the homeopathic remedy acts. The remedy activates the vital force when the immune system and other psychophysiologic factors need stimulation, as in the case of colds, influenza, injuries, or depression. The homeopathic remedy also acts to reduce the activity of the immune or nervous system when they are overly stimulated, as in the case of allergies, rheumatoid arthritis, or anxiety.

HERING'S LAWS OF CURE

Constantine Hering (1800–1880) is considered the father of American homeopathy and was responsible for many valuable contributions to medicine. Based upon his observation of mental, emotional, and physical symptoms as a barometer of the overall health of a person, he was able to measure improvement or deterioration of health. Hering's *laws of cure* state the following:

- Healing moves from the deepest and most vital parts of the person (mental and emotional states, and vital organs such as the brain, heart, or kidneys) to the most superficial and least vital parts of the person (joints, extremities, skin).
- Healing moves from the upper parts of the body to the lower parts.

- As healing progresses, symptoms disappear in the reverse order of their appearance.

Let's look at these laws one at a time. Note, as you read the following, that the reverse of these laws is also true: Disease may progress from superficial and less vital body parts to deeper and more vital organs; disease may spread from the lower parts of the body to the upper parts. Hering's laws demonstrate that the nature of disease is not random or mysterious. Natural laws govern all forms of life, and health is no exception.

Healing moves from the most vital to least vital parts of the person.

The natural direction of cure is always outward or centrifugal, as the organism attempts to establish homeostasis by externalizing disease. Although a person may complain of one or several limiting physical complaints, there are often mental or emotional problems that actually preceded the physical problem. It is uncommon to see a person with a physical problem without a pre-existing or associated psychological or emotional component such as anxiety, depression, or irritability.

Homeopaths believe that physical symptoms often relieve or decrease pressures that build up internally and limit mental and emotional freedom. Seen from this perspective, the physical symptom represents the healing force's ability to externalize the disease process and preserve the integrity of the more vital mental and emotional life. Mental and emotional health may be considered more crucial than physical health. An extreme example is a person who is paraplegic as a result of multiple sclerosis but is relatively balanced in mental and emotional functions. This person may be healthier and more able to enjoy a high quality of life than a schizophrenic with few physical limitations but with a delusional and paranoid mind.

There is also a hierarchy of which organs are more inner and vital. An example is seen in the condition of shock, either due to hemorrhage of blood or massive infection. To sustain life when a person is in shock, blood is shunted away from the less important organs to the most vital ones. The outer skin becomes cold and blue due to the redistribution of blood, and the intestinal tract and kidneys shut down. The majority of blood flow is to the brain and heart—the two organs that are most vital to sustaining human life.

Through its effect on the vital healing force, the homeopathic remedy acts as a channel for smooth, efficient transmission of the disease process from the mind to the body and finally out of the organism. If the first sign of an illness appears in the mental and emotional realm, treatment must take these symptoms into account. The person must first feel better subjectively if cure is proceeding in the proper direction. Physical symptoms, such as a skin rash, may get worse as the cure is taking place and the disease is being externalized to the least vital parts of the organism.

Cure moves from upper to lower parts of the body.
Symptoms move from areas higher in the body to areas lower, during the curative process. For example, eczema that is being treated with a homeopathic remedy often descends from the eyelids to the elbows to the knees before disappearing. Sensations such as pain or tingling also progress in a downward direction when the person is improving. The reverse direction will often be found in cases where eczema or pain worsen.

Symptoms disappear in the reverse order of their appearance.
Detailed analysis of symptom regression has shown that, as the person improves, the symptoms that appeared last are the first to disappear, while those symptoms that appeared earlier disappear later.

SUPPRESSION

If medicinal treatments are given for ailments without a thorough understanding of their origin nor of the whole person and the predictable patterns of disease progression or regression, the natural defense mechanism may be suppressed and a poorer state of health may result. For example, a typical problem often seen by homeopathic prescribers is infantile eczema. Allopathic doctors usually treat these skin eruptions with cortisone creams, but neglect the underlying process and individual symptom pattern. Topical treatment of eczema is often suppressive and forces the problem inward. If the suppression is chronic, the skin symptoms may improve while the destructive force shifts to the internal organs. Classically, the lungs are affected and bronchial infections and possibly asthma result. In fact, homeopaths believe that most cases of asthma and eczema are the same disease. The eruptions and skin appearance so characteristic of eczema can be pushed further inward, affecting the mental state of the child, resulting in symptoms such as irritability and temper tantrums. The centrifugal healing response is suppressed, and there is an inward progression of disease. The deeper organs, and finally the mind, are affected because there is no way to release the disease through less harmful areas such as the skin. The original process becomes more deeply entrenched (as the eczema is suppressed and the disease spreads from less vital areas to more vital ones). In the process of cure, the homeopathic prescriber carefully observes the progression of symptoms. True cure occurs only if the mental state first improves and then the asthma is relieved. The external skin symptoms may reappear and then improve later in the course of treatment, as the centrifugal healing response is re-established.

A disease can be viewed as an obstacle, similar to a wall that a hiker must climb to continue a journey. As the hiker attempts to climb the wall, a boost may be given and the obstacle easily overcome, just as the homeopathic remedy assists the vital force's attempt to overcome obstacles to health.

On the other hand, a person can be pushed to the bottom as he or she attempts to climb the wall. The force is applied in a direction opposite to the desired movement. This is similar to the dynamics of allopathic drug actions. Although it may temporarily reduce the discomfort of the climb, being pushed to the bottom of the wall does not help the hiker continue the journey—he or she is simply avoiding the problem. Similarly, an allopathic drug will not help the defense mechanism overcome challenges—that wall may have to be met sooner or later. If pushed to the bottom repeatedly, a person may become weak and frustrated, and the wall may become insurmountable. When this analogy is applied to health, it is seen that after repeated suppressions the defense mechanism becomes progressively weaker, the symptoms of illness are continuously present, and a chronic disease state exists.

The idea of suppression is very important in understanding homeopathy, especially when treating chronic illness. While this book and CD deal mostly with acute illnesses, the concept is important to explain for a more complete understanding of homeopathy.

ALLOPATHIC VIEW OF DISEASE

Allopathy is the form of medicinal treatment that is used by most doctors in this country. It is a system for prescribing medicinal substances according to principles other than the law of similars. Allopathy is derived from the Greek root *allo,* meaning other or different, and means "other treatment of disease." Hahnemann coined the word to describe treatment based on the law of contraries and all other treatments not prescribed strictly in accord with the principles of homeopathy.

The forerunners of today's allopathic doctors were certain physicians of Greek and then Roman eras. They gradually replaced the importance of the abstract and indefinable vital healing force of the organism with an emphasis upon understanding the individual in terms of physiochemical laws. They began to view the body as a material and mechanical entity and sought to understand it through the laws of physiology, chemistry, and physics. The role of the vital healing force was neglected because it could not be measured with these tools.

Galen was a second-century physician whose extensive work and writings did much to establish allopathic theory as we know it today. Galen developed a concept of disease based upon his knowledge of the body obtained through anatomical study. He postulated that the vital healing force existed only as it was expressed in the various organs of the body, with each organ having its own behavior and manifesting certain qualities that could be rationally studied. This approach downplayed the functioning of the organism as a whole and instead focused on the many parts. Galen's teachings, with emphasis on the organ systems of the body as the key to understanding and treating disease, are easily recognized in modern allopathic medicine. Modern medicine is a highly subdivided profession with kidney, heart, or lung specialists who study disease processes as they appear in these organs, and who use the physical laws of the scientific method.[7]

Allopathic medicine has traditionally tried to understand the cause of disease by examining its effects. Bacteria, tumors, and toxic products of metabolism, which are found in diseased tissues, are seen as causes of disease, whereas they might actually be the result of disease when viewed from the homeopathic perspective. Experimental science, using the same laws of chemistry and physiology as allopathic medicine, supports the allopathic approach as truly "scientific." However, the subtle factors that influence the appearance of disease, such as the individual's lack of internal resistance to environmental stresses, are disregarded in this methodology. In other words, factors that are important in the cause of disease but that cannot be studied by rational and reductionistic methods are overlooked by allopathic medicine. Also, since allopathy is oriented toward diagnosis using pathology as a guide, diagnosis and treatment of many states of ill health are vague or nonexistent when tissue studies and laboratory tests are normal.

The body's innate intelligence, expressed through the symptoms it produces, is ignored as, instead, the body's physiochemical properties are analyzed. The symptoms are not viewed as a reaction to disease but as the result of disease. They are considered abnormal by the allopath and, in accord with the law of contraries, medicinal substances that have an opposite effect are administered to eliminate the symptoms. From the homeopathic view, medicines applied according to this principle go "against the grain of the wood" in that they oppose or suppress the person's healing response. Repeated exposure to these treatment principles, or even their occasional application in an individual with weak powers of resistance, may lead to further weakening of the individual's defense mechanisms.

Psychiatry is one branch of traditional allopathic medicine that has some appreciation of the problems that may result from suppressing symptoms. Psychotherapists contend that thoughts, feelings, and emotions arising from the conscious and subconscious mind represent the person's reaction to psychological trauma. Greater mental and emotional health ensues as these thoughts and feelings are recognized, accepted, and integrated with greater understanding into the person's life. On the other hand, denial of strong feelings leads to the development of defenses, which may suppress these feelings into deeper layers of the conscious and unconscious mind and eventually lead to more severe mental and psychological limitation.

Allopathy's real strengths are in the same areas where this system has focused its emphasis. Anatomy, physiology, biochemistry, and pathology are highly developed. Technical aspects of surgery and laboratory diagnosis are highly sophisticated. The weakness of the system is its lack of attention to the dynamic and energetic nature of the human organism in disease progression and regression. Ultimately, the result has been the adoption of a fragmented system of medicinal therapeutics.

In traditional medical training in this country, the approach to therapy is generally considered to be medicine first (that is, allopathic medicine) and surgery second. This means that since medicine is relatively less invasive than surgery, medicine should always be the first choice to control a health problem. Those practicing homeopathic medicine try to use homeopathy first, allopathic medicine second, and surgery third. The reason for this is that homeopathy actually strengthens the sick person, which is preferable to drugs that do not enhance the person's resistance to disease but merely strive to reduce or eliminate the most distressing symptoms.

Obviously, surgery remains the first choice for injury from accidents, gunshot wounds, and other such forms of trauma. It can also be helpful as an adjunct to managing chronic disease (for example, replacement of scarred heart valves resulting from rheumatic fever, total hip replacement in advanced arthritis, or removal of a cancerous tumor). But, although the surgery may be successful, it may be naive to consider the person cured without carefully assessing lifestyle, eating habits, and ways of coping with stress, which may have lowered the person's resistance and allowed the heart disease, arthritis, or cancer to begin.

Allopathic medicines can be helpful in the nonsurgical management of disease. Some examples include the drugs used to resuscitate people in cardiac arrest, medicines used to treat advanced pathologic diseases (for example, insulin in diabetes and digitalis in heart failure), and antimicrobial drugs such as penicillin used in bacterial meningitis or other life-threatening infections.

Health care should selectively include *all* therapy that is available and appropriate. The first choice should be modalities that strengthen the person, resulting in less susceptibility and more resistance to disease.

WHEN TO SEE A DOCTOR

It is important to recognize when problems are serious and should be seen by a doctor. This may include a very high fever, serious injury when there is loss of blood or suspicion of a broken bone or head injury, or an ongoing problem that does not seem to be helped with simple first aid measures or homeopathic remedies. Immunizations need to be done by a health care professional, as do diagnostic and preventive tests like blood tests, sigmoidoscopies, chest X-rays, or mammograms. One should also see a physician if there are wounds that do not heal, unexplained bleeding, any kind of chest pain or shortness of breath, or any of the following signs of cancer:

- Change in bowel or bladder activity
- Sore that does not heal
- Unusual bleeding or discharge
- Thickening or lump in a breast or elsewhere in the body
- Persistent indigestion or swallowing difficulty
- Obvious change in a wart or mole
- Nagging cough or hoarseness

Illnesses that can be treated at home include sore throats, fevers, digestive problems, and coughs. These are relatively common ailments seen in most families and are often treated either at home or in a doctor's office. Another category of conditions that can be treated at home are minor injuries like stings, bruises, mild burns, cuts, sprains, and strains. Injuries like broken bones need to be treated by a physician, but remedies can help the healing process. Aggravations of chronic illnesses can also be treated at home; these can include skin problems, joint pains from arthritis, or mild breathing problems from asthma.

HOME PRESCRIBING ATTITUDES

Openness
To appreciate and effectively use homeopathy, a person needs an open mind and an interest in exploring different forms of treatment. This openness can stem from concern with the limitations of conventional medicine or from an interest in the philosophy of other forms of treatment.

Belief in the Body's Healing Potential
People using homeopathy must understand that human beings react in totality to illness. Both mental and physical symptoms reflect the body's attempt to re-establish balance and equilibrium. For example, people who practice homeopathy recognize that fever represents the body's reaction to bacteria, viruses, or inflammation. Fever is the body's attempt to heal itself; thus it represents a positive force that should be encouraged while at the same time helped to decrease its intensity of reaction. Suppressing symptoms with antibiotics or medicines to bring down a fever is working against the total system's need to re-establish balance and heal.

Understanding that Homeopathy Is Person Centered
Homeopathy is person centered, which means that homeopathic remedies are used to treat the total person. Good remedy selection can often require an understanding of:

- Physical problems and pain
- Emotions, attitudes, and behavior
- Work stresses
- Home stresses

- Relationship stresses
- Weather changes
- Sleep patterns
- Eating patterns
- Major life events
- Physical activity
- Desires and aversions

Understanding that Remedies Are Safe

People who use homeopathy understand that remedies are effective if they match the right symptoms, but do no harm if the symptoms do not match. Also, there are no side effects to homeopathic remedies.

Persistence

Prescribers need to be patient with homeopathy. Remedy selection can require practice, and prescription skills will improve with steady effort.

There might be times when it is difficult to find the right remedy. A person may feel the need to give up looking for the right remedy, and then contact a doctor or turn to a familiar allopathic drug. This should not be considered a failure. The person should remember what was learned and try homeopathy again the next time.

It is important to give a remedy time to work. Sometimes the results come more slowly than with allopathic medicine.

Finally, prescribers learn not to use homeopathy with a trial-and-error approach, trying one remedy after the next in hopes of finding the right remedy by chance.

Knowing When and When Not to Treat

Home prescribers should not treat conditions that are beyond their knowledge and ability. The person needs to be careful to recognize when illnesses can be treated at home using homeopathy and when problems are serious and should be seen by a doctor. When there are doubts or concerns, consulting a health care professional is necessary.

Having a Good Relationship with the Physician

It is important to continue to work with a physician (whether or not the physician is familiar with homeopathy). The partnership between a person and his or her physician is an important one and needs to be strong.

When working with a physician who is not familiar with homeopathy, it is important for home prescribers to communicate that they are using homeopathic remedies. Hopefully, the physician will be supportive of the attempt to treat problems at home. Honest communication is vital. It is important to let the physician know if any obstacles develop or if the illness does not respond in an appropriate time.

Being Observant

It is important to be observant and make note of any mental symptoms that go along with an illness. Home prescribers may find it difficult to recognize themselves or their immediate family members in the remedy descriptions. It might be useful for home prescribers to have others read the remedy pictures to help match remedies.

Being Non-Rigid

Homeopathy is not an exclusive therapy; other forms of treatment can complement it. Some problems are best treated with allopathic medicines or surgery. Others are best treated with acupuncture, herbal medicines, physical therapy, exercise, or simply with diet.

Keeping Good Records

It is helpful to remember what remedies have worked well in the past for a particular person and situation (keeping a journal is helpful). This information may be useful in the future.

UNDERSTANDING REMEDIES

How Remedies Are Made

Potentization is a very important concept to understand when starting to use homeopathy. When a remedy is potentized, the energy in a substance is released for use by the human body. Core to this process are the steps of dilution and succussion. Both must be present for the remedy to work.

The following is a simple example of the steps that have been used since Hahnemann's time to produce remedies. Today the process is often completed by modern equipment, but the basic steps are the same as they were two hundred years ago.

1. The substance of a plant, mineral, or biological entity is steeped in alcohol. This steeped mixture is the mother tincture.

2. One part of the mother tincture is added to 99 parts of a mixture of distilled water and ethyl alcohol. This is the first dilution.

3. The bottle containing the diluted mixture then goes through the potentization process. The general idea is that the mixture is subjected to vigorous shaking (succussion), which has the effect of enhancing the effects of the dilution. This is called the first succussion.

   There are various opinions about how many times the mixture is subjected to this downward shaking. Some classic practices suggest more than fifty times, while some modern practices of succussion recommend twenty to forty times. To do the succussion, the dilution can be struck against the palm, as was done in the 1800s, or it can be hit against a firm surface. Other procedures have also been developed using automated techniques.

4. At the end of the first dilution and succussion, the tincture is a 1c potency.

5. By adding one part of the 1c potency to 99 parts of a mixture of distilled water and alcohol and succussing again, the 2c tincture is made. The process could be continued to further potentize the remedy.

The general idea here is that with each dilution, potential unwanted side effects are lessened. Then, at the same time, the succussion part of the process increases the curative action of the remedy.

X and C Potency Scales

Two potency scales are commonly in use today: the centesimal (c) and decimal (x) scales. These are expressed here in lowercase letters, but you will also find them shown as capital C and X.

The decimal scale is based on dilutions of 10. When one part of a mother tincture is diluted and succussed with 9 parts of a mixture of distilled water and alcohol, it becomes a 1x potency. When the process is repeated 6 times, it becomes a 6x potency. This might also be written D6 or 6D or 6DH—the continental, or European, form of referring to the decimal scale.

The centesimal scale is based on dilutions of 100. When one part of a mother tincture is diluted and succussed with 99 parts of a mixture of distilled water and alcohol, it becomes a 1c potency. When the process is repeated 6 times, it becomes a 6c potency. This might also be written C6 or 6CH.

When using low potencies in home treatment, either scale can be used. Generally, more classically oriented homeopaths prefer the centesimal scale. Dr. James Tyler Kent recommended use of the centesimal scale in the following potencies: 6c, 12c, 30c, 200c, 1M, 10M, and CM. In this scale, M is 1,000c, 10M is 10,000c, and CM is 100,000c. Europeans use a variety of low potencies, including 5c, 7c, 9c, 12c, or 15c.

Please note that, in homeopathy, high-potency and low-potency have the opposite meanings we assume for standard medications. The more often a remedy is diluted and shaken, the higher its potency and the stronger its healing action, while a low-potency remedy actually has more of the original substance. Look below at the section "Which Potency to Use" for more pertinent information.

Dispensing Forms

Homeopathic remedies come in several forms. In all cases, follow the dosage guidelines listed on the bottle or package.

Powders. These are individually wrapped packets of dry powder with the remedy dropped into it. One packet is a dose. Powders are taken directly under the tongue and allowed to dissolve. Often they are used for the higher potencies (1M, 10M, and CM).

Pills or tablets. Looking very much like traditional aspirin, pills and tablets are allowed to dissolve under the tongue. Often lower-potency remedies are made in this form (6x, 12x).

Globules. These small round balls are allowed to dissolve under the tongue. The medium- to high-potency remedies are often prepared in this form (6c, 30x, 30c, 200x, 200c).

Tinctures. Supplied in dropper bottles, tinctures can be taken directly under the tongue or in four ounces of water.

Ointments. These are usually made with a petroleum derivative, which helps moisturize the skin and is difficult to wash off. It does, however, not allow the skin to breathe easily. Ointments are particularly useful on hand injuries, when other applications may be washed off easily.

Lotion. This thin cream or liquid helps to moisturize the skin.

Gel. This non-petroleum-based product is less greasy than an ointment. Gels can be washed off more easily and allow the skin to breathe better.

Remedy Storage and Expiration

Homeopathic remedies will last forever as long as they are kept in a cool, dry spot away from sunlight, high heat, or extreme cold. If a remedy has been sitting for a long time, tap the bottle against the middle of the palm about forty times to reactivate the substance. Here are some guidelines for keeping and storing remedies:

- Keep handling to a minimum. Remedies should be kept in their original containers. If necessary, remedies can be placed in folded pieces of clean paper for transportation.

- Avoid potential contamination by quickly replacing the cap on the bottle.

- If any of the remedy falls to the floor, throw it away rather than place it back in the bottle.

- Avoid storing remedies where they might be exposed to temperatures higher than 100 degrees Fahrenheit, long-term direct sunlight or intense light, or strong odors like camphor, perfumes, and mothballs.

Safety and Toxicity

Almost all potentized homeopathic remedies are safe and nontoxic. Some remedies, especially those made from more toxic substances like mercury or snake venom, in very low potencies (such as 1x or 2x) could still have enough of the original substance to cause side effects. These remedies, however, cannot be sold by homeopathic pharmacies to the public because of FDA restrictions.

The process of repeatedly diluting and shaking in an alcohol-and-water solution or diluting and grinding in milk sugar eliminates the toxic poisonous nature of some of the original substances. After the remedy has been potentized to 12c or 24x potency, there are statistically no molecules of the original substance left in the remedy. This means that there is no possible toxic effect from the substance. What is left is the energy of the substance itself.

If the remedy is correct, there is improvement. If the remedy is not correct, generally nothing at all happens. Two other uniquely homeopathic reactions that can occur are:

- A proving, where symptoms are generated from the remedy. This means that the remedy does not match the person's symptoms and is not initiating healing. Provings are generally mild and stop quickly when remedies are discontinued.

- An aggravation, where physical symptoms worsen slightly while mental symptoms improve. This type of aggravation is a sign that the remedy is working and is very short and transitory. It means that the person has responded in a healing way to the remedy.

Drugs and Homeopathy

The relationship of drugs and homeopathy is complicated. Generally, one should consult a homeopathic physician to determine whether homeopathic medicines can be used with prescription medicines.

Some homeopaths will not give remedies when people are using drugs, but many practitioners believe that there are times when homeopathic remedies can actually help drugs work more effectively.

This is sometimes true when treating problems like ear infections, when the condition seems to respond more quickly to antibiotics after remedies are used. The immune system is stimulated and often fewer antibiotics are needed in the future if remedies are given between ear infections.

Some drugs suppress the immune system, and remedies do not work well under these circumstances. This is especially true of steroids like cortisone or prednisone. Usually, antibiotics are not mixed with homeopathy; the general rule is that one system at a time is the wisest course.

Certain medications do not seem to act as antidotes; that is, they do not interfere with remedies. These include things like ibuprofen, aspirin, and acetaminophen for pain. Inhalers for asthma can also be used along with homeopathic remedies, although one should always discuss this with a physician.

CHOOSING THE REMEDY

Choosing the remedy that most closely matches the person's mental and physical symptoms is the key to successful use of homeopathy. The right remedy has the power to profoundly affect overall health and well-being. The wrong remedy does no harm. This section includes some basic principles to remember when analyzing symptoms.

Match the Symptoms and the Remedy

The idea in homeopathy is to match a person's symptoms to those listed for a remedy. The goal is to find the closest match, but it does not need to be a 100-percent match. The majority of the person's symptoms should be listed for the remedy, but the person does not need to match all of the symptoms listed in the Materia Medica or the Repertory. There are sometimes thousands of symptoms associated with each remedy, and it would be impossible for a person to match all of these symptoms.

The prescriber should begin by making a complete list of everything that is bothering the person. A professional homeopath would call this "taking the case." It is important that the list be very detailed and that the prescriber make absolutely sure that any mental and emotional symptoms are included.

Rank the Symptoms

Symptoms should be ranked according to the following hierarchy. The symptoms ranked as causative are most important to match and treat; the symptoms that are localized are the ones that might not need to be matched if most of the others are.

Causation. Things or events that caused the condition, such as exposure to cold air leading to earaches, injuries, or grief resulting in crying spells and depression, are considered the first-rank determinants of symptoms.

Mental. This includes behavior and attitudes. Is the person anxious, fearful, angry, violent, sad, weepy, in shock, irritable, or confused? Does the person like to be alone, or does he or she prefer company? These are general ideas on what to look for in order to analyze the mental picture.

Strange, rare, and peculiar. Symptoms that either appear seldom in people or are very unusual in the human experience are listed as strange and rare. Is there a tendency, for example, to sip only very small amounts of water even though there is great thirst? Is there burning pain that is relieved by warmth?

Generalities. These symptoms describe a person's response as a whole, rather than how a person feels in one specific part of the body. With generality symptoms, a person might say he or she does not like being exposed to cold air, or feels miserable all over in hot, damp weather. Other examples are which position is most comfortable and which causes aggravation, or what time of day the person generally feels worse.

Modalities. Expressed with the same kind of language as the general symptoms, modalities, however, qualify specific body parts. For instance, a sore throat might be made better by drinking cold water. Here, the better-by-cold-water part is the modality for the specific sore throat symptom. Another modality is a headache that is better by wrapping the head tightly. Wrapping tightly is the modality qualifying the type of headache. A time modality is expressed when, for example, a person feels that stomach pains are worse from 4:00 to 8:00 P.M. Being worse from 4:00 to 8:00 P.M. is the modality in this situation.

Particular. The obvious symptoms that describe the case tend to be more localized. Examples are back pain or throat pain.

Narrow the Pool of Remedies

There are more than 2,000 homeopathic remedies, and the CD and this book include 105 of the ones most commonly used. *The Complete Homeopathic Resource* provides two ways to narrow down the field of remedies for consideration: the Clinical Repertory here in the book and on the CD, and the Repertory module on the CD.

The Clinical Repertory (Chapter 2 in the book) lists remedies for specific illnesses or conditions, organized by the problems. In the CD Repertory, symptoms are presented in alphabetical order and accessed by name of body part or function. Remedies that can help the symptom are listed next to the symptom. The CD Repertory allows a person to select a unique set of symptoms; the program then analyzes these symptoms to find possible remedies. If there are many different types of symptoms, such as a headache, food cravings, emotional symptoms, and a skin disorder, the CD Repertory may be the best path. When there is a specific problem, such as a headache, the Clinical Repertory here may be most useful.

Refer to the Help section of the CD or Chapter 3 of this book for directions on using the program tools. Sometimes after using these tools, one remedy will stand out as the clear best choice. It is also quite possible that three or four remedies may match fairly well. In this situation, a home prescriber will need to study the Materia Medica to make a final remedy choice.

Study the Materia Medica

Once the field of remedies has been narrowed down to a few close matches, the Materia Medica entry for each remedy (on the CD) should be carefully studied to determine which remedy picture most closely matches the illness.

It is important to keep in mind the rank of the symptoms. All symptoms matter in the total picture. In general, however, causative, mental, generalities, and modalities tend to be the most important categories when selecting a remedy. Strange, rare, and peculiar symptoms are also very useful in narrowing the field of remedies under consideration. Though they are helpful in describing the case, particular symptoms do not generally determine the final selection of a remedy.

TAKING THE REMEDY

Administration of Remedies

Homeopathic remedies should be taken when the mouth is clean and dry. The mouth should be free of food, drink, tobacco, and toothpaste for thirty to sixty minutes before and after the remedy is taken. This allows the remedy to be absorbed into the bloodstream without interference from substances in the mouth.

Because the remedies are uncoated, they should not be touched. Generally the remedies come in a bottle with a cap. The globules or tablets are tapped from the bottle into the cap and dropped directly onto or underneath the tongue. Discard globules or tablets that spill on the floor. Because the remedy is absorbed through the bloodstream, the tablets or globules should be allowed to dissolve in the mouth. They should not be chewed and definitely should not be swallowed before they have dissolved significantly.

For children, the remedy can be crushed between two clean spoons and the resulting powder can then be placed in the mouth.

Certain foods that contain volatile oils may antidote homeopathic remedies. This includes things such as coffee, camphor, and very strong oils like pure, concentrated peppermint. Toothpaste is not a problem since there is usually very little peppermint (and it is usually artificial). It is the very potent and concentrated oils that cause problems. Neither regular nor decaffeinated coffee are recommended, as it is the oil and resin in coffee that antidotes the remedies, not the caffeine. Tea and chocolate, which are other forms of caffeine, are acceptable since they do not seem to antidote homeopathic remedies.

Which Potency to Use

In homeopathy, the more often the remedy is diluted and succussed, the higher its potency and the stronger its healing action. When a homeopath speaks of a *low* potency, he or she is actually talking about a remedy with more of the original substance. A *high*-potency remedy has less of the original substance but more pure energy to stimulate the bio-electrical energy and immune system of the body and mind.

Potencies are classified as follows:

- Low—up to 6c or 6x
- Medium—12c to 30c, or 12x to 30x
- High—200c, 1M, 10M, or above

Low potencies are used when the prescriber is not totally sure that the remedy closely matches the illness. In general, if you are less than 75 to 80 percent sure, use a low potency. Also use a low potency when the symptoms are mild and the person is not very ill.

When the person is very sick and the vital force and immune system are not working to their full capacity, higher potencies may cause the immune system to react too strongly for such a fragile situation.

Low potencies are also appropriate when a deep-acting remedy was previously used.

Finally, use a low-potency remedy for an acute problem such as an injury. Higher potencies generally are not used for acute prescribing conditions.

High-potency remedies become appropriate when:

- The prescriber is very sure the remedy picture matches the symptoms precisely.
- The symptoms are of rapid onset, such as when a cold wind causes a person to be suddenly chilled and then come down with an upper respiratory infection. In this case, a remedy such as *Aconite* 200c can be used because of the rapid onset.
- Lower potencies help the person feel better, but do not seem to hold the person's improvement long enough.

This book generally recommends the 30c potency for home prescribing, although there are several other possibilities. Other low potencies such as 6c, 9c, 12c, or 15c as well as 12x or 30x can also be used. Remedies that are also tissue salts like *Kali mur, Silica,* and *Calcarea sulph* are most often used in the 6x potency. Some remedies are commonly used in the 200c potency for acute problems, especially when there are injuries. *Arnica* 200c is commonly used after injury or surgery to help initiate healing. *Ruta* 200c is often used for tendonitis problems. Refer to the Clinical Repertory and especially to the Materia Medica on the CD for more specific potency information.

Frequency

Remedies can be repeated anywhere from every fifteen minutes to every week or longer, depending on the type of problem that exists. As soon as there is a positive response, generally, the remedy is stopped.

For rapidly progressing problems or those that come on very suddenly, remedies can be taken every fifteen minutes until there is a positive response. For conditions like a cough, nausea, vomiting, or asthma, remedies are taken from every fifteen or thirty minutes to every three to four hours. For certain types of joint pain that tend to be more chronic, remedies are often repeated every twelve to twenty-four hours.

Frequent repetitions are helpful when using low-potency remedies for illnesses that progress quickly and are accompanied by great pain or when there is an intense physical reaction, such as excessive sneezing or drainage from the eyes. Less frequent repetitions are useful when higher potencies are used or when there is a rapid, sustained improvement after the first dose. In this case, remedies are repeated only when the remedy is no longer helping and the symptoms either return or new symptoms appear.

Observing the Reaction

After taking a homeopathic remedy, careful observation is necessary to decide if a person is getting better, staying the same, or getting worse.

If there is improvement in the physical and emotional symptoms, the remedy does not need to be repeated. The remedy acts as a catalyst, stimulating the body's immune system, defense mechanisms, and emotional state. Once this process begins, healing will continue on its own, and it is not necessary to repeat a remedy.

General Improvement

In acute illnesses there is often an improvement without an initial aggravation. Sometimes this improvement can be instantaneous; at other times it is more gradual. As long as there is improvement, no further remedy is indicated. People are showing signs of improvement when:

- They feel emotionally better. They are less anxious, less irritable, less fearful, or less depressed.
- They are able to communicate more effectively and directly.
- They feel like their old self.
- They are able to make decisions more easily, have more self-confidence, and are more productive at school or work.
- Their relationships with other people improve.
- They are more creative and initiate new ideas.
- They have more energy and feel more alive.
- They have more dreams, which are richer and have clearer meaning. The dreams seem to help resolve feelings that may have been causing emotional pain and suffering.
- They fall asleep after taking a remedy, especially after there has been a high fever, agitation, or irritability.
- They vomit after having indigestion, then feel better. Or their cough may become loose, making the shortness of breath characteristic of problems such as asthma feel better.

These signs of improvement or cure represent mental, emotional, and energy level improvements. Even if there is little or no improvement (or even a slight worsening) on the physical level, as long as some of the signs of improvement are present, they indicate that the person is getting better. A watch-and-wait attitude is then the best approach.

Homeopathic Aggravation

One sign of improvement is the homeopathic aggravation. Sometimes this is an emotional aggravation, where a specific trauma or event seems to be more intense. This is very short lived and mild compared to the original event. It will quickly pass, and the person will soon feel emotionally better. At other times, the aggravation occurs on the physical level and the physical symptoms worsen for a short period, especially in acute illnesses. For instance, a fever may go up slightly, or a runny nose may discharge more freely. This represents the body trying to heal itself or rid itself of bodily waste products or toxins. When this type of aggravation occurs, no other remedy should be used.

Temporary Return of Old Symptoms—Hering's Laws of Cure

A temporary return of old symptoms that were suppressed in the past is a sign of improvement, especially in the case of chronic problems. This return of symptoms follows Hering's laws of cure—that symptoms recur and do so in the reverse order of their appearance and start from the more serious to the least serious, from internal organs to the external organs, from inside to the outside, and from above downward.

For example, a person may see that after taking a remedy a headache improves, followed by pain moving to the lower parts of the body, then to the hands and fingers, and finally disappearing all together. A deep cough may improve by becoming laryngitis and then a runny nose. This represents the body improving in its respiratory function because the illness has moved from the deeper organs like the lungs to the least important organs like the nose. One might also see that as asthma gets better, allergies begin, and as this gets better, a skin rash appears. This represents the body healing itself because in allergic conditions, the most important organ is the lung and the least important is the skin.

The progression from inside the body to the outside and from more important to least important can occur either in the progress of cure in chronic cases or as a temporary return of symptoms that have been suppressed in the past.

If symptoms reappear according to Herring's laws of cure, a second remedy is not prescribed and a watchful wait is recommended.

Initial Improvement, but Symptoms Return
One type of reaction is when the condition gets better for a while, but then improvement stops or the condition worsens slightly. If the symptoms are still the same and the remedy still matches, the same remedy should be repeated.

Initial Improvement, but Symptoms Change
Another type of response is when the symptoms change after the remedy is given. In this case, the remedy was not the correct one, and a new remedy should be selected to match the new symptoms.

Failure to Improve or Worsening of Symptoms
A person may fail to improve or actually get worse. This may be due to an incorrect remedy match, a more serious chronic problem, or a problem that is too severe for homeopathic remedies to help.

Improvement, but Sudden Lapse
The person may improve slightly, and then suddenly worsen. In this case, a new remedy should be prescribed because the first remedy was not the correct one.

Physical Improvement, but Mental Aggravation
If the person improves physically but emotionally and mentally seems worse, the correct remedy was not taken. The prescriber should select a new remedy based upon the current symptoms. An example of this might be when a person has loose bowels that improve with the remedy, but the person feels more agitated and angry.

Progressive Worsening of Symptoms
A person may progressively get worse after taking a remedy. This can occur on the mental, emotional, or physical level. In this case, the prescriber should determine whether the person needs a different remedy or whether a physician should be contacted for medical attention.

Reversal of Hering's Laws of Cure

Another type of reaction is when the laws of cure are reversed. This happens when symptoms move from the less serious to the more serious, from exterior parts of the body to the interior, or from the lower part of the body to the upper part of the body. An example of this might be when a skin problem such as eczema improves, but a person experiences more intense headaches. Another example is when a sore throat feels better, but the person gets dizzy or loses self-confidence.

In this case, a person should use no more remedies and allow the effects of the remedy to wear off. In extreme cases, it may be necessary to antidote the remedy with coffee, camphor, or sometimes with another remedy. This generally does not happen in acute problems, but sometimes appears in chronic, constitutional care. This is a complicated situation and an experienced homeopath should be consulted.

Aggravation of Symptoms but No Improvement in Mind or Body

When there is aggravation of the symptoms but no improvement in either the mind or body, it may mean that the remedy was close to matching but not quite right. A new remedy should be selected based upon the symptoms.

Repeating a Remedy

Another dose of a remedy can be repeated after an appropriate period of watching and waiting. Subsequent doses of the same remedy can be used when any of the following are true:

- The original symptoms return
- When discomfort is intense
- When the improvement reaches a plateau and, although the person feels better, improvement seems to be stagnant

One common mistake is repeating the remedy too often. In allopathic medicine, the approach is to give as much medicine as possible to wipe out bacteria or decrease fever as long as the side effects are tolerable. In homeopathy the minimum dose is the best, meaning the optimum situation is to use as small an amount as possible to catalyze a reaction. Once the body's defense mechanisms are set in motion, there is no need for additional remedies. The body has an innate ability to heal itself if it is directed in a correct way; the homeopathic remedy is the initiator and director.

Several remedies can be used in a row, especially if the symptoms change rapidly and a new remedy is indicated because of these changes. Sometimes in the process of cure new symptoms become apparent, and a different remedy is necessary. This is particularly true if illnesses occur with sudden onset and symptoms progress rapidly. Sometimes when the wrong remedy is used or the person is impatient and does not wait for the remedy reaction, one remedy after another is wrongly used. This can cause a mild proving of the remedy or minor aggravations of other symptoms. Eventually it may be difficult to distinguish true symptoms from provings and aggravations.

Sometimes when symptoms change rapidly or many remedies are used because symptoms are unclear, a remedy associated with changeability may be required. Symptoms that call for *Pulsatilla,* for example, are noted for their changeability.

For most conditions, allow two hours between remedies and watch for improvement on the mental, energy, or physical levels. When conditions come on very suddenly or are due to injury, remedies can be used every fifteen minutes or so. This is particularly true of fever that comes on after a cold, dry wind, such as when *Aconite* is the correct remedy. It is also true if a person is stung by a bee and there is swelling. In this case, *Apis* can be used every fifteen minutes. Another indication is if there was an injury with a feeling of great pain or if there are emotional changes. In this case, *Arnica* may be needed, and it can be repeated every fifteen minutes until there is mental improvement and less physical discomfort.

If a remedy is frequently repeated (such as every fifteen to thirty minutes), it is only used this often for the first two to four hours. After this period, the remedy (or another indicated remedy) is usually taken every two to three hours.

USING THIS BOOK AND THE CD

The Complete Homeopathic Resource CD provides three tools for helping people find the remedy that most closely matches, and thus can help, their condition or that of a person for whom they are prescribing. The book version provides only one of these tools, the Clinical Repertory. More information on these modules can be found in Chapter 3, the Help section of this book, as well as in the Help section of the CD.

Common Illnesses and Their Homeopathic Treatment (Clinical Repertory in This Book)

The Clinical Repertory is a listing of specific illnesses or conditions and a description of the remedies that can be used to help the problems. Each remedy under the illness or condition headings is described with its associated symptoms. From the remedy list, a home prescriber may be able to choose which remedy best matches the description of the illness.

Materia Medica (on the CD)

The Materia Medica includes detailed information about 105 commonly used homeopathic medicines. Each description provides an overall picture of a remedy, including the mental and physical symptoms associated with or helped by that remedy. These symptoms have been compiled as the result of provings on healthy people as well as observations of cures when the remedy was given to sick people for other problems. Each remedy description contains the following information:

- Symptoms and conditions associated with the remedy
- A breakdown of the remedy symptoms by parts of the body
- Dosage information
- Relationships between this remedy and other remedies
- Conditions that make the associated symptoms better or worse
- Clinical uses for the remedy

Repertory (on the CD)

A repertory is a book and/or a CD that is essentially an index to the materia medica. It contains a listing of symptoms (rubrics) and homeopathic remedies that are associated with and can treat the symptoms. This program's Repertory is a condensed version of Kent's *Homeopathic Repertory to Materia Medica.*

The Repertory can greatly assist in narrowing the choice of helpful homeopathic remedies. The Repertory is especially useful when the sick person has many symptoms, when the prescriber is unsure of the name of an illness, or when the total symptom set does not describe a single common illness.

The Repertory enables you to select one or more symptoms. The program then analyzes these symptoms to find the remedies that most closely match the symptoms and can therefore treat your condition. To find remedies that best match your condition, the program weights, analyzes, and scores remedies based on the selected symptoms.

SPECIAL CIRCUMSTANCES

Treating Multiple Conditions

It is important to choose one remedy based on the totality of symptoms. For example, a person may have a skin problem and an upper respiratory problem at the same time, and there may also be depression and constipation. The entire person—mind, digestive system, respiratory system, and skin—are all important in choosing the right remedy. Carefully choosing one remedy is often the best approach to treating a problem.

Under special conditions remedies are given in sequence or in alternation, as when someone has a problem with a chronic cough and may have also recently injured the hand or head. In this case the person needs a remedy for the cough along with one to help the body heal from the injury. These remedies can sometimes be alternated every few hours.

What this program does *not* recommend is the use of multiple remedies in combination. This program is based on the proven practice of homeopathy, in which a person takes a single remedy and then observes the reaction. When many remedies are given at the same time, there is no way to prove a match to the true symptom picture. Sometimes the combination works, but it may be only by chance and quite possible that only one of the remedies is helping the condition. Often remedies antidote each other, canceling each other's power to heal. At times combination remedies actually complicate problems, especially if a person suffers from chronic illnesses. This is because new symptoms may result or there may be aggravations from one or more of the combined remedies. In this case, the combination remedy may change the symptoms, which could interfere with the natural progress of the illness or make it difficult for a prescriber to get a clear picture of the condition in order to choose the right remedy.

Pregnancy and Birth

Homeopathic remedies can safely be given to women who are pregnant or trying to get pregnant. Homeopaths maintain that what is good for the mother is good for the child. Midwives and physicians commonly use homeopathy both for labor and post-birth, and for the newborn baby. Homeopathy can aid in the normal progress of labor, it can help the nausea and vomiting of pregnancy, and it can help when breast milk is slow to come. If a woman is pregnant, she should discuss home treatment with her primary care provider, especially if there are complications in the pregnancy.

Homeopathy and Children

Parents clearly see the beauty of homeopathy when their child or infant responds quickly and dramatically to a remedy or when an ongoing illness improves after a child takes a series of remedies. Because infants are not affected by placebo, the true healing powers of homeopathy are experienced. There are many advantages to using homeopathic remedies with children:

- Children tend to injure themselves easily and the remedies are often helpful in accidents and minor emergencies.
- Remedies can speed up the healing process and help to heal a broken bone.

- Remedies are safe and have no side effects. One does not need to worry about the inherent side effects of regular medications.

- Remedies help to avoid the problem of suppression of illness by not using cortisone to treat eczema or other rashes. The child's illness is not driven deeper into the constitution to later turn up as more serious allergies, asthma, or joint problems. Thus, homeopathic remedies can help prevent the development of chronic diseases later in life.

- Because the emotions of a child or adolescent are very important to prescribing, children like the interaction with the prescriber. Their feelings are discussed and acknowledged and given credibility and importance.

- Many of the emotional problems inherent in growing up can be helped by homeopathy. This can include the tantrums that go along with separation anxiety in babies, problems with weaning, night terrors, fear of taking school exams, and a lack of self-esteem.

- Because the remedies are nontoxic, there is no worry that children will accidentally take too much of a remedy.

- Remedies generally taste good because they are dispensed in lactose.

- Because children generally have taken fewer medications over the course of their short lifetimes, they have suffered fewer suppressions and side effects than adults. They also have not had as many emotional traumas and negative experiences that cause deep scars. Therefore the remedies are often very effective and work quickly.

Constitutional Remedies

While the 105 remedies in the Repertory have the potential to treat and cure many acute illnesses, some remedies are more comprehensive and broader in their application. These remedies are also generally deeper acting and quite effective in treating chronic illnesses.

The following remedies are the most comprehensive:

- *Anacardium, Antimonium crud, Argentum nit, Arsenicum alb, Calcarea carb, Cuprum met, Graphites, Ignatia, Kali carb, Lachesis, Lycopodium, Magnesia carb, Mercurius sol, Natrum mur, Nitric acid, Nux vomica, Petroleum, Phosphorus, Pulsatilla, Sepia, Silica, Staphysagria, Sulphur, Thuja*

These remedies are mentioned much more often in the Repertory, and have more illnesses associated with them in the Clinical Repertory. The Materia Medica is more detailed and covers more organs and their problems. In the Materia Medica, the mental symptoms are more developed and a clearer picture of emotional attitudes and characteristics are seen.

Because these remedies are more comprehensive, they are used to treat the person's underlying immune and metabolic systems, also described by homeopaths as their basic *constitution*. These remedies are often referred to as constitutional remedies. There are many more of these remedies in homeopathy, but this book and CD include only the ones that also treat acute problems.

There are several reasons why there are a greater number of symptoms listed for these remedies. Sometimes this reflects the nature and reactivity of the substance itself as determined by the provings on healthy people as well as problems that improve when the remedy is given to treat a sick person who has other symptoms. Another reason is that some remedies have been proven by more people and at more times.

This book and CD are not designed to treat and cure chronic illnesses. Indirectly, however, they may help chronic problems because they include suggestions for treating acute flare-ups of chronic illnesses. The book and CD do not include treatment of serious diseases like heart disease, diabetes, cancer, pneumonia, emphysema, AIDS, or multiple sclerosis. They do include suggestions on treating exacerbations, side effects, or problems that are associated with these illnesses. For instance, the book recommends remedies for emotional reactions to illness and for treating the side effects of medication. The book does not recommend remedies to treat uterine fibroids, but it does recommend remedies that may help control heavy blood flow or pain associated with this problem. It does not offer treatment suggestions for lupus, but it does recommend remedies for associated joint pains.

SETTING UP A HOME REMEDY KIT

How to Begin

While individual remedies are quite inexpensive, collecting remedies for a comprehensive home kit can be a bit costly. Many suppliers offer beginning remedy kits at a substantial discount, so it is a good idea to check these sources before building a kit from scratch. It is, however, also possible to build a comprehensive home kit by purchasing a few key remedies at a time.

This process can be approached in several ways, or in stages. One method is to start with a set of basic remedies that are useful for acute problems like diarrhea, fever, and mild ear problems. A person could then choose additional remedies that are useful for the family's situation. For example, if someone in the family suffers from allergies, it is important for the prescriber to have the set of remedies that are particularly useful for allergies. Another approach is to purchase remedies that are consistent with the prescriber's level of expertise. In this case, a person could first purchase only those remedies that are useful when treating simple conditions, and then add remedies as prescribing skills improve.

Basic Remedies

Basic remedies include those that are useful for injuries, coughs, colds, digestive problems such as diarrhea and nausea, fever, poison ivy, teething, croup, and mild ear problems. In general, these are the first remedies a home prescriber should think of when building a kit. They are broken into three levels according to their importance to the home remedy kit:

- First-level remedies: *Aconite, Arnica, Belladonna, Bryonia, Chamomilla, Colocynthis, Hepar sulph, Ignatia, Ipecac, Ledum, Nux vomica, Pulsatilla*
- Second-level remedies: *Apis, Arsenicum alb, Carbo veg, Ferrum phos, Gelsemium, Hypericum, Mercurius sol, Rhus tox, Spongia*

- Third-level remedies: *Cocculus, Dulcamara, Eupatorium perf, Kali mur, Magnesia phos, Natrum mur, Phosphorus, Podophyllum, Rumex, Ruta, Silica, Sticta, Sulphur, Symphytum, Veratrum alb*

Remedies for Athletes

Certain remedies are useful for the treatment of injuries, sprains, strains, and wounds. (Note that * means the remedy is included in the recommended basic remedies.)

- *Apis*, Arnica*, Calcarea carb, Gelsemium*, Ignatia*, Ledum*, Rhus tox*, Ruta*, Symphytum**

Remedies for Allergies

Homeopathy is especially helpful for treating allergies. The following remedies are useful for respiratory allergies. This does not include eczema, asthma, and hives, which are also considered to be allergic conditions. (Note that * means the remedy is included in the recommended basic remedies.)

- *Allium cepa, Apis*, Arsenicum alb*, Arsenicum iod, Arum triphyllum, Arundo, Gelsemium*, Kali bich, Kali iod, Lachesis, Natrum mur*, Natrum sulph, Nux vomica*, Sabadilla, Sticta*, Wyethia*

Remedies for Children

Two groups of remedies are useful for children. The first group is for acute conditions like sore throat, fever, diarrhea, and nausea and vomiting. The other group is for emotional problems, which are often associated with more chronic conditions. Remedies for emotional concerns are listed in the following section. There is overlap between the two groups. (Note that * means the remedy is included in the recommended basic remedies.)

Remedies for children with acute illnesses include:

- *Aconite*, Allium cepa, Antimonium crud, Antimonium tart, Apis*, Arnica*, Arsenicum alb*, Bryonia*, Calcarea carb, Calcarea phos, Carbo veg*, Chamomilla*, Cina, Colocynth, Drosera, Equisetum, Eupatorium perf*, Ferrum phos*, Hepar sulph*, Ignatia*, Ipecac*, Kali bich, Kali mur*,*

Ledum*, Magnesia phos*, Mercurius sol*, Natrum sulph, Nux vomica*, Phosphorus*, Podophyllum*, Pulsatilla*, Rhus tox*, Rumex*, Ruta*, Silica*, Sponga*, Sticta*, Symphytum*

Children's Emotional Concerns

The following remedies are associated with emotional concerns. (Note that * means the remedy is included in the recommended basic remedies, and ** means that it is included in the list of remedies for children's acute ailments.)

- *Arsenicum alb* **, Baryta carb, Calcarea carb**, Calcarea phos**, Causticum, Chamomilla* **, Cina**, Graphites, Lycopodium, Natrum mur*, Nux vomica* **, Phosphorus* **, Pulsatilla* **, Silica* **, Sepia, Staphysagria, Sulphur**

Remedies for Women

These remedies are particularly effective for women and their specific health care needs. (Note that * means the remedy is included in the recommended basic remedies.)

- *Arnica*, Bellis, Calcarea carb, Calcarea phos, Caulophyllum, Cimicifuga, Cocculus*, Gelsemium*, Helonias, Ignatia*, Kali carb, Lachesis, Natrum mur*, Phosphorus*, Pulsatilla*, Sabina, Sepia, Sulphur*, Thuja, Zincum met*

CHAPTER 2

Common Illnesses and Their Homeopathic Treatment (Clinical Repertory)

The Clinical Repertory is very useful in narrowing the choice of helpful remedies. It is most useful when the name of an illness is known, or a complete set of symptoms describe a common affliction such as an injury, a cold, or a sore throat.

The Clinical Repertory does not include chronic or complex conditions that are more difficult and complicated to treat. It also does not include serious diseases like heart disease, cancer, and multiple sclerosis. Some diseases like chronic fatigue syndrome and mononucleosis can be helped by homeopathy, but are not listed as separate conditions in this program. Because homeopathy emphasizes the symptoms rather than the disease, try reviewing specific symptoms associated with this type of disease. For example, you could try reviewing the Clinical Repertory sections associated with sore throat or fever for help dealing with the symptoms of mononucleosis.

ABDOMINAL PAIN

Many different types of abdominal problems cause pain. Most are minor and easily treated with natural methods, but some require a physician. The location, intensity, and association with other gastrointestinal problems, such as nausea, vomiting, diarrhea, and fever, are all important in determining whether homeopathy can help.

Pain in the upper right area of the abdomen can be gallbladder problems, especially if pain radiates to the back or shoulder blades. Gallstones are common, especially in women who are over the age of forty and overweight. Liver problems, such as hepatitis, can often be similar to and confused with stomach, spleen, or large colon problems, especially before jaundice has occurred. Burning or gnawing pains near the navel are associated with ulcers, gastritis, or pancreatic problems. In these cases, antacids or drinking milk usually give short-term relief. Pain in the lower left abdomen can be associated with diverticulitis or colitis. Lower abdominal pains on the sides of a woman's body may represent ovarian problems. Lower center abdominal pain may be due to a bladder infection if there are urinary tract symptoms, an increase in urination, or pain when urinating. In women, lower center abdominal pain may be associated with uterine problems. Appendicitis is usually worse at the point midway between the navel and the right front tip of the pelvic bone. The pain is intense and worse from any movement. Stomach pains are serious and a physician should be consulted as soon as possible.

Most instances of abdominal pain are not serious; these problems are caused by viral illnesses, constipation, intestinal gas, stress, irritable bowel syndrome, or muscle tension associated with growing or athletics. Irritable bowel syndrome is a disorder associated with cramping and alternating constipation or diarrhea.

Natural methods such as pressure, warmth, eating high-fiber foods such as whole grains, fruits, and vegetables, drinking plenty of water, cutting down on caffeine and alcohol, chewing carefully, and using bulking agents can be helpful for abdominal pain.

Aconite. Useful for the relief of a sudden onset of intense abdominal pain. The pain forces the person to double over, but unlike abdominal pain relieved by *Colocynthis,* doubling over does not relieve the discomfort. The abdomen is sensitive to touch and feels hot, tense, and, in some cases, burning. A fear of dying may be experienced.

Aloe. Useful for relieving abdominal pain that is often associated with a large accumulation of gas. The gas presses downward, causing distress in the lower bowels, which leads to diarrhea. The abdomen feels full, heavy, and bloated, especially around the navel. These symptoms feel worse from pressure. A weak feeling in the abdomen extends to the rectum, and the person feels like diarrhea will come on suddenly. There is also a sensation of a plug between the pubic bone and the tailbone, with a constant urging to have a stool.

Anacardium. The abdominal pain treated with this remedy feels as if a dull plug was pressed into the intestines. The person wants to have a bowel movement, but feels plugged up and cannot have a stool.

Arnica. When the stomach has been punched, hit, or bruised, *Arnica* helps heal injured muscles and organs. The pressure in the abdomen feels like a stone is pressing against the spine. Gas moves both upward and downward from the center of the abdomen.

Arsenicum alb. Useful for relieving a burning pain in the pit of the stomach. The pain feels like fiery coals. Warm drinks relieve the burning. Coughing triggers a pain in the abdomen. The liver and spleen are sometimes enlarged and painful.

Belladonna. Useful for treating severe abdominal pain that is worse from the slightest touch, jarring motion, and lying on the back. Bending forward may bring relief. The transverse colon tends to protrude. The left side of the abdomen hurts, especially with coughing, sneezing, or touching. In general, the person has very hot, dry skin, a high fever, a red flushed face, and dilated pupils. Mental agitation and irritability are also common. These symptoms often come after the use of *Aconite* and when inflammation has localized to a specific spot. *Belladonna* may also be useful in the very early stages of appendicitis. Appendicitis is characterized by intense pain midway between the navel and the tip of the right hipbone; it is worse from touch or movement and may be associated with vomiting and fever. Appendix problems are serious and a physician should be contacted immediately.

Bellis. Useful for soreness of the abdominal walls and uterus. It is especially useful after surgery or trauma to the deeper tissues of the organs or large muscles. Symptoms are similar to the stomach problems associated with *Arnica,* but are more specific for injury to the organs, especially in the abdominal and uterine area.

Berberis. Useful for treating gallbladder pain or kidney pain, especially when associated with gallstones or kidney stones. Pain located in the upper right abdominal area may be due to gallstones. Pains that radiate from the kidneys around to the abdomen and possibly into the hips and groin may be due to kidney stones. Standing or exercise may make these radiating pains worse; pressure does not necessarily make the pain worse.

Bryonia. Useful for treating throbbing or sharp, stitching pains that seem localized in one area. The person lies perfectly still on the painful side; any kind of touch or movement causes great pain. Large amounts of cold water are desired, and the tongue tends to have a thick, white coating. The person is irritable if disturbed and wants to lie alone in the dark. A fever and constipation are common symptoms. *Bryonia* can be helpful in early appendicitis. (Appendicitis is characterized by intense pain midway between the naval and the tip of the right hip bone. The pain is worse from touch or movement and may be associated with vomiting and fever.) If appendicitis is suspected, *Bryonia* may help relieve discomfort as the person is transported to the doctor's office or a hospital.

Calcarea carb. Useful for treating an abdomen that is swollen from trapped gas and sensitive to the slightest pressure. Pains in the gallbladder are sometimes felt, especially when there are gallstones, and the pain is worse after eating a fatty meal. The person cannot bear tight clothing around the waist because the abdomen is distended and hard. This remedy is often useful for a person who has a large amount of fat in the abdomen, tends to be overweight, craves sweets, and feels better when constipated.

Calcarea phos. Useful for treating cramping pain in the abdomen that occurs at every attempt to eat. It is especially useful for children with symptoms that include irritability, cold extremities, and digestive difficulties. Children who have chronic stomach problems and grow quickly find *Calcarea phos* useful. Adolescents and young girls who are first getting their menstrual period may also find relief with this remedy.

Carbo veg. Useful for abdominal pains from gas accumulation, usually located in the upper abdomen. (Abdominal pains associated with *Lycopodium* are located in the lower part of the abdomen; with *China,* pains are located in the entire abdomen.) The pressure from a greatly distended abdomen is relieved from passing gas or belching. Tight clothing around the waist or abdomen is intolerable.

The abdominal pain, similar to the pain from lifting a heavy object, is worse when riding in a car.

Chamomilla. One of the most important remedies for colic of infants and children. Anger may trigger abdominal pain. Abdominal pains are often seen in teething infants and in children who have had a temper tantrum. The abdomen is distended and a gripping pain around the navel extends to the small of the back. The pain is improved, but not relieved, by applying local heat and by passing small amounts of gas. With this type of abdominal pain, the child may have hot cheeks, with one red cheek and one pale cheek. Perspiration often precedes the attack. This stomach problem may be associated with diarrhea that resembles chopped spinach, especially during teething.

China. Helps abdominal pain that is associated with much gas, is located all over the abdomen, and is relieved from bending over. Sometimes belching of bitter fluid or regurgitation of food occurs, which does not bring relief. Movement may help the bloating.

Cina. Bloating, a twisting pain around the navel, and a hard abdomen are typical symptoms of abdominal pain that *Cina* helps. This type of problem is often seen in children who have pinworms.

Cocculus. Associated with nervousness and anxiety, *Cocculus* is especially helpful for treating stomach pain caused from the anxiety, stress, and late night hours of helping other people (such as taking care of sick people). This remedy can also be used to treat abdominal pain and nausea caused from riding in cars or on boats. The abdomen is distended with much gas. When the person moves, the stomach feels like it is full of sharp stones. Lying on one side lessens the pain. Abdominal muscles are sore and weak, as if an object is being forced out through them.

Colocynth. Useful for cutting, sharp pains in the abdomen that cause the person to double over. The person presses against the abdomen to relieve the pain. The agonizing pain feels like stones are being ground together in the abdomen. The person is often restless and sometimes twists and turns for relief. The intestines feel bruised. Pain may be brought on by anger and may be associated with cramps in the calves. Each attack of pain is accompanied by great mental agitation and chilliness. Hard pressure and passing gas bring relief. (Stomach pain associated with *Belladonna* is not relieved with pressure.) Diarrhea that resembles jelly often occurs after eating or drinking even small amounts of food.

Cuprum met. Useful for treating pain after childbirth, especially for women who have had many children. Cramping pain is the primary characteristic. Spasmodic pains start and stop suddenly. Cramps in the lower legs or hands may cause the person to scream out. The person may experience violent pains that feel as if a knife is penetrating through the navel to the back. These pains cause fearful and distressing screaming. They are relieved by pressure and cold drinks.

Gratiola. Similar to *Nux vomica,* this remedy is often useful for women who are irritable and hard-driving. Symptoms include cramps and abdominal pain after dinner and during the night, swelling in the abdomen, and constipation.

Ipecac. Useful for relieving abdominal pain located in the center of the abdomen. The pain feels like a hand is clutching the intestines and is almost always associated with severe nausea and vomiting. Generally, vomiting does not relieve the nausea. Even the pain itself tends to nauseate the person. There is little thirst. *Ipecac* is also a good remedy for amebic dysentery, especially when traveling to foreign countries. Symptoms of nausea, vomiting, and rectal spasms with diarrhea are common. There is a great deal of salivation occurring with the constant nausea and vomiting. Oddly, the tongue looks clean and pink.

Iris. Burning and cutting pains in the abdomen with large amounts of gas may be relieved by *Iris.* The entire intestinal tract burns. Profuse, watery diarrhea burns, especially in the anus, and contains undigested fat; it is typically worse in the morning. Useful for pancreatitis, especially when symptoms include a sweet-tasting vomit. Saliva is profuse and tends to have a greasy taste.

Kali carb. Helps abdominal pain that is often associated with women who have backaches and weak extremities (especially the legs, which seem to give out), and who perspire excessively. Anxiety is felt in the stomach and abdomen. The person is cold and cannot tolerate cold weather. The abdomen is distended. The pain sometimes moves from the upper left portion of the abdomen through the stomach, causing the person to turn on the right side before getting out of bed.

Lachesis. Probably the most important remedy for abdominal pain that is characterized by an intolerance of anything around the waist (such as a belt or clothes). The liver region is very sensitive. The abdomen is distended, sensitive, and very painful to touch. The person is generally worse after waking up. A person with abdominal problems and liver discomfort from too much drinking may find this remedy helpful.

Lycopodium. Helps abdominal pain that occurs immediately after a light meal. The abdomen (especially the lower portion) is extremely bloated and full. A constant sense of fermentation is present in the abdomen, like yeast working. The liver may be sensitive. Pain shoots across the lower abdomen from the right to the left side. This pain is generally better from passing gas. The pain often begins at 4:00 P.M. and eases in the early evening around 8:00 P.M.

Magnesia phos. Useful for treating gas pains around the navel that are improved by drawing the legs up or bending double. This remedy is especially useful for colic-type pains of newborns from trapped gas in the abdomen. Passing gas or belching relieves the discomfort. Symptoms generally feel better from warmth. This remedy may also be helpful for treating the pain associated with gallstones. *Magnesia phos* can be helpful while en route to the hospital or doctor's office with gallbladder pain. A 6x potency is recommended; dissolve twenty tablets in one cup of warm water and sip this mixture continuously.

Natrum phos. Useful for treating colic of infants and children, especially when there are signs of excess acid in the stomach (such as vomiting curdled milk or passing green, sour-smelling stools). This type of colic is often associated with the inability to pass gas or belch, and may occur soon after eating. The back of the tongue and roof of the mouth often have a yellow, creamy coating.

Natrum sulph. Useful for treating sharp, stitching pains in the liver area. This area is very sensitive to touch; tight clothing around the waist is intolerable. The abdominal pain is worse lying on the left side. The gas tends to build mostly in the ascending colon and is often worse before breakfast. The person experiences much acidic belching, and the tongue has a brown coating. Morning stools can be loose, especially after spells of cold, damp weather. Stools can be passed involuntarily when passing gas.

Nux vomica. Helpful for abdominal pains caused by overindulgence in foods and stimulants (such as alcohol, coffee, spicy foods, or meat). The person is usually irritable, gets angry easily, and is hypersensitive to noise, touch, or light. The abdominal walls feel bruised and sore and the abdomen is extremely sensitive to touch. The abdominal pain often has an upward pressure causing shortness of breath and the desire for a stool. The abdomen also tends to be hard and drawn in. Several hours after eating, the person may feel pressure. The pain is generally worse while in motion and better while sitting or lying down. *Nux vomica* is also useful for abdominal pain due to the sudden stoppage of hemorrhoidal bleeding.

Phosphorus. A very important remedy for acute hepatitis and pancreatitis. The person feels a weak, empty sensation in the entire abdominal cavity and sharp, cutting pains in the abdomen. The abdomen feels cold. Stomach pains are relieved by cold food or drinks, especially ice water. These cold drinks, however, may be vomited up when they get warm in the stomach. Note that a person with these conditions should be under the care of a physician.

Podophyllum. Used to treat abdominal pain associated with a weak or sinking feeling in the stomach. The liver region is painful, but feels better from rubbing. Great amounts of gagging and vomiting are sometimes experienced. A thirst for large amounts of cold water (like problems associated with *Bryonia*) is common. Gurgling in the intestines is often followed by profuse, putrid, gushing stools that do not cause pain. This kind of diarrhea often occurs in the early morning, causing the person to wake up suddenly. This remedy is especially useful for teething babies with hot, glowing cheeks. The stool tends to be watery and profuse and contains a jelly-like mucus.

Rhus tox. Used when gas rumbles after first rising up out of a seat or from a bed, but disappears with motion. Abdominal pains compel the person to walk around. Eating even a small amount causes abdominal distention and pain.

Sepia. Helpful for the relief of abdominal pain with a bearing-down sensation, especially in women who have problems with the uterus. Great amounts of gas and headaches are common characteristics. The liver tends to be sore and painful. The pain is relieved by lying on the right side.

Staphysagria. Useful for treating severe pain in the abdominal skin and tissues, especially from a clean, incised wound after an operation. *Staphysagria* is also helpful for trapped gas in the intestines. This stomach pain often occurs after being disappointed and suppressing any angry feelings. This remedy is particularly helpful for children who have pent-up frustrations. Abdominal pains are often seen in a person who has spongy and tender gums, pyorrhea, and dark-colored teeth.

Sulphur. Useful for treating abdominal pain in which the abdomen moves as if something were alive inside it (similar to problems associated with *Thuja*). The person is red-faced, irritable, disorganized, and talkative. The abdomen is very sensitive to pressure and feels raw and sore. Drinking too much alcohol sometimes causes this type of pain. The person feels faint and wants to eat. The abdominal pain is often worse in the late morning around 11:00 A.M.

Thuja. Abdominal problems often associated with gas and constipation are relieved by *Thuja*. Extremely violent pains cause the stool to recede into the rectum. The stomach is distended, tends to protrude in different areas, and feels as if something were alive inside it. These movements are generally painless. Chronic diarrhea is worse after breakfast and is accompanied by a great deal of gas and abdominal discomfort.

Zincum met. A person with abdominal pain who is very restless (especially the legs, which are in constant motion) can be helped with *Zincum met.* The abdominal pain is worse after eating just a small amount. Drinking wine often aggravates or causes abdominal pain. The person is very sensitive to noise and does not like to work or talk.

ABSCESSES AND BOILS

An abscess is a small area of inflammation that generally starts out as an area of redness, followed by swelling and pain. Fluid collects and pus forms and gathers at the center of the abscess. The abscess may break open and drain until no pus remains; it is then that healing takes place. If the abscess does not break open, several measures are taken to help bring the boil to a head to facilitate drainage. One method is to apply warm, moist packs on the boil for ten to twenty minutes two or three times a day. The temperature of the moist pack should be similar to body temperature so it does not burn the area. Another method is to lance the abscess or boil with a sterile needle, although this should be done only by a health care practitioner or physician. A third method is to use homeopathic remedies to help either bring the boil to a head and drain or reabsorb the fluid internally.

It is important to never squeeze the abscess to drain the pus, since this may make the inner borders of the abscess break and spread the infection inward. This can cause a systemic infection. Before the abscess drains or comes to a head, it should not be covered. Only after the abscess is draining should a person cover it with porous material, such as cotton gauze. The gauze allows the site to breathe and soak up the draining pus.

Homeopathic remedies can be used to treat boils and abscesses, but certain situations should be treated by a physician: One circumstance is when a person has a fever, headache, or fatigue, or there are multiple sites of infections; another is when there are red streaks extending from the abscess upward or toward the center of the body. This means that the infection could be spreading along the blood or lymph system.

Apis. Useful only in the early stages of an abscess or boil. The affected area of the skin feels and looks like a bee sting—it shines, swells, and becomes pink and then pale. Cold applications relieve the symptoms somewhat; heat and touch aggravate them. There is itching and a bruise-like soreness. Useful for infections that occur in areas with loose tissue (such as the eyelids and genitals) where much swelling can occur. Cold compresses relieve the swelling. The person is not thirsty and may alternate between perspiring and having dry skin.

Arnica. Useful for treating extremely sore boils that come in crops and do not mature. The boils shrivel up before they come to a head, and another crop of boils returns. This remedy may also be used for very sore boils that are full of blood. *Arnica* helps ripen the abscess, causing the discharge of pus. The whole body feels sore. *Arnica* should not be used topically because it aggravates and irritates boils.

Arsenicum alb. Useful for treating boils that are often filled with blood or have a bluish-black base surrounded by a red discoloration. This type of boil may quickly degenerate into an ulceration surrounded by dry, rough, scaly skin. The burning pain is accompanied by putrid discharges, especially after the skin breaks down and begins to bleed. Despite the burning, the person feels better with warm applications on the boil or abscess. Cold drafts make the person feel worse; warmth makes the person feel better. The skin is usually cold and dry and the person is always restless, fearful, anxious, cold, and thirsty.

Belladonna. Most useful for treating the beginning symptoms of an abscess. The affected area swells rapidly, becomes red, and has intense, throbbing pain. Pus develops quickly. The swelling increases, and the redness radiates from the center of the infection. This remedy is especially helpful for tooth and gum abscesses, as well as abscesses on the glands around the neck (such as the tonsils or lymph glands). Symptoms come on suddenly and include shiny, red skin, throbbing pain, and intense heat that radiates with a burning sensation. The person is generally agitated and may experience nightmares or delirium if there is a fever.

Calcarea sulph. Useful for an abscess where the pus seems to continue indefinitely. Before this remedy is useful, the pus must find a vent and be draining. *Calcarea sulph* often is used after *Silica* to help the body heal from within and encourage the drainage to continue.

Ferrum phos. Useful for generalized inflammation (such as fever or multiple sites of inflammation). *Ferrum phos* should only be used in the early stages of inflammation before the boil or abscess has developed.

Hepar sulph. Useful for abscesses that form on unhealthy skin from scratches or irritation. An important symptom is excessive sensitivity in the area of the abscess. The person is always chilly.

The area of the abscess throbs, and sharp, stick-like pains are worse at night and from cold. The boil may begin as a small pimple that rapidly enlarges and quickly ulcerates. A large, putrid ulcer surrounded by small pimples may form. The pus, which may be bloody, often smells like old cheese. If *Hepar sulph* is given in a low potency when pus is threatening to drain, pus continues to form. If this remedy is given in a higher potency, the pus-forming process is often stopped. High-potency remedies are not recommended for home prescribing. Consult a physician or skilled homeopathic consultant for potencies above 30c.

Kali mur. Useful after *Ferrum phos* for the second stages of inflammation and infection of an abscess. This abscess is characterized by swelling and pain without pus formation. *Kali mur* is often used in the 6x potency.

Lachesis. Useful for treating an abscess. The discharge from the abscess is thin, very dark and purplish, and offensive. The symptoms are worse from touch and any pressure. The pain is better after the pus has started to form and discharge, and is always worse after sleep. The person may be extremely restless and talkative; he or she speaks rapidly and changes quickly from subject to subject.

Mercurius sol. Useful after *Belladonna* when pus has actually formed. The pus is green, thin, and watery, and forms more slowly than the pus associated with *Hepar sulph*. If pain accompanies the abscess, it is worse at night. Perspiration, increased saliva, and a putrid odor (either from the perspiration or the abscess) are common symptoms. When boils form in the mouth, the tongue is often thick, wide, and thickly coated with a yellow substance. The imprint of the teeth is seen on the sides of the tongue. The gums are spongy and bleeding, and the person shivers and is very thirsty. Symptoms are aggravated by any extremes of temperature (either from being too hot or too cold). Increased perspiration at night does not make the person feel any better. This remedy is especially helpful for abscesses in the roots of the teeth. In a lower potency, it helps pus form so that it will drain. In a higher potency, *Mercurius sol* helps stop the boil from forming (especially in tonsillitis). This remedy is also very helpful in pyorrhea. *Mercurius sol* should never be given after *Silica*. High-potency remedies are not recommended for home prescribing. Consult a physician or skilled homeopathic consultant for potencies above 30c. Note that these symptoms should be evaluated by a doctor or dentist.

Pyrogenium. Useful for abscesses that spread quickly. Often, a red streaking line moves from the abscess toward the center of the body or toward the head. The person has a high fever, is very weak, and looks extremely sick. If this situation occurs, a physician should be consulted. The boils or abscesses may quickly ulcerate and become very offensive and foul smelling (like those associated with *Arsenicum alb*). The person cannot lie still. A constant change of motion helps for a while (like symptoms associated with *Arsenicum alb*). The person may be talkative (like symptoms associated with *Lachesis*) and very anxious. This remedy is of particular help for ulcers of the elderly that do not heal, especially when these ulcers begin to spread.

Rhus tox. Useful for quick-forming abscesses. This remedy is especially helpful for abscesses in the area around the eye, the parotid glands, and the axillary glands underneath the armpit. The pus is often bloody, the pain is intense, and the swelling around the abscess is often dark red. The person is extremely restless and thrashes around or paces the floor. This remedy is often helpful in septicemia and was used before antibiotics when infection entered the bloodstream. If the person is very sick with a high fever and the abscess or boil seems to spread, a physician should be contacted immediately.

Silica. One of the most important remedies for boils and abscesses that are slow to heal. The pus is thin, watery, and offensive. An irritating discharge causes the surrounding skin to itch and to be sensitive to touch. When given, *Silica* helps thin the pus and encourages the formation of granulation and other healing tissue. Once the tissue begins to heal, this remedy should be stopped. If given too often, *Silica* may often cause another abscess to form. The boils are sensitive to cold and better from warmth. *Silica* is particularly helpful for abscesses that occur at the site of a vaccination or immunization. Ingrown toenails are also aided by this remedy. Often useful for fistulas, *Silica* helps to heal the tissue from within. *Silica* is also useful after an abscess has been lanced or opened to help the skin heal. It helps the pus form and helps the painless boil come to a head. In 6x potency, *Silica* should be given every two hours until the boil begins to drain. As the swelling goes down, the dosage should be gradually tapered down over a few days. If painful swelling occurs, a different remedy is generally required. *Silica* should never be used with *Mercurius sol.*

Sulphur. Useful for treating chronic boils, especially when recurrent crops of boils form in various parts of the body. Pus from these boils causes irritation, burning, and itching of the skin around the affected area. Generally, these people are unclean, disorganized, and often unaware of the problem's severity because they do not pay attention to themselves.

ACNE

Acne is a skin disorder that results from pores being clogged, eventually forming small infections known as pimples, whiteheads, blackheads, or cysts. There is often redness, inflammation, and pus formation within the pimple. Inside the pimple is generally sebum, carotene, and bacteria. The bacteria produces enzymes, which break down fatty acids in the sebum to form free fatty acids that irritate the hair follicle wall. Deeper cysts form when these follicles dilate and rupture.

Acne can occur on the face, neck, upper back, chest, and shoulders. It generally begins during adolescence and disappears by early adulthood, but in some cases may continue throughout life. It is particularly a problem for women because of their hormonal cycles, and sometimes women in their thirties and forties develop acne, especially around the time of their menstrual period. Heredity also seems to play an important role, especially among people who have oily skin. Generally, acne gets worse when the androgens, the male sex hormones produced by both the testes and ovaries and the adrenal glands, begin to increase in amount during puberty. These androgens stimulate the oil glands to produce increased amounts of sebum, which is the lubricant of the skin.

The face should always be washed gently using a mild soap. The face should not be scrubbed too hard since the bacteria that causes acne is deeper in the skin and not on the superficial layer that is washed off. Whiteheads should not be squeezed unless the pus has turned yellow or white and the top of the pimple is soft. The area should only be squeezed gently after it has been softened with warm water. Blackheads are plugs of oil that darken upon contact with the air and should also be removed carefully. Since blackheads are not dirt, scrubbing will not help; in fact, it will only make them worse. An extractor, which can be found at any drugstore, can be applied to the pores after a warm compress. Fingernails should never be used since they can leave scars on the skin.

Topical lotions that may be helpful come from tea tree oil (used topically once a day), *Calendula* tincture (especially when there are many blackheads and the skin is oily), and benzoyl peroxide. Benzoyl peroxide as a medicated lotion dries and reddens the skin, so it is important to start with a 5 percent concentration to minimize irritations. If moisturizers, makeup, or suntan lotions are used, it is important to make sure they are hypoallergenic, because sometimes allergies to these can aggravate the acne.

Allopathic medications used to kill acne infection include oral antibiotics, antibacterial skin medication, and derivatives of vitamin A, such as Retin A and Accutane. Consult a physician or pharmacist for further information. There may be side effects to these medications, as well as interactions with homeopathic treatment.

Homeopathic remedies can be used to control acne. There are also useful natural methods based upon dietary changes, supplementation, and cleansing. Important factors include a low-fat diet with no more than 18 to 20 percent of calories from fat, high fiber content with whole grains, and fresh fruits and vegetables. Some people find that eliminating dairy products from their diet helps decrease pimple formation. Certain vitamins are known to relieve acne.

Antimonium crud. Ueful for treating small, red pimples on the face. There is excessive thirst and a very thickly coated, white tongue. Often, indigestion accompanies this type of acne. This remedy is also useful when acne forms after a person has been near a fire (such as a camp fire or a fireplace). This type of acne is common in people who drink too much alcohol or who are overweight.

Arsenicum alb. Useful for pimples that emit an odorous discharge and burn and itch intensely. These symptoms are relieved by warm applications and are worse from cold. The person tends to be very fastidious, orderly, and concerned about appearance. The pimples cause extreme distress, and the person becomes very anxious and restless.

Belladonna. Useful for the treatment of bright red pimples on the face. The face is hot and flushed. Pimples often form on the temples, the corners of the mouth, and the chin. A bright red inflammation is the most important symptom.

Calcarea phos. Useful for the acne of a girl around the time of puberty who is growing rapidly. *Calcarea phos* is particularly helpful for a girl who tends to be anemic during the early phases of the menstrual period, has headaches, and has a distended abdomen from gas. These symptoms are usually better by eating.

Causticum. Itchy, red pimples on the face that are worse on the nose can be treated with *Causticum*. These pimples appear after becoming overheated.

Graphites. Useful for treating pimples that tend to ooze a sticky, thin discharge. Cracks may form around the acne, and eczema on the face may generalize in one area. There is a peculiar sensation of cobwebs on the face. The person is generally constipated and has large, difficult stools with mucus threads in them. This type of acne is generally worse around the time of the menstrual period, especially if the menstrual period is late.

Hepar sulph. Useful when pimples form whiteheads and pustules. To help promote drainage, the remedy should be given in a low potency. To help stop the formation of the pustules, the remedy should be given in a high potency. A characteristic symptom of this type of acne is extreme sensitivity to pain and cold. The person does not like drafts on any parts of the body, especially in the area of the pimples. The person is also sensitive to touch. Often these pimples appear on the forehead. Discharges from the pimples often smell like old cheese. (Note that high-potency remedies are not recommended for home prescribing. Consult a physician or skilled homeopathic consultant for potencies above 30c.)

Hydrastis. The type of acne that occurs on the chin can sometimes be helped by *Hydrastis.* The skin is unhealthy and the affected person tends to perspire profusely. Discharges from the acne are often thick, yellow, and sticky.

Ledum. Useful for red, pimply eruptions (especially on the forehead and cheeks) that sting when touched. This acne is better from cold applications and worse with warm applications and at night. *Ledum* is also useful for treating the acne of people who drink too much alcohol.

Nux vomica. May help relieve acne for people who drink too much alcohol, smoke too many cigarettes, and generally abuse or overwork themselves. People affected with this type of acne often have stomach problems (such as increased acid or constipation). Cheese aggravates the acne.

Pulsatilla. A woman who has acne (especially around the time of the menstrual period, when the period is late or absent) may respond to *Pulsatilla.* The person is weepy, chilly (but likes the open, cool air), thirstless, and desires comfort and consolation.

Sepia. Helps relieve itchy pimples on the face that are worse when the menstrual period does not appear. *Sepia* is also an important remedy for acne during pregnancy. Eating too many sweets and chocolate aggravate the acne. These pimples are often located on the forehead and nose.

Silica. Especially when used in low potency, *Silica* is useful for very cystic acne to help drain whiteheads. Given in high potency, this remedy helps stop the formation of the boil. *Silica* is a very important remedy for healing the area after the boil has drained; it helps form stronger, healthier tissue. This remedy also helps prevent scars after a large, cystic acne has formed. High-potency remedies are not recommended for home prescribing. Consult a physician or skilled homeopathic consultant for potencies above 30c.

Sulphur. One of the most important remedies for acne, especially if the acne tends to be chronic and recurrent. The area around the pimples burns and itches. The skin of the face is rough, dry, and hard. The acne is often associated with large comedones and boils.

Any kind of water touching the skin is aggravating. The person tends to be constipated and looks dirty and disheveled.

AFTER-CHILDBIRTH BLEEDING

> **Take special care.** While homeopathic remedies are safe during pregnancy, labor, and breastfeeding, a pregnant woman should confer with her obstetrician or midwife to coordinate treatment.
>
> A physician should be contacted if there are any signs of bright red blood or increase in the normally dark uterine blood after childbirth.

After a baby is born, the placenta passes out the vaginal opening. The placenta is the tissue that nourishes the baby and is the connection between the mother and child. A physician or midwife should always help gently extract the placenta. Homeopathic remedies can help control the bleeding that occurs as the placenta is being expelled.

Arnica. Can help prevent excessive bleeding if used during and after labor. *Arnica* is useful when the uterus and vagina feel sore and bruised.

Belladonna. Useful when the after-birth blood is hot and coagulates or clots very quickly, which may actually cause the placenta to be retained longer than it should. The person is hot, flushed, and irritable.

China. Useful after childbirth for heavy uterine bleeding that causes the person to feel weak, debilitated, and possibly faint.

Ipecac. When the after-birth blood is not clotted, but is fluid and gushing, *Ipecac* may be helpful. This remedy may be associated with nausea and vomiting that accompanies severe after-birth bleeding.

Kali carb. Useful for postpartum bleeding due to the inability of the blood vessels to contract and close off; this can occur up to one week after childbirth. The person tends to feel weak and weary. The legs tend to give out easily, and the back feels very sore. The person may feel anxious and will feel this anxiety in the pit of the stomach.

Sabina. Useful when after-birth blood is red and has very dark clots. The after-birth pain is severe and, when present, tends to move from the back of the uterine area to the front of the abdomen.

AFTER-CHILDBIRTH PAIN

The uterus contracts after the birth of the baby to expel the placenta. This can cause excruciating pain in the uterus and is sometimes as painful as the birth of the baby. With subsequent births, the after-birth pains can actually intensify with each delivery.

Nursing often increases the intensity of the pain because nursing helps contract the uterus. This contraction helps to bring the uterus down in size more quickly, but it can cause increased cramping. Gentle massage or sitting in a bathtub can be helpful to relax the intense uterine contractions.

Arnica. Used routinely after childbirth to help speed healing of the uterus and vagina, which feel sore and bruised. *Arnica* is also useful for pain and discomfort after a cesarean section or episiotomy to help heal the tissue quickly.

Bellis. Especially useful for deep tissue damage during delivery, especially in the uterus. *Bellis* can also be useful when the bladder or intestines are irritated and sore after childbirth. This is also an important remedy for healing the uterus after a cesarean section.

Bryonia. Useful for after-birth pains in the uterus that are aggravated by movement or deep breathing and are relieved when the person lies still. The person is comfortable if left alone, but if bothered by family or friends will become irritable and easily angered. The person is thirsty for large amounts of cold water and eats at infrequent intervals.

Calendula. Used as an ointment, may be applied directly to an episiotomy scar or to a tear in the vagina that occurred during childbirth. *Calendula* may also be used to help heal the tissue on a cesarean scar.

Caulophyllum. Useful after a prolonged and exhausting labor, especially for pain that moves quickly between the lower abdomen, chest, and groin.

Chamomilla. Useful for pain experienced as the placenta is being expelled; the pain drives the person frantic and extends to the back and down the legs. The person is extremely irritable and angry, and lashes out. *Chamomilla* is also helpful when the uterus contracts after childbirth and when the baby first starts to nurse, especially when the woman cries out in pain and becomes irritable and angry.

Cimicifuga. Helps intolerable after-birth pain that tends to move into the groin and across the pelvis from hip to hip. The person is often depressed and fearful, and may be claustrophobic, especially if in a small room. There may also be a headache that feels intolerable.

Cocculus. Useful when after-birth pain is located in the intestinal area, especially if it has been a hard labor and the intestinal wall is irritated. The person tends to feel better with firm pressure on the abdomen, when doubled up, and with warm applications. *Cocculus* is also useful for after-birth pain that continues and is associated with angry feelings.

Coffea. Useful for extremely intense after-birth pains accompanied by a fear of death. There is less irritability and anger than with *Cocculus* or *Chamomilla*.

Cuprum met. After-birth pain accompanied by cramps in the legs, calves, and thighs is helped by *Cuprum met.*

Hypericum. Useful after a surgical procedure (such as a cesarean section or episiotomy) when there is shooting pain along the nerves in the skin. *Hypericum* can be taken orally or used as an ointment applied directly to the irritated nerve tissue. This remedy can also be used as an ointment in conjunction with *Calendula.*

Nux vomica. Useful for after-birth pain that feels like it is in the rectum or bladder. *Nux vomica* is also helpful when the person feels the urge to urinate or have a bowel movement, but nothing seems to come. There is general irritability and hypersensitivity to noise, and even the presence of other people.

Sabina. Useful for after-birth pain that shoots from behind the uterus to the front of the abdomen. This remedy may also be useful for bleeding when the placenta is expelled. The blood is bright red with thick, dark, odorous clots.

Sepia. Useful for after-birth pain that tends to shoot up from the vagina into the uterus (or even higher). There is a sensation of great weight in the pelvis, and it feels as though the uterus will drop out of the vagina; the sensation disappears when crossing the legs. The person may feel totally indifferent toward the family and wants to get away and find quiet. Both depressed and irritable, the person cries if shown any sympathy. There is nausea, especially if food is being cooked nearby.

AIR TRAVEL PROBLEMS
(INCLUDES FEAR OF FLYING AND JET LAG)

Problems experienced when flying include anxiety, fear, motion sickness, and pain in the ears when ascending or descending. Another problem is jet lag. People who travel long distances, especially those who frequently cross many time zones, experience fatigue, weakness, and sometimes confusion and depression; these conditions are worsened if people are unable to sleep.

Aconite. Fear is always the most characteristic symptom of *Aconite.* Useful when a person is extremely apprehensive and fearful prior to or during an airplane flight.

Argentum nit. Can be used to treat the fear of flying, especially when the person experiences terror while anticipating an upcoming airplane flight. Nervous anticipation and a constant irrational fear that the airplane will crash or fall out of the sky are key symptoms. Nervous anticipation of an upcoming ordeal brings on diarrhea. The person feels severely claustrophobic, and the thought of being in an airplane and being unable to get out and walk is terrifying. The person will often choose a seat on an aisle for quick escapes. Looking up or down increases the anxiety. Those who need *Argentum nit* often try to hide their irrational thoughts from others.

Arnica. Helps when the entire body feels sore and bruised after a long flight. Difficulty in sleeping leads to soreness and a feeling that the person has worked too hard.

Arsenicum alb. The person is extremely anxious (but is not terrified or fearful), restless, and paces in anticipation of an upcoming airplane flight. Defense mechanisms against the anxiety often include becoming orderly and fastidious in preparing to leave (such as packing a suitcase perfectly).

Calcarea carb. Particularly helpful before airplane flights. There is a feeling that something bad is going to happen. These people are scared of losing their minds and that others will notice their confusion. Having a heart attack on the airplane and being unable to reach a hospital or get help is a particular fear; restlessness accompanies this fear. Claustrophobia is also experienced. Anxiety increases as the plane ascends. This remedy is also useful for those who fear high places, such as a hill or mountain, or fear looking down from a high place. There is great fear of looking down, which causes anxiety and dizziness. Even the sight of another person looking over a ledge can cause great anxiety. Dreams of being in a high place and looking over the edge actually reflect this anxiety. Altitude sickness occurs, especially as the plane ascends. Looking down causes an empty sensation in the stomach.

Chamomilla. The person experiences sharp ear pain during the ascent or descent of an airplane. This pain can be excruciating, causing the person to cry out. Irritability is common.

Cocculus. This remedy for motion sickness is especially useful on long flights. The person is not able to sleep, and it seems as though the flight goes very slowly. Abdominal problems, nausea, and vomiting are typical. The person feels adverse to any kind of food or drink, and especially does not like the smell of cooking food. A desire for cold drinks, which may help the nausea, is sometimes experienced.

Gelsemium. Helpful for the fearful anticipation of an upcoming airplane flight, especially when this apprehension results in poor sleep. Frequent urination from anxiety is a common symptom. The body is weak and aching, especially the back and limbs. The person feels dull, heavy, and tired upon arriving at the destination and does not want to be active, especially after a long overseas flight. Even when the person should be excited to be in a new city or place, there is a desire to sleep and not be disturbed.

Kali mur. The most characteristic symptom is ear pain due to fluid in the middle ear, without the excruciating pain associated with *Chamomilla.* The person has trouble hearing and sound is muffled.

Natrum mur. The person worries and broods over past airplane flights that did not go as expected (such as a bumpy flight or rough landing). The person believes the upcoming flight will have the same problems.

Phosphorus. There is nausea from the exhaust odors of an airplane. The person is often irritable and high-strung.

ALCOHOL AGGRAVATION (INCLUDES HANGOVER)

Alcohol is a poison that affects the entire system. It destroys nerve and brain cells and especially affects the liver and kidneys. Alcohol in small amounts (one to two drinks a week) is considered relatively safe, but even small amounts of alcohol in susceptible people can have serious side effects. Alcohol in large amounts leads to alcoholism, which is a psychological and physiological dependence on alcohol. Many factors make some people more susceptible to alcoholism, such as heredity, stress, and learned behavior from a family member who drinks too much.

Alcohol has a disinhibiting effect on the psychological and emotional state of a person. This can cause a person to do things he or she normally does not do—driving too fast, talking too much, being impulsive in behavior. The subsequent effect of alcohol, after the initial disinhibiting effect, is depression. The person becomes tired, lethargic, and emotionally withdrawn. A person also may have outbursts of anger.

Alcoholism is a disease that must be treated on a long-term basis by a competent clinician, skilled in the many aspects of how alcohol affects people's lives. Alcohol is considered a problem if a person does not participate in normal duties, such as going to work, or if a spouse or family member feels that alcohol has had a negative effect on the person's life.

Often a support group, such as Alcoholics Anonymous, can help a person abstain from alcohol. Counseling, family intervention, good diet, and exercise also help the person avoid alcohol. Chronic overuse of alcohol can be treated by a homeopathic physician, who can help integrate good nutrition, homeopathy, and psychotherapy support to help the person avoid alcohol.

The homeopathic remedies listed here have been useful to both help decrease the craving for alcohol and treat people for the side effects of drinking too much.

Arsenicum alb. Useful when the person drinks too much and experiences burning in the stomach that gets better when drinking warm liquids. The person is restless, anxious, and constantly changes positions. A marked fearfulness accompanies *Arsenicum alb,* and the person is easily irritated. There may be hallucinations of sight and smell. Diarrhea burns in the rectum and anus as it comes out. Headaches are relieved by cold applications, and a burning in the stomach is relieved by warm drinks. This remedy is particularly useful when drinking causes breathing problems or asthma. Extreme sensitivity to any commotion or disorder is common. The hangover is worse when wine is consumed.

Bryonia. Useful when the person drinks too much and there is dizziness, especially when the person moves. The person is thirsty and wants to lie still and be left alone. The tongue is coated white.

Carbo veg. Useful for the person with a hangover who feels fullness and heaviness in the abdomen. Excessive belching temporarily relieves abdominal fullness. Belching is sour and burning. Nausea is excessive, especially in the morning. The person feels chilly and wants to be fanned because of not getting enough air. *Carbo veg* is useful for the person who is particularly affected by the consumption of liquor.

Ipecac. Associated with excessive vomiting after drinking too much.

Nux vomica. The most important remedy for drinking too much. Excessive irritability occurs when the person stays up late drinking too much. The person also tends to desire other stimulants such as coffee and cigarettes. The person tends to be irritable and cannot tolerate noise, odor, or light after drinking. The person tends to find faults in others and is critical of them. *Nux vomica* is useful for a nauseous feeling that occurs in the morning after drinking, especially after eating. A weight and pain in the stomach worsen after eating.

The stomach region is sore when pressure is applied. An intoxicated feeling in the head is accompanied by vertigo. The person feels worse from trying to think, and feels worse in the open air. *Nux vomica* is useful for the person who is aggravated by the consumption of beer, brandy, and wine.

Pulsatilla. Useful for the person who reacts to drinking too much by becoming emotionally sensitive, crying easily, and needing attention and consolation. A strong, bitter taste in the stomach is accompanied by abdominal distention. The person feels a weight (such as that of a rock) in the stomach area. Belching is accompanied by an extremely bitter taste from food previously eaten. Symptoms are worse in the morning upon waking. Lack of thirst and chilliness are experienced, but the person wants the windows open to feel the cool breeze, despite the chills.

Sulphur. Drinking too much causes irritability and a quick temper in the person. This remedy is best indicated when a person becomes dirty and messy after drinking and cannot keep clean. The body feels hot, and the person often feels worse around 11:00 A.M. The person sleeps for short periods of time. The person may have an offensive odor. There may be a sensation of heat on top of the head. The person tends to desire beer, brandy, and wine.

Zincum met. Useful for the person who is sensitive to wine and becomes depressed, fearful, and hypersensitive to noise. Headaches are common after consuming the smallest amount of wine. There is occasionally a feeling that the person will fall to the left side. The person becomes easily intoxicated after consuming even a small amount of wine. Drinking too much can also lead to weakness and restlessness of the legs, with the feet constantly in motion. The person cannot keep the feet still, even at night in bed. The body jerks during sleep after excessive drinking.

ALLERGIES (INCLUDES HAY FEVER)

Allergies are caused by the body's hypersensitivity to foreign substances such as pollen, animal dander, dust, and foods. Irritation of the mucous membranes along the upper respiratory system is common. Symptoms are sneezing, a runny nose, itchy eyes, irritation of the roof of the mouth, a stuffy nose, congested sinus areas, and a headache. Allergies are not simple to treat; they generally represent a chronic problem that is genetic, although they may skip one, two, or three generations.

Homeopathic remedies can help in the acute stages of allergies to help relieve the symptoms, but usually a more constitutional approach to help the underlying condition is necessary for permanent relief. Homeopaths believe there is an association between allergies, skin problems (such as eczema and hives), and asthma. It is best not to suppress the symptoms of the skin or mucous membranes since that can actually drive the process of irritation further into the system, creating such conditions as asthma or perhaps joint problems. It is always best to start with homeopathic remedies to see if the symptoms improve.

Allergies that occur in the wintertime are generally due to allergens such as dust from heating systems and molds that accumulate in basements, humidifiers, and furnaces. Allergies in the springtime are often due to tree pollen; in late spring or early summer, grass pollens are usually the cause. Later in the summer, problems are often due to ragweed, goldenrod, and dust during the dry season. Molds, especially those from trees and leaves, are usually the allergens during early to late fall when the weather is damp.

Natural treatments that can help allergies include using eyeglasses or sunglasses to avoid getting pollens in the eyes and washing the eyes out with water after being outside and exposed to irritating pollens. Rinsing the nose with salt water can be helpful to wash out pollens. The use of a HEPA filter in the furnace can help take out mold, animal dander, and dust in the air. Keeping dogs and cats out of the house while children are suffering from allergies is also very important. Keeping the basement dry can reduce mold accumulation. Having hardwood floors and avoiding carpeting is helpful, especially when the person is allergic to dust. If the person has a sensitivity to feathers, pillows made from foam rather than down should be used.

Other helpful hints are avoiding cigarette smoke, car exhaust, and alcohol, since they inflame bronchial tissues. Not storing newspapers and magazines and making sure that old rugs, carpets, stuffed animals, and upholstered furniture are clean are also helpful. House-plants can be a source of pollen and should be avoided in the homes of people who have allergies. Venting clothes dryers outside is impor-tant, as is removing damp clothes from the washer quickly so mold does not accumulate. Keeping windows closed during the summer and fall when the allergen counts are high can help. Running a clean air conditioner in the summer months may also help take mold out of the air. A low-fat diet is recommended and avoiding foods that are mucus producing, such as dairy, yeast, and sweets, is important. If the person is allergic to a specific food, that food should also be avoided. Aspirin and ibuprofen should be avoided in people who have allergies. Certain vitamins and herbs are known to help allergies.

Allium cepa. The eyes burn, sting, and swell and are sensitive to light. Tears are profuse but do not irritate the skin around the eyes (*Euphrasia* is the opposite with irritating eye discharge and non-irritating nasal discharge). An important characteristic is that the nose and eyes stream with great amounts of watery discharge. The person sneezes frequently. Acrid nasal discharge burns, making the nose and upper lip sore. Post-nasal drainage makes the throat raw. The person is extremely thirsty. A headache often accompanies the allergies and may be felt in the back of the head or in the forehead in the sinus area. Symptoms associated with *Allium cepa* seem to get better in the open air, especially when the air is cool. However, the cough that accompanies this illness may get worse when cool air is inhaled. Symptoms seem worse indoors or in a warm room.

Arsenicum alb. Asthma is often associated with this type of allergy. Mental agitation, anxiety, and restlessness occur. The eyes burn, and tears are hot and acrid, stinging the face and cheeks. Sneezing can be extreme. There may be a tickle in one spot inside the nose that is not relieved by sneezing. Heavy mucus drainage from the nose alternates with blockage of the nose. Nasal discharge is thin and burning and is not yellow or green, but watery. The upper lip is irritated and raw from the discharge. There is extreme thirst for warm drinks, which are sipped rather than gulped. Often, breathing is labored. The person is chilly and intensely intolerant of light. Warm applications to the face and nose, elevating the head, and wrapping the body seem to help the symptoms. Sitting up is often the best position. Wet weather, weather changes, and being by the ocean aggravate the symptoms. The allergies tend to get worse from midnight until 2:00 A.M.

Arsenicum iod. The person has a constant desire to sneeze with irritation and tickling of the nose. Watery, irritating, and excoriating discharge comes out the front of the nose and runs down the back of the throat. If the allergy continues for a long period of time, the thin discharge changes to a thick, yellow, hanging discharge that becomes a post-nasal drip, irritating the back of the throat. There is a feeling of blockage within the head and eustachian tubes. Often, the person has trouble hearing because of this fluid blockage. The person seems better outside in the open air. Sneezing aggravates the condition, as do dry and cold weather, windy and foggy weather, and tobacco smoke. Symptoms are also aggravated from exertion and being indoors.

Arum triphyllum. Nasal discharge is extremely acrid and excoriating, producing raw sores on the front of the nose and upper lip. (Allergies associated with the *Arsenicum iod* remedy produce irritation but do not produce sores.) The nose can be obstructed, causing the person to breathe through the mouth. There is pain over the top part of the nose, with large scabs often forming on the right side. The person constantly picks at the nose and lips until they bleed. The lips, roof of the mouth, and palate are often sore or raw and burning; the lips are also chapped. The corners of the mouth can become raw, chapped, and cracked. There is profuse saliva. The voice becomes hoarse, and gets worse from overuse and talking a lot. The face may feel chapped, as if a cold wind were blowing on it. Cold and wet winds, lying down, and the heat of a room aggravate the allergies.

Arundo. The roof of the mouth is extremely itchy, and the eyes and ear canals itch and burn. The nostrils itch annoyingly. Much sneezing and loss of smell are also common with these allergies.

Dulcamara. Especially suited for the person who lives or works in a damp, cold home or office. Symptoms can result from sitting on cold, damp ground or with sudden changes of temperature, especially from warm to cold. The nose stuffs up with a cold rain; otherwise, there is constant sneezing and a profuse, watery discharge from the eyes and nose. Eye discharges get worse in the open air. The person is thirsty for cold drinks. Diarrhea and joint pain can come on, especially in cold weather. Symptoms are often worse on hot days and cold nights (toward the end of summer and in early autumn). Symptoms are better with external warmth or by moving around.

Euphrasia. The eyes water constantly, causing itching and burning. Sometimes a sticky mucus on the eyes can be removed by winking or wiping them. Eye discharge is acrid, burning, and often thick (this is the opposite of *Allium cepa*). Nasal discharge is profuse and watery, but does not irritate the nose or upper lip (this is the opposite of *Allium cepa*). A frontal headache may accompany nasal discharge. Frequent sneezing that gets worse at night is common. However, if a cough is present, it is actually better at night and worse during the day. Allergies are worse in the sunlight and the wind. Staying in a dark room is helpful.

Gelsemium. There is violent sneezing and nasal discharge. The face is hot and the nose tingles and often has a burning discharge, especially in the morning. Thirstlessness accompanies the allergies, even though the mucous membranes are dry. Eyelids become so heavy that the person can hardly open them. Common symptoms also include a dull headache and slight fever. Legs may ache, and a chill may run up and down the spine. A peculiar symptom is profuse urination that accompanies a headache. Allergies are often worse in humid, foggy weather and can be aggravated by sudden emotions, bad news, and surprises. Allergies tend to be worse in the summer and in the morning around 10:00 A.M.

Kali iod. A profuse, watery, nasal discharge burns the nose and lip. The tip of the nose is often red. Frontal sinus pain is common. Pain in the sinuses and head may make the person anxious and irritable. When the sinuses are full, the nose is dry and does not have discharge. There is extreme thirst with violent sneezing. The person feels alternately cold and hot.

Natrum mur. A common symptom of this type of allergy is excessive, watery nasal discharge (similar to the raw white of an egg). This thin discharge often lasts from one to three days, and then the nose may become stuffy, making breathing difficult. Sneezing is also common. The tongue has a frothy, bubbly coating, especially around the edges. Sometimes canker sores develop on the lips and the corners of the mouth. A salt craving is a particular symptom associated with this type of allergy. The mouth is dry, and the thirst seems unquenchable. The person often loses the senses of smell and taste. Sometimes, a hammering headache accompanies these allergies, which can be worse over the eyes. Allergies are worse in the morning from 9:00 to 11:00 A.M. and in the sun when it is warm outside. Symptoms improve in the open air and when bathing in cool water. Perspiration also seems to relieve the allergies. The person often feels better wearing tight clothes or a tight wrapping around the body or face.

Nux vomica. Prolonged sneezing spells occur, especially when first awakening in the morning. Nasal discharge is runny during the day, but the nose is stuffed up at night and outdoors, and the stuffiness alternates between nostrils. There is itching all the way from the throat to the larynx and trachea. Itching is also felt in the eustachian tubes. Uncovering, noise, odor, and touch can sometimes initiate sneezing. The person is chilly and irritable and often stays up late at night with the bothersome allergies. The allergies can get worse after eating a meal, in the cool and open air, in drafts, and in the wind. The person feels better when the nose begins to run. Symptoms are better from rest and napping, warm drinks, and moist air.

Sabadilla. The most common symptom of this type of allergy is excessive sneezing with a runny nose. Prolonged sneezing attacks can cause nosebleeds and severe headaches. Severe frontal sinus pain is a common symptom. The person can be particularly sensitive to the smell of apples. The eyes have a watery discharge, and there is great itching in the nose. The roof of the mouth itches and is relieved by rubbing the tongue on it. (This palate itching is less intense than seen with *Arundo* or *Wyethia.*) The eyelids are hot, red, and burning; however, the tears do not redden the skin around the eyes. Sometimes the person has difficulty hearing due to eustachian tube blockage. The mouth is dry, yet the person is not thirsty. There is a general body chilliness and a sensitivity to cold air. Symptoms are often worse from the odor of strong foods such as garlic and onion and certain flowers. Allergies are relieved with warm food and drinks.

Sticta. The back of the nose has a feeling of fullness with a dryness of the nasal membranes. The person sneezes often and constantly needs to blow the nose, but there is no discharge. Dry scabs form, especially in the evening and at night. There is a feeling of floating in the air. Sometimes the neck is stiff. A dry, hacking cough comes on at night, and gets worse on inspiration. Allergies tend to get worse with sudden changes of temperature.

Wyethia. The back of the nose and roof of the mouth itch intensely (similar to the allergies associated with *Arundo*). The throat is dry and has a sensation of being swollen, causing difficulty with swallowing and clearing the throat of mucus (*Arundo* has fewer throat symptoms).

ANAL AND RECTAL PROBLEMS

The most common problem is rectal fissures, small tears usually in the back part of the anus. They cause great pain and bleeding, sometimes filling the toilet with bright red blood. This is particularly true if the stools are large, causing the cut to reopen. The rectal fissure often lies close to the internal sphincter muscles; after a stool is passed, which irritates the fissure, the internal sphincter muscles contract. This keeps constant pressure on the fissure, causing burning that can last for many hours after passing the stool. Fissures are usually associated with hemorrhoids, and the hemorrhoids may also bleed.

Rectal fissures can be prevented by keeping the stool soft, having regular bowel movements, and drinking plenty of water. If a fissure does appear, it is often helpful to dab the rectum with toilet paper saturated with cool water after a stool. This helps to contract the tissues around the fissure, which slows the bleeding and decreases the burning. Homeopathic remedies can help heal the tissue and relax the spasms of the internal sphincter muscles.

Other types of rectal problems are ulcers, inflammations as in Crohn's disease, ulcerative colitis, or fistulas. These conditions should be treated by a physician.

Aloe. Can relieve a burning anus and rectum. The rectum is hot, sore, and bleeding, and the person feels a constant bearing-down sensation. Cold water brings relief. The sphincter muscles feel weak, especially when passing gas, and the person is unsure whether gas or a stool will come. The stools contain mucus. Hemorrhoids are sore, tender, and protrude like grapes. These hemorrhoids feel better with cold water. Rectal pain is often worse during the menstrual periods and while sitting.

Arsenicum alb. If the rectum and anus have feelings of burning and pressure that are relieved by warm applications, *Arsenicum alb* is the best remedy. The rectal pain is worse during and after a stool and particularly bad at night. The person is restless and paces often. The burning pains are better after passing gas.

Causticum. Can relieve burning pains around the rectum that are worse from walking. The area feels sore and extremely irritated. The person rubs the area until it is raw. The pains in the rectum are worse after long hours of study or work. Rectal fissures burn like fire and bleed after a stool and when walking.

Graphites. Useful for relief of sharp, cutting rectal pain during a stool, followed by constriction and aching of the rectum for several hours. This problem is usually associated with people who are very constipated and develop rectal fissures. A sticky moisture from the anus causes the anus to itch. This moisture is more excessive after stools and may be associated with eczema around the anus.

Nitric acid. Rectal pain relieved by *Nitric acid* is characterized by a sensation of splinters or sticks in the anus. The anus and rectum are burning and raw. Rectal fissures bleed after a stool. Stinging pains occur during and after a stool.

Sepia. Useful for the relief of shooting pains that run from the rectum into the abdomen. These pains are usually associated with bleeding hemorrhoids. Rectal pain is worse from sitting, especially in the middle of the morning. Movement seems to relieve the symptoms.

Silica. Rectal pains, usually due to rectal fissures, that last for several hours after a stool are relieved by *Silica.* Partially expelled stool tends to recede into the rectum.

Sulphur. Helps when the anus itches and burns, but is relieved by cool compresses. The area around the anus is extremely red, usually from painless diarrhea. The person wants to have a bowel movement immediately after waking up early in the morning.

ANESTHESIA SIDE EFFECTS

Anesthesia is used for several reasons. When there is a great amount of pain, anesthesia medications may help dull the pain. Injection of topical anesthetics can also help diminish pain, especially when injected into joints. Another type of anesthesia is used to create a level of consciousness where a person is unaware of procedures, such as surgical procedures, that would cause great discomfort if the person were awake. These medications are usually administered through intravenous solutions. Some create a very deep level of unconsciousness and others have more superficial results. Reactions or side effects from anesthesia may occur immediately after the procedure, although some people may not experience them for several days or weeks.

Homeopathic remedies can be helpful for a person who has problems after the administration of anesthesia.

Carbo veg. The person feels nauseated after awakening from anesthesia. Belching improves the feeling of nausea and bloating in the stomach. The person cannot get enough air in the lungs and wants to be fanned, despite feeling cold. The skin feels cold and has a bluish tint.

Nux vomica. There is extreme irritability following anesthesia, and the person easily loses his or her temper. The person is oversensitive and cannot bear noise, light, odor, and being touched. Because of nausea and vomiting, the person is unable to eat. When finally able to eat, the person gets indigestion, stomach pain, and the sensation that the weight of a stone is in the stomach. There is unusual bloating after eating small amounts of food, and the stomach area is extremely sensitive to pressure.

Phosphorus. The person can be mentally confused and emotionally oversensitive. Since the anesthesia was used, a greater fearfulness of disease and death is experienced. The person feels that the energy has left the body after the anesthesia, and there has been no return to a normal state. Burning in the stomach is relieved by drinking cold liquids. As soon as water gets to the stomach, however, it is often vomited up.

ANTIBIOTIC SIDE EFFECTS

Antibiotics serve an important role in today's health care. Many conditions have been helped by antibiotics, which prevent bacterial spread. Unfortunately, antibiotics are often overprescribed, and there are certain conditions when they are used on a chronic basis. Antibiotics should not be used when there are viral infections since they have no effect on the virus. There are also side effects with antibiotics. Homeopathic remedies can be used for certain types of infections and can sometimes be used in place of antibiotics.

Apis. A useful remedy for an allergic reaction to antibiotics (various body parts swell and puff up). If the person has difficulty breathing, seek emergency treatment immediately. A red, rosy appearance is sometimes accompanied by soreness and stinging pains. The pain and itching are worse from heat, slight touch, and in the afternoon. The person experiences constricted sensations in the swollen areas. Irritability and angry feelings are often present.

Arsenicum alb. Useful when antibiotics cause digestive upsets (such as burning in the stomach) that get better after warm liquids are consumed. *Arsenicum alb* is also useful for the person experiencing diarrhea that is burning and excoriating to the anal tissues. Restlessness and anxiety often accompany the symptoms.

China. Useful for excessive diarrhea from antibiotics that is painless and which gets worse after eating and during hot weather. The person experiences excessive flatulence and a feeling of weakness. There may be dizziness when walking, a blue face, and a cold body.

Lycopodium. Useful for antibiotic sensitivity experienced by people who are weak, thin, and full of gas (especially helpful for the elderly). The abdomen is extremely distended, and there is excessive flatulence. Apprehension, oversensitivity, and fearfulness of breaking down under stress are experienced. Aggravation often occurs between 4:00 and 8:00 P.M. The person wants to drink only warm liquids, which seem to help settle the stomach.

Natrum phos. Useful for the person who experiences a sour taste in the mouth. The vomit is acidic, and there is a yellow, creamy coating on the tongue and in the back of the mouth. *Natrum phos* is helpful for vaginal infections caused by antibiotics, especially when vaginal discharge is cream- or honey-colored and sour smelling.

Nitric acid. Useful for the person who experiences a strong reaction to antibiotics. Blisters and ulcers that bleed may occur in the mouth and on the tongue. Diarrhea may be experienced. Extreme cutting pains after a bowel movement leave the person feeling irritable and exhausted. Abdominal pains appear and disappear quickly. In the past, this remedy was often prescribed for the overuse of mercury in the treatment of syphilis.

Nux vomica. Used to help the effects of taking any drugs, especially antibiotics. Useful for the person who is overstressed and overindulges in food, alcohol, or tobacco, or for the person who stays up too late at night. The person often takes antibiotics or other medications to calm the stomach and feel better, but then actually feels worse after taking them. The person is irritable, nervous, hypersensitive, and cannot bear noise, odor, or light. There may be constipation or diarrhea; in either case, the person feels that some stool always remains unexpelled. A weight and pain in the stomach are experienced that are worse after eating and after excessive vomiting. The region of the stomach becomes sensitive to pressure.

Thuja. Useful for the side effects of antibiotics that seem to linger for a long time; the person never feels quite right after taking antibiotics. It is generally used after other, more acute oriented remedies have not completely eliminated the problems. The person has excessive flatulence, abdominal distension, and a feeling in the abdomen that something is moving and alive but causes no pain. *Thuja* is useful for chronic vaginal infections that occur with the use of antibiotics. Vaginal discharge is thick and yellow or green.

ANXIETY (INCLUDES FEARS AND PHOBIAS)

Anxiety disorders or feelings of anxiety can be defined as a state characterized by feelings of dread, accompanied by physical symptoms that indicate a hyperactive nervous system. Anxiety can be differentiated from fear because fear is a response to a known cause while anxiety usually has no predisposing stimuli.

Physical signs of anxiety include shakiness, trembling, backache, headache, tension in the muscles, shortness of breath, easy fatigue, being startled easily, flushing of the skin or paleness, heart palpitations, cold sweats, diarrhea, dry mouth, increased urination, numbness, tingling in the extremities, or difficulty swallowing. Psychological symptoms include feelings of dread, difficulty concentrating, inability to sleep, decreased sex drive, and a feeling of a lump in the throat or anxiety in the pit of the stomach.

There are several types of anxiety disorders. Panic disorders are characterized by spontaneous panic attacks that are often associated with agoraphobia or claustrophobia. Generalized anxiety disorder is expressed as ongoing anxieties for at least a one-month duration. Phobic disorder is an irrational fear of a situation or object and the need to avoid it. This can be a social phobia such as a fear of public speaking, a phobia of taking tests, or a simple phobia of objects such as heights, animals, or needles.

Obsessive-compulsive behavior is another form of anxiety disorder. An obsession is present when recurrent intrusive ideas, impulsive thoughts, and patterns of behavior are unpleasant, time consuming, and interfere with the person's normal routine. For example, a person may have feelings of wanting to injure a loved one or use language that is against religious beliefs. The thoughts and ideas are usually senseless and the person often wants to ignore and suppress them, but has difficulty doing so. Compulsions, the other characteristic of the disorder, are repetitive and intentional behaviors that form a response to the obsession according to certain rules that a person makes up. The person's behavior usually neutralizes and prevents discomfort of some dreaded situation. The person also realizes his or her behavior is excessive and unreasonable, but cannot help doing it.

The final type of anxiety state is called post-traumatic stress disorder. It is usually a response to some intense or extraordinary major life stress, such as an accident that has occurred in the past, a sexual assault, or the experience of war by soldiers.

Symptoms of post-traumatic stress disorder include recurrent and distressing memories and dreams of the event and feeling as if the event is actually recurring. This includes flashbacks and psychological and emotional distress from exposure to an event that symbolizes or resembles the traumatic event. There is difficulty falling or staying asleep, outbursts of anger, difficulty concentrating, exaggerated startled responses, and physiologic responses, such as perspiring when exposed to events that symbolize or resemble an aspect of the traumatic event.

People with this kind of anxiety try to avoid stimuli, feelings, and thoughts that are associated with the traumatic event or activities that arouse memories of the trauma. They may sometimes have amnesia about some important aspect of the trauma. They also may have diminishing interest in activities that they enjoyed before the trauma, have problems forming attachments with other people, and have difficulty showing loving feelings.

One form of treatment for anxiety problems is medications prescribed by doctors to induce emotional and physical relaxation (such as benzodiazepines, which include Valium or Xanax); consult a physician or pharmacist for further information. Psychotherapy and antidepressants, if the problem also has a depressive component, may also be recommended by a physician. Specific types of psychotherapy are psychoanalytical, group therapy, cognitive therapy, and behavioral therapy. Behavioral therapy has many components involving positive and negative reinforcements. Special techniques of relaxation therapy can also be helpful, such as breathing techniques, biofeedback, meditation, and prayer.

Homeopathic remedies can be very effective for anxiety and fear. Reference to the Repertory will show that there are many specific types of fear, such as fear of open spaces or animals, and specific symptoms of anxiety, such as anxiety about being alone at night. Carefully matching the anxiety, along with other mental and physical symptoms, with the specific remedy will help minimize the feelings of stress, anxiety, and fear. If anxiety is prolonged or incapacitating, a professional skilled in psychotherapy should be contacted to evaluate the person's condition.

Aconite. For treating a person who experiences fear and anxiety when ill, however minor the illness. *Aconite* is an important remedy for panic attacks and panic disorders and is useful for the beginning stages of fever (such as with an upper respiratory infection or influenza) when the person feels fearful. There may be a fear of death and the belief that death is imminent; the person may actually predict the date and time of death. These symptoms are common when the person has a high fever. The person has feelings of foreboding and tends to worry. Useful for agoraphobia and other phobias (such as airplane flights, getting hit by a car, crowds, or fear of the dark). The person fears death during illness, as well as dying from heart disease, heavy work, and during pregnancy. There is a fear of ghosts, especially at night. A woman may experience fearfulness before her menstrual period begins. *Aconite* may help claustrophobia in subways, elevators, and other enclosed spaces. Anxiety also occurs at night, during a fever or chill, in a crowd, during a headache, and when pain is experienced anywhere in the body. The person also fears earthquakes, tornadoes, and other natural disasters. *Aconite* is often used before a person rides in an airplane or subway to help lessen the fear.

Anacardium. Helpful for the person with a lack of self-confidence and an inferiority complex from fear of not being liked by others. The *Anacardium* person is generally insecure and tries hard to be liked. A feeling of powerlessness may cause the person to avoid others. The person may fear something unfortunate may happen to him or her, and fears possible paralysis or death. There is despair of recovering from an illness. The person is afraid of hurting others and of disappointments in life. If feelings of self-worth continue to decrease, the person may become angry, bitter, and possibly insensitive, aggressive, and violent.

Apis. Useful when the person is afraid of dying and has premonitions of death. A fear of dying may be accompanied by the sensation of an inability to breathe. This is particularly true when fluid is retained, and the person feels heavy, bloated, and short of breath or when the person experiences an allergic reaction to hives or swelling in the throat. A person needing *Apis* may be afraid of others not being honest, which may lead to jealousy, loss of temper, and possibly screaming. The person may experience the peculiar symptom of feeling poisoned.

Argentum nit. Helpful when the person feels anxiety about

performing or speaking in front of others. This remedy may also help a person who has claustrophobia or agoraphobia. Because of the anxiety, the person is always in a hurry and becomes more anxious and walks faster. The person may be afraid of missing a deadline or arriving either too late or too early for an engagement. There is fear of being left alone and abandoned and of beginning new tasks and not doing them correctly. The person may be afraid of being alone (especially because of the fear of dying), going to church, walking past certain street corners, being in public places or in a crowd, or dying when alone. The person may predict the dates and times of future happenings (such as an impending disease, evil occurrence, fainting spell, convulsion, or robbery). Useful for panic and anxiety attacks (such as when the person is ready to go to a movie or a religious service and develops diarrhea). There may be a fear of heights. For example, the sight of a high building may cause the feeling that buildings on both sides of the street will move together and crush the person; when looking down out of an airplane window there may be a feeling that the airplane will crash; or when on a bridge or other high place, the person may have the impulse to jump off.

Arnica. Useful when a physical injury or severe mental trauma causes stress, shock, anxiety, or fearfulness; it is as though the mind, as well as the body, is bruised and sore. Because of this vulnerability and soreness, the person is afraid of others touching him or her and causing additional injury. In fact, the person may feel like a wounded animal and be fearful of anyone's approach, or being bumped or jostled in a crowd. There may be fear of sickness, dying at night, sudden death, doctors, buildings or high walls falling on the person, and heart disease. Useful for emotional shocks, especially when accompanied by physical injury. The person may be a victim of rape, robbery, or child abuse. *Arnica* is helpful for head injuries or strokes that affect mental functioning and for those who are overworked, exhausted, anxious, and fearful. The person has not felt well since being frightened, injured, or emotionally traumatized. Sudden fears may arouse the person during the night, especially after an accident. The entire body feels sensitive, and the person is nervous and cannot bear additional pain. Curiously, despite these symptoms, the person often says that nothing is wrong and wants to be left alone.

Arsenicum alb. Helpful for anxiety and fearfulness stemming from deep-seated feelings of insecurity. Vulnerability causes a desire for control, and in order to feel secure the person may become obsessively orderly, clean, and tidy. Fastidiousness is seen in every aspect of the person's life. The person gains security by controlling others and being possessive. Selfishness and self-worry are present, and the person is mainly interested in how he or she is affected personally (for example, when a friend or loved one dies, the loss is overshadowed by the main concern of whether he or she will also die). The person needing *Arsenicum alb* may also be dependent, not because of needed interaction with others, but because the person needs others close by for reassurance and support. The person may be surrounded by possessions as well as people, and may be miserly and greedy, often hoarding money and collecting valuable objects. If the person donates money (such as to a charity or a political organization), the motivation is not selfless, but rather out of concern for what will be given in return. On a physical level, typical symptoms are nighttime aggravations (especially between midnight and 2:00 A.M.), burning pain that is improved by warm drinks or warm applications, great chilliness, and nighttime restlessness. If insecurity increases and fastidiousness, greediness, and selfishness are not checked by homeopathic remedies or psychotherapy, the problem of anxiety gets worse, and the person becomes extremely anxious and fearful about health and death. These symptoms get worse at night, especially after midnight, and the person fears getting sick and dying alone. The person becomes agitated and restless and may actually move from place to place or bed to bed throughout the night. The person may seek reassurance from others when these symptoms occur, often going from one person to the next and possibly becoming unpleasant and demanding help. There may be fearfulness of a fatal disease (especially cancer), and the person often sees several doctors to confirm the presence of the disease; if the fear is not confirmed, the person becomes aggravated, angry, and anguished. The person may feel sure of death, and this fear represents the deepest form of insecurity and loss. The person becomes inconsolable and even more afraid of being alone; as this cycle continues, the person may become angry, critical of others, and mean-spirited.

Baryta carb. Useful for those who are shy, especially children who have difficulty learning new things and are slow to walk and talk, often falling behind in school. These children may have problems clearly understanding what is happening in the world and often stay by themselves. They may feel uncomfortable in new surroundings and with new friends, and are fearful of others, especially strangers. These children do not like to travel or leave home and are afraid of losing their parents. This remedy is helpful for small children who hide behind furniture or behind their parents when meeting a doctor and who often want to stay at home where it is safe and familiar. As adults, the person needing *Baryta carb* may exhibit child-like behavior. These people often perform daily activities adequately, but do not like the complication of learning new skills. The person may experience anxiety and difficulty in making decisions. This remedy is helpful for the elderly who have memory trouble and for those who feel anxious taking on new tasks.

Belladonna. Useful when anxiety and fearfulness are accompanied by extreme agitation. The person has dilated pupils and wild eyes, a flushed face, and heat coming from the body. This can be seen when the person is feverish and delirious, especially when falling asleep. There may be frightening visions (such as of animals, dead people, ghosts, and monsters). The person may become wild, run around the house, and tear at clothing. Speech and actions are extremely quickened. *Belladonna* is also a remedy for those who experience acute problems with mania in manic-depressive syndrome; these people may become violent, sing, swear, and do ridiculous things. A physician should be contacted if these symptoms are exhibited. Useful for the mental changes associated with high fevers. The higher potency is often used by homeopathic physicians, especially when the person is delirious.

Borax. Helpful for the person who experiences extreme anxiety from motion that has a downward direction, such as when children are carried downstairs or when they are being laid down or rocked.

This is particularly true for infants and young children. The child becomes anxious when being set in the crib or bed and may throw up his or her hands as if afraid of falling. The person who needs *Borax* is nervous, easily frightened, and sensitive to sudden noises (especially thunder).

Bryonia. Useful when the person is fearful and anxious while sick with fever, respiratory problems, or gastrointestinal problems. The person is afraid of business failures or losing money while sick and generally feels fine if left alone. As soon as the person is disturbed, these feelings intensify and activate anxiety about business and finances.

Calcarea carb. Useful for the person who is apprehensive and fears losing control of emotions and mental capacity. There may be fear of misfortune, cancer, infectious diseases, and especially heart disease. The person may feel constant fear of death and is concerned and anxious that others will discover or observe these fears. The person is generally afraid of the future and is not caught up in brooding or dwelling on past or present disappointments, but tends to worry about what will happen in the future. Generally the person is fearful of the unknown. The person is strong willed and able to handle stress fairly well; however, if stress and demands of life become overwhelming, these fears surface. Children who need *Calcarea carb* are very sensitive and particularly affected by sad or scary movies. They worry about what will happen when they die and whether God or any other supernatural beings exist. This remedy is generally associated with children and adults who are overweight, chilly, tend to perspire (especially children around their head), and crave sweets, cold drinks, ice cream, salt, and sugar.

Carbo veg. Helpful for anxiety accompanied by weakness and chilliness and for those who have never recovered from a past illness. The person's vitality is low, often due to loss of blood or a serious disease. Anxiety may be accompanied by trembling and a feeling of exhaustion. There may be fear of the dark and of ghosts or of committing a crime the person cannot remember. The person tends to be slow thinking, irritable, unhappy, and indifferent. There also may be anxiety during and after eating, especially when gastric problems and bloating are present. Anxiety generally gets worse in the evening (particularly during twilight).

Causticum. Helpful when the person is anxious and worries about others (especially friends, children, and injustice and exploitation in the world). The person may control children and often does not let them do anything that could get them in trouble or that represents danger. The person is extremely cautious and often becomes rigid because of the need to be careful. The person may be compulsive in thought and action, and often worries about such things as whether the stove was left on or the doors were locked. Anxiety becomes particularly severe at night (especially during twilight) and when falling sleep. The person may experience anxiety while straining during a bowel movement. Children who need this remedy may not want to go to bed alone, may cry when alone, and may fear darkness upon closing the eyes. These children may also fear dogs, ghosts, something happening to them in bed, and noise (especially at night) both inside and outside. There is a particular fear of strangers. These people are anxious and worry about the poor or those who are exploited. They may become revolutionaries, anarchists, or activists with strong moral opinions.

Cocculus. Helpful for the person who experiences extreme anxiety while caring for others; the person often stays up late at night taking care of the sick or dying. This leads to physical problems such as stomach cramps, abdominal distention, and diarrhea. There is anxiety from riding in a car, boat, or airplane because motion sickness comes on easily. The person may become anxious from looking at food, drink, or tobacco because he or she becomes faint and nauseated from them. The person may feel that time passes too quickly and is absorbed in thought.

Croton tig. Useful when the person is fearful of personal misfortune. There is an inability to express feelings. This causes frustration because the person is unable to release thoughts or concerns.

Cuprum met. Helpful for children who are afraid of falling and of others approaching them. Children who need this remedy are afraid of the dark and of strangers. The child may shrink away from an approaching stranger and cling tightly to a parent. There may also be anxiety before a coughing spasm and an irrational fear of the police.

Drosera. The person may have a fear of ghosts, being poisoned, and being persecuted. These symptoms get worse when the person is alone at night and upon awakening at night. *Drosera* is associated with the person who has coughing spasms and is short of breath, which causes fear and anxiety.

Gelsemium. Helps the person who experiences extreme apprehension and dread of appearing in public (such as singing or speaking, attending a class, or flying in an airplane). The person dwells on the upcoming event a long time and may develop diarrhea. There is great fear of lightning, and possibly a peculiar fear that the heart will stop beating unless the person remains in constant movement. There may be a fear of losing self-control, especially when in public.

Graphites. Helps anxiety that is accompanied by shyness and the inability to make decisions. The person is afraid and easily startled. Fearfulness makes the person lazy and not want to work. Because of the anxiety, the person is indecisive. Anxiety before the menstrual period gets worse while sitting and being inactive. The person becomes anxious at the thought of manual labor. When the person is warm, the anxiety seems to lessen. The person also feels better when crying. There is a constant fear that misfortune will happen, especially in business. Restlessness and anxiety are experienced while at work.

Hypericum. Often helps alleviate emotional and mental consequences of injury, shock, or extreme fright. *Hypericum* is useful for confusion and fear that results from a head injury. Agitated depression may follow the injury. Depression that is helped by this remedy is associated with anxiety, and those affected fear making mistakes in writing or forgetting what they want to say.

Ignatia. Useful for the effects of sudden loss, shock, disappointment, or grief (such as the death of a loved one, the loss of a relationship, or disappointment at work). The person does not like to cry and tends to keep feelings inside. Repressing these feelings often causes anxiety and fear. There may be a fear of burglars (especially at night upon awakening), doctors, death (especially upon awakening from an afternoon nap), or of others approaching the person. Fear and anxiety are often experienced during the menstrual period as well as when in enclosed spaces (claustrophobia). As the person attempts to hide fears and anxieties, anger and irritability may be experienced. The person does not want consolation for the grief or irritability. The person may become angry and upset if criticized.

Kali carb. Useful when anxiety is felt in the stomach area. The person is full of fear, especially the fear of dying while alone. The *Kali carb* person has an active imagination, is afraid of disease and death, and may experience anxiety when hungry. As a defense mechanism, the person becomes inflexible and rigid in behavior and in the expression of emotions. The person may become stoic and closed and may become extremely conscientious and conservative in action. There is often a great amount of bottled-up anxiety, but the person does not show it because he or she wants to remain in control. The *Kali carb* person may find it difficult to express feelings, especially to a doctor. The need to control feelings and anxieties often causes nighttime restlessness and sleeplessness when natural barriers and defenses weaken. The person may awaken around 3:00 A.M. feeling anxious and overwhelmed. Along with inner anxiety and the defense mechanism of being extremely conscientious and proper, the *Kali carb* person is often sensitive to drafts, experiences nighttime aggravation between 2:00 and 4:00 A.M., has swollen upper eyelids, craves sweets, and feels anxiety in the pit of the stomach.

Kreosote. Helpful for anxiety and fear, particularly when a man fears having sexual intercourse with a woman. The person may be anxious and sad and even may cry when listening to music. Children who need *Kreosote* may cry out when having a bowel movement. They may want to be given things but will discard them when they are received.

Lachesis. May be helpful when anxiety and restlessness occur at night. Depression and anxiety increase as the day progresses. There is anxiety about the future, personal salvation, and guilty feelings. There is a particular fear of dying at night. After a nightmare, the person is afraid of dying upon return to sleep. There is also fear of infectious and contagious diseases, robbers, snakes, water, and being poisoned.

Lycopodium. Useful when there is a fear of failure and making mistakes. There is a particular fear of giving speeches or presentations, especially in teachers, lawyers, religious leaders, and business people; however, these people usually perform well. Insecurity results in the need to control their world, and they are critical of themselves and the mistakes of others. They may be domineering, controlling, and extremely concerned about maintaining power and authority. Also, because of the insecurity, they may feel incapable of fulfilling responsibilities and thus may avoid emotional responsibilities. They may exaggerate their importance to others and hide feelings of inadequacy. There is a dislike of being around people or crowds and of being watched while working. They like to be alone but may be afraid to be alone. They want people nearby who are quiet and mind their own business; this is particularly true when they are ill. People needing *Lycopodium* become particularly anxious in the late afternoon around 4:00 p.m., and begin to relax after 8:00 P.M. They tend to feel better in the open air, are anxious about their health, possibly hypochondriacal, and worry about religion and personal salvation. There is a fear of being alone, darkness, noise, undertaking new things, and when awakening from nightmares. Children who need this remedy often have learning disabilities or dyslexia, and tend to use the wrong word, transpose letters, and write or read letters backward. These children are often afraid of people, especially strangers, and of being alone. They may also fear not reaching destinations (such as getting to school). People who need *Lycopodium* usually have some digestive problem (such as excessive flatulence, internal rumblings in the abdomen, and indigestion from foods such as beans, milk, onions, and cabbage). There may be a desire for sweets and sugar, as well as hot foods and hot drinks.

Magnesia carb. Useful for the effects of shocks, injuries, and mental stress, especially when the person feels extremely nervous afterward. The person is sensitive to the lightest touch and worries excessively. This remedy is particularly helpful when the person is constipated and has heaviness in the body. Nighttime anxiety gets better when the person goes to bed. The person tends to perspire often and tremble. There is a fear that accidents will happen. When under stress, there may be a peculiar symptom of feeling dazed. The person may do things such as packing and unpacking suitcases. This nervousness and anxiety tend to accompany the person to bed in dreams that are full of anxiety and woe and are about the dead, fire, long journeys, misfortune, robbers, and of being in water or being in danger. This is a useful remedy for women who are anxious, especially those in menopause who feel worn out and overwhelmed.

Natrum mur. May be beneficial for the person who, when healthy, is very emotional, sensitive, sympathetic to the problems of others, and feels responsible for helping others. Doctors, therapists, social workers, and religious leaders are often helped by *Natrum mur.* The person tends to be a good parent who cares for children and is very watchful and cautious. Because of vulnerability, however, the person fears being hurt and rejected. This causes anxiety and, as a defense mechanism, the person becomes highly organized, concerned about details, fastidious, and fussy about cleanliness. Hypochondria is common, and the person may become extremely concerned about diet, environment, and catching infections. Women who need *Natrum mur* often experience anxiety before and during the menstrual period; these women have many fears and premonitions that something bad will happen. There may be a fear of robbers, thunderstorms, evil, crowds, enclosed spaces, and possibly ghosts (especially at night). Children who need this remedy are often anxious because they are sympathetic, kind, and afraid to hurt the feelings of others. They try hard to please others and hide their anxiety and vulnerability. They often act older than they are and are sometimes called little adults.

Natrum phos. Helpful when the person experiences the unusual fear that something bad will happen at night. The person has an active imagination and in the dark may believe that a piece of furniture is a person or hear footsteps in the next room. Listening to music may cause anxiety and sadness.

Nitric acid. Helpful for anxiety that is experienced during a thunderstorm, after a bowel movement, and before a menstrual period. The person has the peculiar symptom of becoming anxious when ascending steps to a high place and when thinking about problems. There is extreme anxiety when the person stays up late at night caring for people who are sick. When the person loses sleep, the anxiety increases. There may be a fear of death.

Petroleum. Helpful for people who are anxious and afraid that death is near and must hurry to settle affairs. Anxiety is felt when in a crowd or in the company of many people. They become anxious, confused, and worried about getting lost on familiar streets; they may forget which side of the street their house is on. They tend to have a lot of worries but cannot determine why they are so fretful.

Phosphorus. For the person who is sensitive, friendly, open, and creative, but, when stressed, becomes hypersensitive and oversympathetic to the problems of others. There may be a tendency to overlook one's own needs to help others, and the person may become emotionally run down. Anxieties and fears about the health of others may develop, and the person may be afraid of the dark and of being alone at night. The person may become gullible and vulnerable and get hurt when others take advantage of a relationship. If not helped, the person who needs *Phosphorus* may become paralyzed with fear, highly excitable, and overwhelmed. A fear of naturally occurring events like thunderstorms may develop, as well as panic attacks and a tendency to hyperventilate. The person may often look to doctors, friends, or family for reassurance. Children who develop anxieties and need *Phosphorus* are similar to the adults in that they are intelligent, artistic, and have many friends. These children work quickly but sometimes make careless mistakes. Adolescents like to attend parties and have many friends, but sometimes get burned out trying to care for others and may become anxious, fearful, and afraid of failing in school.

Pulsatilla. Helpful for people who are anxious, kind, and sensitive to others, and who are easily hurt. They feel better after crying and, when consoled, tend to hide true feelings, suffering in silence and self-pity. There may be anxiety when in an unhealthy relationship, and this anxiety may take the form of jealousy and dependency. They may be extremely protective of their children and want to shield them from the loss and pain they themselves experienced as children. When these people hold their feelings in because they fear hurting others, anxiety is experienced.

Rhus tox. People taking *Rhus tox* experience anxiety that is often accompanied by restlessness and continual changes of position. The anxiety and apprehension get worse at night, and they are unable to remain in bed, often moving from place to place and room to room, talking to people, in order to find a comfortable spot. This continual motion seems to relieve general aches and pains. There are many fears, especially when a fever is present. They may feel as if being poisoned. They tend to be extremely anxious about their children. There is a tendency to exhibit anxiety, especially during twilight hours, and to worry about business and the future; these symptoms generally get worse after midnight. Anxiety decreases when they walk outside in the open air or when moving about.

Sepia. The person who needs *Sepia* often feels anxious and fearful that something horrible will happen, of catching an incurable disease, or of going crazy. This fear is based on an inner feeling of being emotionally dead inside. This is a result of the person's sad, quiet, and withdrawn nature. The person may seem to take no joy in life and becomes hardened, stern, and unfeeling.

Silica. People helped by *Silica* are shy, reserved, and like to please others. They avoid conflict, become easily discouraged, and have a strong fear of failure. There is anxiety because of the inability to cope with new situations and new tasks. They experience particular anxiety about giving a speech. This is often true of business people who have to give speeches or communicate in public but experience fear each time it must be done. Because of a generally conscientious nature, these people are able to rise to the occasion and perform well in public. There is a peculiar fear of pins, needles, and sharp objects and a definite fear of shots, vaccinations, and drawing blood. The thought of seeing a person get a vaccination, draw blood, or visit an acupuncturist causes a terrifying reaction. Ironically, they are attracted to pins and feel compelled to count them, as long as they are not harmed by them.

ASTHMA

Asthma is a common disease of the bronchial tubes and lungs. While asthma can usually be controlled and treated with relatively simple measures, there has been an increase in severity in recent years.

Asthma symptoms include coughing, wheezing, shortness of breath, chest tightness, and excessive mucus production. There are often allergy symptoms associated with asthma including rhinitis, sinusitis, sneezing, nasal polyps, and eczema. In children, eczema behind the ears and in the bends of elbows and knees and recurrent episodes of bronchitis or pneumonia can often be associated with asthma.

Asthma is usually an inherited condition, and sometimes skips one or multiple generations in a family. Asthma can occur at any age, from shortly after birth to age seventy and older. Approximately 80 percent of children with asthma greatly improve in adolescence and adulthood but will generally continue to be susceptible to the symptoms.

Asthma is associated with three main problems: spasm and irritability of the muscular wall of the bronchial tubes; inflammation of mucous membranes along the respiratory system; and production of thick, sticky mucus inside the bronchial tubes.

Asthma is often worse at night because lying down allows the bronchial tube secretions to pool and not be coughed up. Also, the body's natural adrenaline drops (normally, adrenaline keeps the bronchial tube's muscle wall more relaxed), and there is greater anxiety at night, which can make the asthma worse.

There are several common triggers for asthma, including viral respiratory infections, exercise, inhaled or digested allergies (pollen, mold, animal dander, spores, dust mites, cockroach droppings), weather changes (hot to cold or cold to hot), humidity (either hot or cold), inhaled irritants (air pollution, strong odors, tobacco smoke), chemicals (food additives, toxic substances at work or home), medicines (aspirin or beta-blockers, such as Inderal, used for blood pressure problems), emotional stress (anger, fear, anxiety), and gastroesophageal reflex.

Asthma can be prevented or better controlled by avoiding triggers such as pollens, animals, chemicals, and smoke; avoiding heavy exercise in extremes of weather or humidity; receiving prompt treatment of respiratory infections; learning ways of handling stress; and avoiding oversecretion of acids in the stomach. Also, milk products contain an enzyme that thickens mucus, so milk should be avoided during upper respiratory infections or allergic conditions in people prone to asthma.

A diet that avoids chemicals and additives is important since these can trigger reactions. Natural, unprocessed foods are often best, although very allergic people should be attentive to reactions to such foods as peanuts, true nuts, eggs, fish, and shellfish, which can cause immediate reactions. Other foods that can cause delayed asthma reactions are dairy products, chocolate, wheat, and citrus fruits. Avoidance of food dyes, especially orange, red, and blue, is important. Other chemicals known to trigger asthma are food chemicals and preservatives such as sodium benzoate, sulphur dioxide, and sulfites; these are used to keep the food's color, flavor, and freshness.

A vegetarian-type diet is recommended since a very potent stimulation of bronchial constriction is the fatty acid, arachidonic acid, found only in animal products (meat, eggs, and dairy). Cooking foods slowly is helpful since the heat breaks down chemicals and makes digestion easier. Nonglutenous grains such as brown rice, millet, buckwheat, and corn often help decrease mucus in the system. Dairy products can thicken mucus so they should be avoided during asthma. Wheat, oats, barley, and rye often increase mucus production and should also be avoided during asthma.

Exercises, physical stimulation, and relaxation techniques are helpful with asthma. These include: aerobic exercises, such as slow running, walking, and sports that can build up the strength of the respiratory system; swimming, which is perhaps the best way to exercise for people with asthma, especially if the water is not too cold, because the moisture helps relax the bronchial tubes; yoga and Tai Chi for stretching and relaxation; massage; acupuncture; and breathing exercises.

Generally, the above preventive approaches are supportive and helpful with homeopathy. Asthma is a chronic disease and usually needs constitutional treatment by a homeopathic physician. However, mild to moderate attacks of asthma can be helped by using the correct homeopathic remedies.

Aconite. Useful for asthma that comes on after being in a dry, cold wind or after a sudden emotional experience. The person experiences anxiety, fear, and great restlessness. The remedy is most useful in the first three to six hours after onset and can be repeated every ten to twenty minutes. A painful, dry cough is common.

Antimonium tart. Most useful for children and the elderly. A great rattling of mucus cannot be expectorated. The person cannot get enough air into the lungs. Often gagging, retching, or vomiting occur with the cough. When there is expectoration, the asthma is relieved. If this remedy is correct, relief will occur within minutes. The remedy can be repeated every ten to twenty minutes.

Arsenicum alb. The person is restless and fearful, especially fearing death by suffocation. Symptoms of asthma tend to come on during sleep, generally between midnight and 2:00 A.M. This type of asthma can emerge after extreme anger, especially if it is suppressed. Breathing is oppressed, and the person might need to spring out of bed at night. At times, it feels as if the person is inhaling dust. A dry, burning cough is accompanied by a soreness in the chest. There is little expectoration and, if present, it tends to be bubbly. The person is thirsty for warm drinks, which seem to help, and tends to sip them. Although chilly, the person may want the windows open. Symptoms often become apparent when skin eruptions, like eczema, are suppressed with cortisone creams. Damp and wet weather, nearness to the ocean, and cool night air often make the symptoms worse. Generally this type of asthma is better by bending forward, applying warm applications to the chest, and drinking warm drinks.

Arsenicum iod. Useful for asthma caused by allergies or hay fever, especially when pollen is the allergen. Asthma attacks associated with this remedy tend to occur between 11:00 P.M. and 2:00 A.M. The person fears suffocation and cannot lie down. Symptoms are often worse when lying on the back. There is less burning than with *Arsenicum alb* and less restlessness and fear.

Bromium. Especially useful for a person who sails or travels on the ocean and experiences asthma after coming ashore. Dust may also cause asthma. The person has great feelings of suffocation and rattling of mucus, especially in the larynx. Sometimes it feels as if the air passages are full of smoke.

Carbo veg. Especially useful for the elderly. Asthma is also associated with allergies. Attacks usually come on in the evening or after an upper respiratory infection or cold. Long coughing spells cause a burning sensation in the chest. Coughing can include gagging or vomiting of mucus. Excessive flatulence is trapped in the abdomen. The person is chilly, but wants to be fanned with cool air; there is a sensation of not getting enough air.

China. This type of asthma often occurs in a person who has lost a lot of body fluids through diarrhea or bleeding. Excessive flatulence in the abdomen can aggravate the symptoms. Symptoms are worse in damp weather and seem to get better every other day. Symptoms are often worse at 3:00 A.M. and in the autumn.

Cuprum met. Helps asthma when chest spasms are predominant and the cough is often spasmodic. There may be cramps in the calves. Symptoms for this type of asthma both come on and ease suddenly. The person feels suffocated and the face may become blue. Attacks are worse at 3:00 A.M. and are often better after drinking cold water. Walking against the wind makes the asthma worse.

Hypericum. Symptoms of asthma occur during foggy weather, before a storm, or when the weather changes. *Hypericum* is also useful after a spinal injury that triggers an asthma attack. Sweating improves the asthma.

Ipecac. Asthma is associated with gagging and vomiting, and the person is extremely anxious. The wheezing is accompanied by a lot of saliva in the mouth. This remedy is especially appropriate for plump children and adults who are not strong and catch cold easily, especially in warm, moist weather. Unlike *Arsenicum alb,* there are no burning pains in the chest; *Ipecac* is often used before *Arsenicum alb* is needed. Coughing is incessant and violent, often with each breath. Sometimes a person coughs until the face becomes blue. The person cannot cough up much phlegm; it is only when vomiting that the person can get any phlegm out. The person has a feeling of a suffocating weight on the chest. A sudden onset of wheezing is made worse by movement. Often, the tongue is clean. Cold perspiration covers the extremities. A physician should be contacted when symptoms are this intense.

Kali bich. Asthma is associated with a thick, sticky, stringy, green and yellow mucus that is coughed up, providing relief to the person. Symptoms tend to return in the winter or in chilly summer weather. Symptoms begin at 2:00 A.M. and are worse between 3:00 and 4:00 A.M. The person must bend forward and sit up in order to breathe.

Kali carb. The guiding *Kali carb* asthma symptom is its time aggravation. Symptoms are worse between 2:00 and 3:00 A.M. or 3:00 and 4:00 A.M.; around 3:00 A.M. is the most characteristic time. Anxiety is often felt in the stomach. The person is often quite chilly and may have heart palpitations. The person feels a sense of weakness, especially in the legs or extremities. Puffiness of the upper eyelids (between the eyebrows and the lids) can occur, especially after excessive coughing. There is much phlegm (unlike the dry wheezing associated with *Arsenicum alb*), and the person wants to stay immobile (a person with *Arsenicum alb* symptoms is restless). Rocking the body may help relieve the wheezing. The wheezing person must bend forward and sit up in order to breathe.

Kali mur. A person with this type of asthma experiences stomach problems and indigestion. A white mucus is hard to cough up. The tongue is often coated white.

Lachesis. The *Lachesis* type of asthma is defined by its characteristic modalities. The asthma begins or is aggravated upon waking in the early morning or from a nap. Anything around the chest or throat (such as a turtleneck or tight collar) is intolerable to the person and may make the asthma worse. The person can be quite talkative during the attack. Symptoms tend to get worse from touching the throat or moving the arms. This type of asthma often occurs with allergies and hay fever with much sneezing. The person is thirsty, chilly, and craves warm drinks. Talking or eating also makes the symptoms worse. Sitting bent forward and coughing up large quantities of watery phlegm provide relief.

Natrum sulph. Helps asthma symptoms that are aggravated by damp or rainy weather. It is also helpful for asthma that gets worse from bodies of water, especially inland lakes that tend to have moldy vegetation. Asthma is often aggravated or can begin between 4:00 and 5:00 A.M. This type of asthma is associated with allergies, especially when the weather is wet; therefore mold can be an important trigger. Children often benefit from this remedy. During an attack, the person must sit up and hold the chest in order to breathe. Vomiting after eating or during an attack is common. After an attack, bowels tend to be loose. These loose stools are sometimes worse when the person arises from bed in the morning. There is a productive cough, and the sputum tends to be greenish.

Nux vomica. Asthma is most characteristically brought on by either sudden bouts of anger or from eating, especially if the person has overeaten or has indigestion. Other important aggravations are staying up late, studying or working too hard, or drinking or smoking too much. The person is irritable, critical, and quite volatile. This type of asthma can also occur with allergies, especially if there is overwork or indigestion. Symptoms tend to be worse in the evening. Cold air aggravates the asthma. The person feels quite chilly and avoids the cold weather. Loosening clothing or belching may bring relief when the asthma is associated with indigestion. Stomach disturbance is common. Often there is an urge for a bowel movement, but the stool is difficult to pass. These symptoms are aggravated by overeating, cold air, and sudden anger.

Pulsatilla. People who need *Pulsatilla* for asthma may be weepy, frightened, and like consolation, comfort, and care. Although they have a dry mouth and a dry feeling in their lungs, they have no thirst. Though chilly, the person wants the windows open. Asthma can occur after eating rich or fatty foods, and it can be aggravated during pregnancy. (Note that while homeopathic remedies are safe during pregnancy, labor, and breastfeeding, a pregnant woman should confer with her obstetrician or midwife to coordinate treatment.) A dry cough in the evening tends to loosen in the morning. The cough produces a greenish-yellow, moderately thick mucus. Symptoms are often worse at night, especially before 10:00 P.M. Symptoms also get worse after eating and after skin eruptions have been suppressed by creams and ointments, especially steroids. The person feels better when sitting upright.

Spongia. Asthma helped by *Spongia* is associated with a dry cough, especially when there is croup or dryness in the larynx area causing loud breathing. An important guiding symptom is that the cough is usually better after drinking or eating, especially warm things. Anxiety is common. The person sometimes grabs the throat while swallowing. Often there is a sensation of a plug in the larynx. Breathing is worse during inspiration and before midnight. Symptoms may get worse after sleep. A person may fall asleep and wake suddenly with a shortness of breath.

Sulphur. May be taken in the late stages of asthma and is useful after many other remedies have been given. Feelings of burning and of oppression or heaviness in the chest are common symptoms. During asthma attacks, the person tends to be messy and will not have changed clothes or taken a bath for many days. The person has a difficult time breathing and wants the windows open. There is a loose cough with much rattling mucus. Symptoms tend to be worse at 11:00 A.M. or during a full moon. The person does not like to stand.

Thuja. Useful for chronic cases of asthma in children, especially for those children who need *Natrum sulph* or *Arsenicum alb* often. The person tends to be better when drawing the limbs toward the body. Symptoms are worse at 3:00 A.M. or 3:00 p.m., in cold and damp air, at night, and in bed.

BACK INJURIES (INCLUDES SPINAL INJURIES)

If not certain about the extent of the injury, it is best to consult a physician or go to an emergency room. When transporting an injured person, it is important not to aggravate the injury. Consulting a Red Cross first aid manual or taking a first aid course can be helpful.

Back injuries are one of the most common problems in medicine today. Back pain causes many missed days of work and is a large cost to the health care system. Most back problems are relatively minor, involving irritation or pulling of the muscles along the spinal cord or in the upper or lower back. Resting, applying ice for the first twenty-four hours followed by heat, and decreasing activity level are enough to heal back strains. Physical therapy or other types of treatment can be helpful for back pain that continues after two or three weeks. A danger sign is pain that travels down from the neck to the fingers; this indicates an irritation of the nerves that come out the cervical vertebrae. Another danger sign is pain that runs down the back of the leg to the foot. This may indicate irritation of the sciatic nerve (sciatica). Numbness in the feet or hands, weakness, or decreased reflexes should always be evaluated by a physician.

Aesculus hippocastanum. An important remedy for pain and soreness of the sacroiliac joint caused by overlifting or overstretching. Pain and soreness in the sacroiliac joint can also occur from viruses. The affected area aches painfully. Hemorrhoids are a possible associated symptom with this problem.

Arnica. Often the first remedy given for an injury. The pain tends to feel bruised and sore and can become black and blue. This remedy is also useful for dislocations of the spine or herniated disks. (A physician's care is necessary for these conditions.) *Arnica* can be helpful for ailments from lifting.

Bryonia. Useful when the back is sore and stiff. The pain is worse from motion and better from lying still. *Bryonia* can be helpful for slipped or herniated disks and ailments from lifting a heavy object. (A physician's care is necessary for these conditions.) The person feels extreme pain and is irritable, especially if bothered.

Calcarea carb. Useful for back injuries that tend to be chronic or for previous injuries that have healed and caused new symptoms after a minor injury. Useful when problems occur after lifting and the back aches painfully. The person is often cold, craves sweets, and is fearful.

Hypericum. If back problems occur after lifting and the person is in great pain, *Hypericum* is a useful remedy. It is particularly useful for an injury to the spine (especially to the neck and lower spine around the coccyx). *Hypericum* is often helpful as a tincture if a wound accompanies the back injury.

Kali carb. Useful for extreme weakness in the small of the back. This remedy is helpful for a severe backache during pregnancy (especially from pressure caused by the growing baby) or after a miscarriage. The pain is often sudden and sharp and tends to extend up and down the back to the thighs. There is a tendency for the legs and back to give out.

Magnesia phos. Helpful for back spasms after an injury. These problems can occur from overstraining and overlifting. Twenty tablets of the 6x potency can be dissolved in one cup of warm water and sipped throughout the day.

Natrum sulph. Particularly helpful for head trauma or injury to the area where the spine meets the lower part of the skull. Often, the person experiences confusion or other emotional changes after this type of injury. Watch for signs of injury, including changes in consciousness or emotions, confusion, seizures, dilation of the pupils, nausea, or vomiting. Watch for twenty-four hours, even waking the person at night to make sure he or she is not having problems with consciousness. If any of these conditions occur, contact a physician.

Rhus tox. Useful for decreasing the pain of a sore back that gets worse from an initial movement, but becomes better after limbering up. This back problem can be caused by sprains and strains of the lower or middle back, as well as the neck. The problem occurs most frequently from heavy lifting or unusual twisting. Symptoms often occur from playing sports. The pain is better with warm applications and worse from cold.

Ruta. Helps relieve the aching that occurs after overlifting. This remedy tends to be most helpful when the tendons and ligaments of the back are sore and strained, rather than the muscles or soft tissue.

BACK PAIN

Back pain is one of the most common reasons why people visit a doctor. It is responsible for billions of dollars in lost wages and productivity in the workplace. There are many causes and treatments for back pain. It can be a result of minor trauma or fatigue such as shoveling snow, sitting in a car or airplane too long, or sitting at a desk. In such cases, rest, changing positions, and simple exercises to stretch the back muscles are usually all that is necessary to improve the symptoms.

Other causes of back pain include degenerative joint disease of the lumbosacral area. Back pain can also occur in the neck area and cervical spine when the vertebrae become weakened with age and form calcium deposits, putting pressure on the nerve root.

Some congenital conditions are associated with lower back and neck pain, such as spondylosis and spondylitis. Lower back pain can also be caused by spina bifida occulta, a congenital deformity that produces an opening from the lower spine toward the surface of the body.

Obesity can be another cause of back pain because of the stretching of the lower back muscles and abdominal muscles. Pregnancy can cause another form of back strain and lower back pain. Lower back and neck pain can also be emotion- or stress-induced. This usually occurs when the muscles that lie alongside the spinal cord and vertebrae spasm, causing tension on the nerves that go out from the spinal cord. More serious injuries can damage the muscles and ligaments in the back and cause fracturing of the spine or rupturing of the disk. A ruptured disk occurs when the soft cushioning of tissue between the vertebrae is pushed forward, causing the vertebrae to put pressure on the nerve as they collapse onto themselves.

Because of the many different types and causes of back pain, there are many different treatments. Most important is ruling out any major problem with the spine or nerves that travel out of the spine. Any prolonged pain, burning, tingling, numbness, loss of reflex, or bowel or urine function should always be considered serious. Consult a doctor in these cases.

Chronic back pain can be handled through exercise, relaxation, stretching, massage, physical therapy, chiropractic care, and acupuncture. Heat can be used to relax muscle spasms, and ice can be used to decrease inflammation after a sudden injury. Posture is very important. Lifting with the knees bent forces the person to use the leg muscles instead of straining the back. When sitting, it is helpful to have the knees higher than the hips by putting the feet on a stool or other object. The back should be straight with the pelvis tucked underneath and the knees relaxed. Any position that puts a person in the sway-back position should be avoided, such as sleeping on the stomach. Certain vitamins, oils, and supplements are known to help back pain.

Aconite. Helpful when numbness, stiffness, and neck pain are experienced, especially when the person is exposed to cold, dry wind; a fever may be associated with these symptoms. Also, the person may experience a bruised feeling between the shoulder blades.

Arnica. Helps any type of back pain that comes on after a back injury or overexertion. The pain gets worse with motion. There is a bruised or sore feeling, and the person does not want to be touched. The pain improves when the person lies down and rests.

Berberis. Useful for pain that travels from the back to the abdomen, especially when there is a kidney stone in the kidney or one is being passed. The pain seems to shoot down the back and around the sides to the abdomen. The pain may also extend from the abdomen, especially if there is a bladder infection, in which case the pain shoots up and around toward the back.

Bryonia. Painful stiffness of the neck and lower back are experienced. The person cannot sit upright, and the back feels worse with movement. The back improves as pressure is applied while the person is lying on the painful side. Any kind of splinting so the painful part of the back does not move at all is helpful. Hot applications also help.

Calcarea carb. Uuseful for problems that occur from lifting too much or overexerting the back, especially after first trying *Arnica*. The person feels like the back has been sprained. The neck is stiff and rigid. Pain between the shoulder blades sometimes impedes breathing. Weakness is felt in the lower part of the back. All pain is worse with exertion and exposure to cold. Back pain may also occur with kidney stones.

Causticum. Useful when the back muscles feel constricted and contracted, as if they are too short. The person experiences back pain that is associated with contracted or tight feelings of the left hip. Back pain can also affect the neck, causing torticollis, where the neck is twisted to one side. Back pain can be triggered by cold and damp weather.

Cimicifuga. Helpful for women who experience extreme aching in the lower back. It is particularly helpful for those who have joint problems and uterine complaints, such as menstrual cramps or premenstrual pains.

Colocynth. Useful for contraction of the muscles causing cramps in the lower back extending to the hip. The pain gets better when hard pressure and heat are applied. The cramping pain in the back can come on after a sudden expression of rage and anger.

Hypericum. Useful after an injury to the tailbone, especially when the person is in extreme pain and cannot walk or stoop. *Hypericum* can also be helpful for an injury to the vertebrae in the neck accompanied by pains traveling along the nerves from the neck to the arms. This remedy helps heal the nerves.

Kali carb. The person has a characteristic stitching pain in the back. Back pain is also sharp and cutting. The back feels weak and there is a feeling it could give out. This remedy is also useful for an elderly person with problems of sweating, backache, and muscular weakness. The pains get worse with any atmosphere change, especially when cold weather sets in. *Kali carb* is particularly helpful for severe backaches during pregnancy and after a miscarriage. Pains may awaken the person at night, especially around 3:00 A.M., compelling him or her to get up and walk around. Lower back pain that shoots up and down the back is experienced, especially in the thighs. Besides back weakness, the legs also feel weak, as if they may give out. Note that while homeopathic remedies are safe during pregnancy, labor, and breastfeeding, a pregnant woman should confer with her obstetrician or midwife to coordinate treatment.

Ledum. Useful when the person experiences stiffness in the back, especially after sitting still for a long time. Back pain becomes worse at night and is better from cold applications.

Lycopodium. Helpful for stiffness and lower back pain, especially when accompanied by excessive abdominal distention and flatulence. The person also experiences burning pain between the shoulder blades.

Magnesia phos. Helps sharp pains in the back that get better from warmth and pressure. This remedy may be used in the 6x potency by dissolving twenty tablets in one cup of warm water and sipping it slowly throughout the day.

Natrum mur. Used to help a person who experiences pain in the small of the back that gets better when pressing the back against something hard or when lying down with the back pressed against something. People who are worriers, who dwell on past disappointments, or who have lost a loved one are sometimes helped by *Natrum mur.*

Nux vomica. Helps backaches that get worse at night, especially while lying in bed. The person must sit up just to turn over. Back pain is felt in the lower back in connection with hemorrhoids. The person experiences morning backaches, and the longer the person lies in bed, the more the back aches. The typical *Nux vomica* temperament of irritability and excessiveness of habits is seen.

Phosphorus. Can be helpful when the spine is extremely sensitive to touch. Burning pain is experienced, especially between the shoulder blades. Weakness is felt in the back, as if it would give out.

Pulsatilla. Useful for lower back pain that becomes worse from stooping or from a sprain. The pain gets better with rest, sleep, and gentle slow motion. The person is weepy, chilly, and feels better when outside in the cool air.

Rhododendron. Useful when lower back pain becomes worse before a thunderstorm.

Rhus tox. Can help back pain that is aggravated on beginning motion but gets better with continual motion. It is especially useful for pain in the deeper muscles of the lower back. The pain feels as if the back is broken. Back pain gets better when pressure is applied and gets worse in bed. Walking and lying down on a hard surface help lessen the pain. Lower back pain is also relieved by bending backward.

Ruta. Useful for pain that stems from the attachments of the ligaments, especially in the lumbosacral area of the lower back. These ligaments get sore to the touch. Pain becomes better when pressure is applied. The pain becomes worse in the morning before the person gets out of bed.

Sepia. Useful for a backache and weakness in the small of the back. Pain is particularly worse in women who have diseases of the uterus and pelvic structures. The pelvic organs have a bearing-down sensation (as though the organs would actually drop out). These sensations extend to the small of the back, which becomes weak when the person walks and worse when the person sits. The back pain, however, gets better when the person walks and exercises (similar to *Rhus tox*). The person experiences sudden pain in the back, as though it were struck by a hammer; this pain is relieved by pressing the back against a hard surface.

Silica. Useful for spinal injuries, especially to the tailbone. The spine generally feels weak and back pain can occur after exposure to drafts.

Staphysagria. Useful for low back pain that causes the person to get up early and move around. *Staphysagria* is especially useful for the person who smokes or drinks too much and suffers in the morning.

Sulphur. Helps back pain that comes on while standing. The person who needs *Sulphur* is always uncomfortable when standing up and needs to sit or lie down to feel better. The back pain can be burning, but it is better when exposed to cold and when lying down. The person experiences an unusual sensation as if the vertebrae were gliding over each other.

Zincum met. Useful for the person whose spine feels very irritated. The person cannot bear to have the back touched and feels a burning sensation along the spine and aching in the upper lumbar area. The pain is aggravated by sitting and relieved by walking around (similar to *Rhus tox*). The legs are often restless and the person has difficulty keeping the legs still.

BITES AND STINGS

Bites from an animal or stings from an insect that inject an irritating substance into the skin are forms of puncture wounds. These wounds can lead to infection or swelling and can be extremely painful. Types of bites that can be treated through homeopathy are bee stings, nonpoisonous snake bites, and mosquito bites. Dog and cat bites can also be treated by homeopathy, but these types of injuries should receive medical attention because of the possibility of rabies. Infections can also occur from the saliva of these animals. Always contact a physician or emergency room personnel after a bite from a stray dog or cat. (See Puncture Wounds for specific information about pain and infection caused by wounds from sharp, penetrating objects.)

Apis. Useful for bee, wasp, yellow jacket, and jellyfish stings. *Apis* often follows *Ledum.* If the person reacts strongly to the sting, use a high potency of *Apis* as prescribed by a homeopathic physician. This remedy may also be used in a lower potency (6c or 30c) every ten to fifteen minutes. The injured area stings, sometimes burns, and swells rapidly. The swelling is rosy (rather than bright red), and the skin is puffy (rather than firm). The injury is quite sore to touch. The person may have difficulty urinating. The frequency of urination may increase, or there may be difficulty initiating the urine flow. Cold applications provide relief, and warm applications aggravate the symptoms.

Arnica. Useful for bee or wasp stings when the area around the sting is bruised and sore.

Belladonna. Useful when the wound feels hot (*Ledum* helps when the wound feels cold) and is not relieved by cold applications. The wound is swollen, red, throbbing, and hot, but pus does not form. These symptoms are often seen in dog or snake bites (especially when there are symptoms of a fever, a hot, red face, dilated pupils, and agitation).

Calendula. Used in lotion or ointment form, *Calendula* helps alleviate pain and reduces the risk of infection in a sting or bite. Also, any combination of *Urtica, Hypericum,* and *Calendula* tincture can be used on the bite to decrease pain and possible infection. Mix equal parts of each tincture used.

Cantharis. Useful for the burning pain of a nettle puncture.

Carbolicum acidum. Used for extensive wasp or bee stings (such as from a swarm), or for a sting in a very sensitive area (such as the mouth, lips, eyes, ears, or nose). *Carbolicum acidum* can also be used for snake bites. The person is extremely lethargic and may even lose consciousness. A feeble pulse and labored breathing may also be seen. The face can be very dull or dark in appearance, and the person may have increased thirst. Symptoms quickly deteriorate. In this situation, the person should be transported to the nearest hospital as soon as possible.

Crotalus horridus. Used for a serious insect or snake bite. Symptoms are similar to those of a bite or sting helped by *Lachesis,* including a blue swelling and dark, oozing blood around the bite. However, *Lachesis* helps bites or stings located more on the left side of the body, and *Crotalus horridus* tends to help bites or stings located on the right side of the body.

Hypericum. Particularly useful for spider, cat, dog, and other small animal bites (especially if the bite is very painful and has jagged edges). This remedy can be used as a tincture, as well as taken internally. A bite in which the pain travels up the limb can often benefit from *Hypericum.* The wound gets worse from cold applications and is sensitive to touch. *Hypericum* can also be used when the bite is located on a fingertip, or after a painful horsefly bite in which the pain seems to travel upward.

Lachesis. Useful for treating snake bites and severe dog bites. The affected part is bluish and swollen. The person may feel worse when awakening from sleep, and dark blood may ooze from the bite. A physician should always be contacted to make decisions on possible rabies exposure, the need for infection control, and tetanus prevention.

Ledum. Tthe first remedy given after an insect bite (such as by a mosquito, wasp, or flea, or a bee sting) and for a bite from a snake, spider, or scorpion. This remedy is also useful for soreness after a puncture by a sharp instrument, an injection, or a vaccination. A shooting, prickling pain is accompanied by puffiness and swelling. The affected part is cold to the touch, although it may actually feel hot to the person. Symptoms are relieved from cold applications, icy cold water, and cold air when uncovering the body. The pain is worse from warmth and any touch. Generally, *Ledum* is the first remedy given for any type of bite. *Ledum* is often followed by *Apis* if the affected area becomes hot and rosy-colored. If the bite does not cause much discomfort, *Ledum* may be the only remedy necessary. For chronic or long-lasting effects from a bite, a high-potency dose of *Ledum* is often useful. A consultation with a physician is helpful in this situation.

Phosphorus. Helpful when profuse bleeding accompanies a bite.

Urtica. Can be used for an allergic reaction to a bite or sting. The area becomes itchy and blotchy. The typical conditions helped by *Apis* (cold applications relieving the irritation of stings and bites, and warm applications causing increased aggravations) are not seen.

BLEEDING

There are many different causes of bleeding. One cause is trauma or injury to the soft tissue, resulting in bleeding that can be slight or serious to the point of hemorrhaging. If an artery is injured, blood will spurt from the damaged tissue. Other causes of bleeding are injuries, dry air, hemorrhoids (especially after a hard bowel movement), and problems with canker sores or gingivitis of the gums.

Blood loss symptoms can range from no symptoms to symptoms of severe anemia. Usually bleeding leads to iron deficiency anemia because the body loses iron when there is a loss of blood. Anemia symptoms are easy fatigue, rapid heart rate, heart palpitations, shortness of breath with exertion, paleness, conjunctivitis, smooth tongue, brittle nails, and an unusual craving for specific foods, particularly ice cubes.

Bleeding may also occur in the lungs, especially with bronchitis or pneumonia. Blood disorders that can lead to bleeding problems include hemophilia and certain types of red blood abnormalities. Nosebleeds can be controlled by pinching the nose and tilting the head backward. If the nosebleed is heavy, allowing the blood to flow out with the head placed forward may be necessary.

Bleeding during the menstrual cycle can range from light to very heavy. Vaginal bleeding that is abnormal can be caused by fibroid tumors, infections, or the effects of birth control devices, such as IUDs or birth control pills. Menstrual bleeding generally is not a major problem unless the bleeding is severe.

The cause of the bleeding should always be ascertained by a physician or a nurse practitioner of gynecology. Bleeding from the respiratory, urinary, or gastrointestinal tract should always be evaluated by a physician. Dark black blood in the stools often represents upper gastrointestinal bleeding such as when a person has a bleeding ulcer. Bright red blood or blood that looks like coffee grounds in the vomit usually represents bleeding in the esophagus, stomach, or small intestine. Passing bright red blood in the stools represents lower gastrointestinal bleeding (colon) and can be the result of colitis, polyps, diverticulosis, hemorrhoids, rectal fissures, or cancer.

Blood loss due to a problem with the blood cells, such as red blood cells or platelets, should always be evaluated by a specialist in hematology.

Treatment for bleeding depends upon the cause. For example, if trauma initiates a hemorrhage, pressure should be applied to the area that is bleeding. Applying firm pressure with a clean cloth or gauze will often stop the bleeding quickly. If there is damage to an artery, a health care practitioner may need to apply a tourniquet to control the bleeding.

An important treatment for bleeding is replacing iron and, in more severe cases, replacing fluid. This can be accomplished by taking iron supplements or, in more serious cases, having intravenous fluids and/or blood transfusions. A medical professional should be consulted in these cases. Iron can sometimes be difficult to absorb, so people who have problems with constipation or digestion should avoid iron sulfate (ferrous sulfate). Ferrous gluconate or chelated iron are often easier to absorb and cause less of a problem with constipation. Eating foods that are high in iron such as lean meats, dried beans that are dark (black beans or pinto beans), dried fruit (raisins), and molasses is also important. Cooking vegetables in a cast iron pan can also increase the amount of iron in the body. Certain supplements are known to help bleeding.

Aconite. Useful for bleeding associated with extreme panic and restlessness. The person is often thirsty for ice-cold drinks.

Arnica. Generally the first choice for bleeding caused by an injury, especially when shock is associated with the bleeding. (The signs of shock include: a rapid, weak pulse; cool, clammy skin; light-headedness; irregular breathing; confusion; or loss of consciousness. A doctor or person trained in emergency medicine should be contacted.) The body parts feel bruised. *Arnica* is often used for a nosebleed in a growing child. Often, this is the first remedy given for bleeding that results from soft tissue damage of any body part.

Arsenicum alb. Useful for bleeding when the person is restless, extremely weak, and constantly changes position. Since these symptoms may indicate a large amount of blood loss, it is important to consult a physician. The person is often thirsty for small sips of warm water. Possible symptoms include burning pain and irritability. *Arsenicum alb* is also useful for recurring nosebleeds.

Belladonna. Useful for bleeding characterized by bright red blood that clots easily. The blood feels hot. The face is red and dry, and the person is often extremely thirsty. Agitation is a common characteristic.

Calcarea carb. Used for bleeding (especially heavy, profuse, menstrual bleeding) that lasts too long and is aggravated by overexertion and excitement. The body feels extremely cold. Often the person craves sweets and salty foods.

Carbo veg. Useful for continuous, slow hemorrhages. The skin is cold and bluish, and the pulse is rapid and weak. The person wants to be fanned. There is extreme weakness and lethargy, and often burning pain in the lower back. The breath, limbs, and perspiration may be cold. There is often a feeling of air hunger (a feeling of needing more oxygen, indicated by gasping for air)—this condition is serious and the person should be transported to the hospital. The remedy can be given on the way to the hospital.

China. Useful for bleeding characterized by dark, clotted blood from any orifice of the body. There is ringing in the ears and the feeling that the person will faint. The person wants to be fanned. This problem is often associated with bleeding after childbirth.

Ferrum phos. Helpful for bleeding of bright red blood that is profuse and tends to clot easily. A nosebleed is common with this type of bleeding. Often no other guiding symptoms or mental symptoms are associated with the bleeding. *Ferrum phos* is especially useful when no other remedies are indicated due to a lack of conditions that relieve or aggravate the symptoms.

Hamamelis. Passive bleeding of dark, venous blood can be relieved with *Hamamelis.* The parts feel sore and bruised, and the person is exhausted by the blood flow. Sometimes small reddish spots associated with platelet problems can be seen on the body. These reddish spots should always be evaluated by a physician. This type of bleeding is often associated with hemorrhoids and nosebleeds.

Ipecac. The bleeding helped by *Ipecac* is characterized by gushing, bright red blood. The person has great nausea, a weak pulse, cold perspiration, and often gasps for breath. The face may be pale with dark rings around the eyes. These symptoms may be seen with a nosebleed, heavy menstrual bleeding, and rectal bleeding (such as from hemorrhoids or internal colon problems). If this type of rectal bleeding is seen, a physician should be consulted immediately, especially if the person has no history of hemorrhoids or rectal fissures.

Kali mur. Useful for bleeding when the blood tends to be thick, clotted, and often mixed with mucus. Common symptoms include vomiting of dark, clotted blood from the stomach and nosebleeds that get worse in the afternoon. (If there is red or dark blood or black material in the vomit, a physician should be contacted.) Few mental symptoms are associated with this remedy.

Phosphorus. Helps a person who has bright red bleeding from any orifice (including the respiratory system, nose, mouth, rectum, or from hemorrhoids). Bleeding starts and stops often, and may be associated with a feeling of emptiness in the stomach and a desire for cold drinks. Bleeding can occur with heavy menstrual periods (especially if the woman has fibroids in the uterus). Useful for a profuse nosebleed (especially after the person blows the nose) and for small wounds that bleed easily and profusely.

Pulsatilla. Useful for a light nosebleed that occurs instead of the menstrual period. The person can be tearful, thirsty, and chilly, yet wants to open the windows or walk outside in the cool air.

Sabina. This type of bleeding is characterized by bright red blood with many clots that is worse from motion. *Sabina* is often associated with heavy menstrual bleeding, post-birth bleeding, or bleeding after a miscarriage. Uterine pain, if it accompanies the bleeding, tends to extend from the pubic bone to the back and down the thighs.

Trillium pendulum. Can be used in tincture form for any type of bleeding, whether it is passive and slow or active and gushing. A nosebleed, heavy menstrual bleeding, or bleeding after the extraction of teeth are particular uses for this remedy. *Trillium pendulum* is especially useful for a nosebleed in a growing child. An important characteristic for uterine hemorrhages is the sensation that the thighs may separate. (This condition should always be evaluated by a physician or nurse practitioner.) This sensation is relieved by a tight bandage around the body.

Veratrum alb. Usually associated with intestinal hemorrhaging, especially when there is profuse diarrhea that contains blood. Note that a person who has blood or black material (old blood) in the stool should always be evaluated by a physician. There is a great sense of internal coldness and restlessness, but no relief from restless movements. The person feels faint and exhausted, has cold perspiration on the forehead, and feels better from heat.

BREAST INJURIES

The most common breast injury is cracks on the nipple from nursing. The second most common type is a contusion, which is often very painful and can sometimes form a firm, irregular mass called thrombosis. The mass can be confused with cancer, so evaluation by a physician is necessary. A lump in the breast should always be evaluated by a doctor who has experience with this condition. Often an ultrasound or mammogram is necessary to differentiate the swelling of simple breast trauma from a more serious problem.

Arnica. The first remedy given after a blunt trauma to the breast (such as from an accident, blow, or fall). It is also given after breast biopsies or breast surgeries.

Bellis. The most important remedy for contusions and injuries to the breast (especially if the injury is deep and extremely sore). This remedy follows *Arnica* well and can be used in a 30c potency or 200c potency three times a day for several days to several weeks. Note that high-potency remedies are not recommended for home prescribing; consult a physician or skilled homeopathic consultant for potencies above 30c.

Conium maculatum. Useful for injuries to the breast from a blow, excessive pressure, or overuse of the arms. The injured area tends to harden and is extremely sensitive. The breasts are painful from even the slightest touch (such as clothing) or movement (such as walking).

Phytolacca. When the breast is injured and pain radiates from the nipple all over the body (especially down the arm from the armpit), *Phytolacca* is a useful remedy. The person is chilly, and the entire body aches.

BREAST PROBLEMS (INCLUDES BREASTFEEDING, LACTATION, MASTITIS, AND NURSING)

Take special care. While homeopathic remedies are safe during pregnancy, labor, and breastfeeding, a pregnant woman should confer with her obstetrician or midwife to coordinate treatment.

Breastfeeding, also known as nursing or lactation, is the most important and natural way for a mother to nourish her child. Soy formula, cow's milk, or other artificial formulas are not as healthy as mother's milk. Breast milk is much easier to digest, lowers the incidence of food allergies, has antibodies that can protect the baby from infectious diseases, and prevents constipation and diarrhea. Breastfeeding is also important for emotional bonding between a mother and baby. It enhances skin-to-skin contact and satisfies sucking needs in a natural way. Breastfeeding causes a release of hormones that contract the uterus and thus decrease the amount of blood lost with the placenta immediately after the baby is born. It allows the mother to rest and helps the uterus contract back to its normal shape and size.

After nursing the baby, it is important to express a little breast milk, massage it on the nipples and areola, and let it air dry. Leave the breasts open in the air as much as possible. It is important not to use soap or alcohol on the breast or nipples; water is usually all that is needed. If the nipples become sore, the mother should limit the nursing time on that nipple. It is important to nurse on the least sore side first. A little milk should be expressed first to stimulate the milk let down. Massaging the breast during nursing can help stimulate the milk flow. Protecting the nipple by using bra pads is also helpful. If the nipple becomes dry and cracked, lanolin cream or *Calendula* ointment can be used. If the nipples become extremely sore, multiple-hole breast shields can be used between nursing. This allows air to circulate and protects the nipples from rubbing on the bra. It is also possible to use a nipple shield to nurse the baby, but this sometimes irritates the nipple. The nipples usually heal in time, especially if the above instructions are followed.

Breast milk for future use can be stored at room temperature for up to six hours. If it is refrigerated, seventy-two hours is considered the maximum, and if it is frozen, six months is the longest time it should be stored. It is important to never refreeze thawed milk.

Several problems can occur with breastfeeding. One of the most immediate problems is breast engorgement, especially during the first week after delivery. This occurs when the colostrum, the creamy milk secretion, changes to breast milk, causing the breast to become full. At first, the baby's sucking reflex may not be strong enough. This causes the breasts to become painful and engorged for the first three to five days. They often feel hot and hard. The breast can also become engorged later on in nursing when a milk duct becomes plugged. This can also lead to a hot, painful, and lumpy breast. The woman may develop a fever, feel chilled, and develop red spots on the breast.

Breast engorgement or breast inflammation can be prevented to some extent by breastfeeding the baby at least ten or twelve times during a twenty-four hour cycle. It is often recommended to breastfeed the baby on demand. The mother should avoid supplements of water or formula for the first month unless there is medical indication. If a feeding has been missed because the baby has been ill or away from the mother, the milk should be hand expressed from the mother's breast. Weaning should be done gradually.

If the breast does become engorged or there is infection or inflammation, it is important to use hot, moist towels on the breast for five minutes or take a shower before nursing the baby. It is often best to hand express some of the milk to soften the nipple area after using the moist heat. This makes it easier for the baby to attach to the breast. Gently massaging the breast before and during breastfeeding can be helpful. The mother should relax and lie down so that the muscles around the breast do not contract and create tension. It is important not to use cold compresses on the breasts. If the breast continues to be engorged and the baby does not suck enough, an electrical pump or hand expression should be used.

If the nipples remain flat, it is often helpful to wear multiple-hole breast shields for thirty minutes before breastfeeding to help draw the nipple out. Pacifiers, bottles, and nipple shields should probably be avoided because this will diminish the baby's need to suck from the breast. When hand-expressing milk, the breast should not be cupped with the fingers and thumb. Instead, the nipple should be grasped with the thumb above the nipple and the index and middle finger below it. It is important not to squeeze the breast, but to gently roll the thumb and fingers, which will compress and empty the milk reservoir without injuring the sensitive breast tissue. Avoid sliding the hand over the breast because it may cause painful skin burns; also avoid pulling the nipple since this may result in tissue damage.

Another common problem is sore nipples that may blister, crack, or bleed. If pain continues during or between feedings, the nipples may be irritated. To prevent nipple cracks and bleeding, it is important to place the baby in a proper position; while the baby is lying down, he or she can be cradled in the mother's bent arm, like a running back cradles a football. The baby should be breastfeeding frequently, every one to two hours. It is important to release the suction of the baby's mouth before removing the baby from the breast; do this by placing a clean finger inside the baby's mouth, between the jaws.

Homeopathy has been used successfully for helping all sorts of breast problems, including nursing problems, lactation, and mastitis. If, however, the fever stays high or a hard spot develops and does not go away and an abscess seems to be forming, it is important to immediately contact a doctor. This can be a serious problem and medical consultation is essential.

Aconite. Useful for acute mastitis in which breast inflammation is characterized by pain, redness, and a fever. Especially useful when the breasts suddenly get painful because the person is exposed to a cold, dry wind and becomes chilled. The breast milk may suddenly become scanty. If *Aconite* does not help the symptoms, *Belladonna* is often needed.

Arnica. Useful for breast problems during nursing, especially when the infant bruises the breast or the woman injures her breast in another way. The breast may have a black or blue discoloration and be extremely sore. *Arnica* may also help sore and cracked nipples, especially after the infant bites down hard and bruises or injures the nipple.

Belladonna. One of the most useful remedies for the early stages of breast infections. *Belladonna* is often useful after *Aconite.* Red streaks radiate from a central point, accompanied by pulsating pain, a headache, high fever, and a general hardness of the inflamed area. The milk flow often stops or is less abundant. This remedy is also used for weaning to help stop the flow of breast milk. It may also be used for a hungry infant who is irritable and angry about being weaned. *Belladonna* may help when breast milk flows profusely without any stimulation at all. *Belladonna* is usually associated with a fever, irritability, and a red, hot, and dry face.

Bellis. Helps when the breast is painful due to deep bruising, especially after a major injury or surgery. The pain and discomfort are similar to *Arnica* in that the person is sore, but the injury itself is deeper and more extensive than *Arnica.*

Borax. May be helpful for thrush in an infant or for a painful, burning yeast infection on the mother's nipple. This remedy is also useful for breast milk that curdles quickly.

Bromium. Helps relieve stitching breast pain that is worse on the left side. Shooting pain travels from the breast to the armpit and gets worse when pressure is applied.

Bryonia. Useful for mastitis accompanied by hard and painful breasts. Breast infections often begin with a chill and are accompanied by stitching pains in the hardened area. There is great swelling in the inflamed area. General symptoms associated with *Bryonia* are headaches, excessive thirst for large amounts of cold water at infrequent intervals, a desire to not want to move (especially the breast), and feeling better when lying perfectly still. The person is irritable if bothered and lies quietly if not disturbed. There is a general aching feeling and a tendency toward high fevers. There may be complete stoppage of breast milk if the person has this type of mastitis.

Calcarea carb. Useful when breast milk is profuse and sometimes flows involuntarily without any stimulation from the infant.

This causes the mother to feel quite weak and, as the mother gets weaker, the breast milk becomes more scanty and she becomes colder. *Calcarea carb* is also associated with breast milk that tastes so disagreeable that the infant cries and does not want to nurse. The person who needs this remedy sometimes gets headaches after nursing.

Calcarea phos. Useful when nursing sometimes brings on breathing problems in the mother, who feels as if she is suffocating. The breast milk seems to taste bad to the infant, who often refuses to nurse. The breast milk may be too thin, salty, and have a bad taste.

Chamomilla. Useful when breast milk stops flowing during fevers or after angry episodes. *Chamomilla* may help cracked nipples, which are quite tender to the touch, that occur during nursing. An unusual symptom in infants is that their breasts are tender. This is a very important remedy for nursing babies who are irritable, colicky, and refuse to nurse. Infants want to be picked up, and when they are, they quiet for just a few moments and then start to scream again. Infants will also have colicky pains and diarrhea that resembles a mixture of chopped eggs and spinach.

Croton tig. Helpful for inflamed breasts when pain shoots from the nipple to the shoulders and back. When the baby nurses and the mother's nipples are cracked and sore, there is pain felt from the breast to the back.

Dulcamara. Useful for suppressed breast milk due to exposure to cold, damp air. (*Aconite* is useful for suppressed milk due to cold, dry air.)

Graphites. An important remedy for cracked nipples while nursing. These cracks are very painful and sometimes ooze a thin, sticky discharge. The person tends to be constipated and depressed about the symptoms. *Graphites* may also be associated with women who have eczema on their breasts, which tend to crack and ooze a sticky discharge making it difficult to nurse. Useful for scars from old abscesses that remain hard and retard the flow of milk.

Hepar sulph. Useful for breast infections when pustules form on the breast or small abscesses form within the breast. The main indications are extreme sensitivity of the breast and sharp, splinter-like or needle-like pains. The person is extremely sensitive to cold drafts and is very chilly. The person is also quite irritable. Higher potencies, such as 200c, are used to prevent pus from forming. When the pus actually has begun, lower potencies such as 3x or 6x can be used to hasten the discharge of pus. High-potency remedies are not recommended for home prescribing. Consult a physician or skilled homeopathic consultant for potencies above 30c. Note that a person with a fever that stays high or a hard spot that does not go away should contact a physician immediately.

Ignatia. Useful for suppressed breast milk due to stress or grief (such as the loss of a loved one).

Kali bich. Useful when an infant refuses to drink breast milk because it tastes bad and is thick and stringy.

Mercurius sol. Useful when a breast infection forms an abscess or when there is an abscess of the nipple. (A physician should always be contacted for this condition.) The person is very sick, perspires excessively, and has very offensive breath and perspiration. The person is thirsty for large amounts of water and generally feels worse at night. The breast milk tastes bad, is bloody, and may contain infected pus.

Natrum mur. Useful when a nursing mother's hair falls out.

Phytolacca. Helps breasts that are extremely sensitive during nursing and have an excess flow of milk. There is a tendency for the breast to cake at the nipple and actually form pus. The person is chilly, and the entire body aches. When the baby nurses and the mother's nipples are cracked and sore, pain radiates from the nipple to all parts of the body, especially down the arm from the armpit.

Pulsatilla. A very important remedy for scanty flow or absence of breast milk in the mother. The person is sad, tearful, and wants consolation. There is a tendency to be chilly, yet the person likes the open air. When the baby nurses and the mother's nipples are cracked and sore, pain is felt from the breast to the uterus. *Pulsatilla* is an important remedy when breast irritation in adolescent girls who are not breastfeeding causes milk to flow. This remedy is helpful when the mother is weaning and the breast tends to swell and feels stretched and sore. This remedy actually helps milk flow from the nipple to ease swelling and discomfort. *Pulsatilla* is also used for weaning infants who are sad, tearful, and want the mother to continue to nurse; the child wants to be held and looks pleadingly at the mother.

Silica. Useful to break up and disperse the hard lumps in the breast after a breast infection. *Silica* is associated with sharp breast pain during nursing. If there are cracks in the nipple, blood may flow from them whenever the infant nurses. There may be a sharp pain from the breast to the uterus while nursing. The infant will vomit breast milk after nursing and sometimes even refuses breast milk altogether. This is an important remedy for abscesses in breast infections, as it will help bring them to a head if they are close to the surface or help absorb them if they are within the breast. A physician should always be contacted in these situations.

Sulphur. Useful for burning breast pain during nursing.

Urtica. Useful for the absence of the flow of breast milk for which there is no apparent cause and no other symptoms.

BROKEN BONES

Broken bones always need to be evaluated by a physician. A cast is usually worn to immobilize the area and allow the bone fragments to grow together. Surgery to put pins in the area is sometimes needed, especially if the break is severe. Certain vitamins and supplements are known to help broken bones.

Homeopathic remedies can help the pain and promote healing of a broken bone.

Arnica. This is usually the first remedy given for a broken bone. The affected part feels sore and bruised. *Arnica* is especially useful if the person is in shock. In the case of a severe accident, homeopaths may prescribe a high-potency dose of *Arnica*. The signs of shock include: a rapid, weak pulse; cool, clammy skin; lightheadedness; irregular breathing; confusion; or loss of consciousness. If any of these signs of shock are present, a doctor or person trained in emergency medicine should be contacted. Note that high-potency remedies are not recommended for home prescribing. Consult a physician or skilled homeopathic consultant for potencies above 30c.

Calcarea phos. Especially useful for a child who breaks or fractures a bone. It is also a valuable treatment for an elderly person who has brittle bones and recurring fractures. The bone heals slowly, and the area around the break has a cold, numb feeling. *Calc phos* can be used several times a day for fairly long periods of time in the 6x potency. This remedy can also be alternated with *Arnica* or *Symphytum* throughout the day at three- to four-hour intervals so that each remedy is taken two to three times daily.

Symphytum. An important remedy for a broken or badly bruised bone. Because it greatly helps the formation of callus, *Symphytum* is useful when bones are slow to heal. This remedy is used for injuries to the periosteum, which cause great pain. It is also used for injuries to the bones around the eyes (such as by snowballs and baseballs). *Symphytum* can be used several times a day in a 30x or 30c potency for several weeks.

BURNS (INCLUDES SUNBURN)

Burns can either be superficial and minor or extremely serious and life threatening. It is important to assess the degree of the burn before deciding to treat with natural methods or homeopathic remedies.

First-degree burns are characterized by pain and redness of the skin; they can be caused by touching a hot stove or frying pan, or by getting sunburned. Covering these burns with gels, such as those made from *Calendula* or *Urtica,* is helpful. Aloe vera gel can also be used externally to promote healing and diminish pain.

Second-degree burns are usually associated with blistering of the skin. They can be covered with *Calendula* or *Hypericum* gel and accompanied by an internal remedy.

Third-degree burns are more severe and cause damage to the layers of tissue below the surface of the skin. They should never be treated with local gels because of the risk of infections. A physician who specializes in burns should be consulted.

The two most serious dangers in severe burns are fluid loss in the areas where the tissues are damaged and swelling around the injured area, which may cut off circulation. The burns should be covered, and the person should be encouraged to drink. Severe second-degree burns or any third-degree burns should always be handled in an emergency room or by a burn specialist.

If a chemical irritant has caused the burning, the substance should be washed off with cool or lukewarm water. It is important not to scrub the area that is burned since this may tear off loose flesh. This is especially true for electrical burns where there can be extensive tissue damage underneath the skin but the surface of the skin shows less damage.

Aconite. Useful for fear and extreme apprehension associated with a burn. If the person is feeling panicky, this remedy may be given first. *Aconite* does not help heal the burn, but it does help the person feel less afraid.

Arnica. If shock is associated with a burn, *Arnica* is a useful remedy. It may need to be given first if the person is not fully conscious, or if weakness from loss of fluids is possible. The signs of shock include: a rapid, weak pulse; cool, clammy skin; lightheadedness; irregular breathing; confusion; or loss of consciousness. If any of these signs of shock are present, a doctor or person trained in emergency medicine should be contacted.

Calendula. When healing of burns has begun, *Calendula* can be used to help prevent scarring, and the ointment can be used on the burn to help prevent infection. This remedy may be alternated with *Hypericum. Calendula* lotion, which acts as an antiseptic, can also be put on the gauze that is placed on the burn area. A physician should be consulted to be sure that no infection is starting.

Cantharis. Useful for first-, second-, and third-degree burns. *Cantharis* is useful if the burn is extensive, blistered, or charred. Note that severe blistering or charring should be evaluated by a physician. *Cantharis* can help decrease the pain. This remedy can be repeated every five to ten minutes in the early stages of a burn.

Causticum. Useful for second- and third-degree burns (especially when burns to the limbs blister). The person feels pain and is restless. The burned skin tissue is still pink. The remedy can be repeated every five to ten minutes, or whenever the pain returns. If the skin is charred or has turned white, *Cantharis* is probably a better remedy.

Hypericum. Particularly useful for first- or second-degree burns accompanied by extreme nerve pain. The ointment form of this remedy can be used on the burn itself, alternated with *Calendula* ointment. A tincture of *Hypericum* may be especially helpful if made as follows: Boil and cool 8 ounces of water. Add fifteen drops of *Hypericum* tincture to the water. Saturate the gauze with this lotion and place it on the burn.

Urtica. Useful for superficial first-degree burns when only the outer skin is damaged and no blistering occurs. *Urtica* is also helpful for a sunburn. It can be used internally or externally. Later on, *Urtica, Hypericum,* or *Calendula* ointment can be used to complete the healing process. The 30c potency can be given every five to ten minutes. To make a lotion (for *Urtica, Calendula,* or *Hypericum*), add ten to twenty drops of the mother tincture to eight to sixteen ounces of cold, previously boiled water. Then soak the dressing or gauze that covers the burn in this lotion. Any type of burn can be treated (such as high heat, chemical, electricity, extreme cold, or radiation).

CHEMICAL HYPERSENSITIVITY

Some people are very sensitive to gasoline chemicals or other chemicals used in cleaning products, perfumes, or industry. A person can develop allergies to chemicals or react very strongly with changes in moods or behavior.

Arsenicum alb. This remedy corresponds closely to the person who reacts strongly to chemicals and has the signs and symptoms of chemical hypersensitivity. *Arsenicum alb* may help progressive weakening of many vital functions of the digestive system, particularly those causing weight loss and weakness. Slow, progressive inflammation of the respiratory tract also occurs, as well as in the mucous membranes of the respiratory tract. There are skin changes accompanied by dryness, scaling, and rashes. The person becomes thin, pale, and sensitive to cold, always wanting to be near a source of heat to keep warm. The person is restless and tires out quickly. The person may become overly meticulous in response to feeling fearful, anxious, and out of control. General burning pains are relieved by heat. Often the sufferer awakens between 1:00 and 3:00

A.M. *Arsenicum alb* is sometimes used for the side effects from pesticides.

Coffea. The person affected by chemicals exhibits hyperactivity of the emotional and mental spheres. Ideas flow rapidly and continuously; the person's thoughts may speed up. There is an increase in mental abilities and a feeling of emotional and mental excitement. The person is hypersensitive to noise, odor, and pain, which result in insomnia.

Mercurius sol. This type of hypersensitivity to chemicals is associated with the person who reacts by perspiring and has extremely foul-smelling body odors, including the breath and sweat. The person may experience increased salivation, the development of ulcerations and canker sores in the mouth, and a general weakening of the body and immune system; these symptoms are aggravated at night. The person is intolerant to slight temperature fluctuations. This hypersensitivity to chemicals can actually result in the formation of boils and skin ulcerations.

Nitric acid. This remedy is associated with long-standing hypersensitivity to chemicals. The person becomes worn out, preoccupied with health, and is irritable, easily angered, and vengeful. These symptoms may be associated with pains that are sticking or prickly, as though the person is being pricked by a thorn. There may be ulcerations, especially in the mouth, throat, anus, and genitalia.

Nux vomica. Often the first remedy given when the person is hypersensitive to chemicals. It is like a homeopathic antidote because it often is given after initial exposure, even if there are no other guiding symptoms. *Nux vomica* seems to immediately help the body metabolize or excrete toxic substances. It is especially associated with the person who is hypersensitive to odor, sound, and visual stimuli.

Phosphorus. This type of chemical hypersensitivity is associated with long-standing intoxication. The person experiences bleeding of the nose or digestive system, as well as fragile capillaries and bruising. The person is unable to focus, has memory trouble, and is hypersensitive to external events. The person alternates between overexcitement and extreme depression. There may be an abundance of energy, but the person weakens quickly. *Phosphorus* is useful for the person who is very tall and thin, is affected by exposure to cold, and is afraid of thunderstorms; these symptoms are often worse when lying on the left side. The person improves when exposed to heat, and after sleeping and eating.

Sulphur. Useful for the person exposed to chemicals, resulting in burning pains that are relieved by cold applications. The chemicals cause itchy, red rashes to form. The person becomes less concerned about hygiene, and is depressed and unable to stay organized. The symptoms often are aggravated around 11:00 A.M., when the person feels particularly exhausted.

CHEMOTHERAPY SIDE EFFECTS

Homeopathy is not a replacement for the treatment of cancer by conventional methods such as surgery, radiation, or chemotherapy. Homeopathic remedies, however, can help diminish pain and some of the unpleasant side effects from the treatment of cancer.

Arsenicum alb. Useful when the person is weak, tired, and irritable. It is useful for chemotherapy that occasionally causes burning diarrhea and burning in the stomach area. All burning pains can be relieved by warm drinks or applications.

Cadmium sulphuratum. One of the most important remedies for the side effects of chemotherapy. *Cadmium sulphuratum* may help extreme weakness and exhaustion from vomiting. The person feels cold even when near heat or wrapped warmly. Vomiting may be so extreme that it tears blood vessels in the stomach lining, causing coffee-colored vomit; stool will appear black and tarry due to this blood loss. There is extreme weakness and vertigo. If there is red or dark blood or black material in the vomit, contact a physician.

China. Useful when there is great purging of the bowels and other types of bodily fluids after chemotherapy. The person feels cold, has bluish skin, and is extremely weak.

Ipecac. Helpful for extreme nausea and vomiting that occurs after certain chemotherapy drugs. The tongue is usually clean. There may be blood in the vomit. If there is red or dark blood or black material in the vomit, contact a physician.

Nux vomica. Often the first remedy given for side effects of chemotherapy. The person is irritable and hypersensitive to noise, smell, and touch. There may be diarrhea accompanied by the feeling that not all of the stool has been eliminated.

CHICKENPOX

In 1995, a chickenpox vaccine became recommended. Before 1995, however, chickenpox was a common illness, often occurring in epidemics in young children. In metropolitan areas, at least 90 percent of the population had chickenpox by the age of fifteen and 95 percent had it by young adulthood.

Chickenpox is an acute viral illness with a sudden onset of fever, headache, and a skin eruption that starts as red spots which become blisters in three to four days. A breakout tends to occur in successive crops with several stages of maturity present at the same time. It tends to be more abundant on covered areas of the body, such as the chest and trunk, although it may also appear on the scalp, face, underneath the armpit, in the mouth and throat, and on the genitals. Breakouts tend to be worse as people age.

Transmission is by direct contact with droplets of mucus from the nose or throat or by airborne spread of secretions from the respiratory tract when the infected person sneezes or coughs. The incubation period is generally between thirteen and seventeen days, and the period of communicability is usually one or two days before the onset of the rash until five days after the appearance of the first crop of blisters.

The most common complication from chickenpox is viral pneumonia, which rarely is fatal. Encephalitis can also occur. Children with acute leukemia, even those who are in remission after chemotherapy, are at increased risk of fatal chickenpox. Reye's syndrome tends to appear after a case of chickenpox, especially when aspirin has been used to bring down a fever; therefore, aspirin should never be used with either chickenpox or influenza. Infection early in pregnancy may result in congenital defects.

Homeopathic remedies are helpful for chickenpox and can help decrease the intensity of the breakout, relieve itching, and help reduce scarring.

Aconite. Useful in the very early stages of chickenpox when the person is hot and thirsty. The person is also restless and anxious.

Antimonium crud. Helpful when the person is irritable (for example, a child does not want to be bathed, touched, or even looked at). The person has a very white, coated tongue.

Antimonium tart. Often useful after *Aconite* for a loose, rattling cough in which no mucus is expectorated. *Antimonium tart* is useful in the stage before eruptions appear and actually can help bring out the eruptions. The person is irritable during this phase (a child may whine). Generally, as the cough improves, the eruptions appear; this is a sign that the person is improving because the illness is moving from more important organs (like the lungs) to less important organs (like the skin).

Ferrum phos. Generalized inflammation is experienced, accompanied by fever and pain. There are few guiding mental symptoms with this remedy and it is sometimes used in alternation with a more indicated remedy. *Ferrum phos* 6x can be alternated with another remedy throughout the day at two- to three-hour intervals so that each remedy is taken three to four times daily.

Kali mur. Use this remedy as soon as eruptions appear to help diminish scarring of the rash. This remedy also may help prevent infection. The tongue is coated white. The 6x potency can be given four times daily until all the scabs have healed.

Mercurius sol. Useful for infected eruptions because it helps when pus has formed and the chickenpox spots tend to ulcerate. The breath and the pus emanating from the chickenpox spots are odorous. There is increased perspiration, and the person feels worse at night. Periods of feeling cold alternate with periods of feeling uncomfortably warm. This remedy is particularly helpful when the chickenpox affects the mouth, making the gums bleed. The tongue is thickly coated with a white or yellow discoloration.

Pulsatilla. Useful when the person is tearful, wants consolation, and is not thirsty. The person feels chilly, yet wants the windows open or to be outside.

Rhus tox. Useful for extreme itching and for the person who is restless and paces the floor. *Rhus tox* helps stop the itching and helps speed the healing of the eruptions.

COLD SORES AND CANKER SORES (INCLUDES HERPES SIMPLEX)

Canker sores and cold sores are two types of eruptions that occur on the lips and in the mouth. Canker sores (also called recurrent aphthous stomatitis) are painful eruptions and ulcers that occur singly or in groups. They appear on the inner lips, gums, and tongue, and generally recur. They may be caused by a virus or bacteria, or they may represent an anti-immune disorder.

Cold sores (also called fever blisters) can be caused by the herpes simplex virus as well as other viruses. They usually occur on the border of the lips where the lip meets the skin (vermilion border). They also can occur on the nose or hard palate. Fever, an upper respiratory infection, stress, diet, trauma, alcohol, dental work, sunburn or sun exposure, allergies, or exhaustion can lead to a breakout. These lesions often recur because the person has the herpes virus chronically in the body. Healing usually takes place in one to three weeks when the blisters break open and scabs form.

Natural approaches to healing cold sores and canker sores include taking lactobacillus acidophilus, which is the bacteria that grows in yogurt. It is also helpful to avoid arginine-rich foods, such as chocolate, oatmeal, nuts, raisins, and seeds. Certain vitamins and supplements are known to treat canker sores and cold sores.

Argentum nit. Helps canker sores and ulcers that occur on the edge of the tongue. The person is nervous and has excessive flatulence. The canker sores are considerably ulcerated, the breath is bad, and there is increased saliva.

Arsenicum alb. Helps the person who has blue or white cold sores that tend to burn and are relieved by drinking warm liquids. In severe cases, the cold sores may become infected and ulcerated.

Baptisia. Can help cold sores associated with extremely putrid breath. The gums may be ulcerated, loosened from the teeth, and dark red or purple. Increased salivation and great muscular soreness in the body are experienced.

Borax. An important remedy for children who have cold sores and thrush at the same time. Pain may cause the child to cry while nursing or drinking from a bottle. The cold sores and thrush tend to bleed easily and occur inside the cheeks and on the tongue. There is extreme heat and dryness in the mouth, and the cold sores are commonly white. A nursing mother will often notice that the infant's mouth is hot during nursing.

Bryonia. Useful for a nursing infant with cold sores and mouth ulcers. The mouth tends to be dry, and the infant may refuse to nurse until it is moistened.

Dulcamara. May help a person when there are canker sores on the lips and the tongue is dry and rough. The person has a sore throat and thick, sticky saliva. All symptoms get worse from any kind of cold, damp weather.

Hydrastis. Helpful for cold sores in nursing mothers. The tongue is yellow, swollen, and flabby, and there are teeth imprints on the sides. An excessive amount of thick, sticky mucus drains from the sinuses and drips down the throat into the mouth.

Kreosote. Helpful for cold sores, canker sores, and mouth ulcers during pregnancy. Note that while homeopathic remedies are safe during pregnancy, labor, and breastfeeding, a pregnant woman should confer with her obstetrician or midwife to coordinate treatment.

Mercurius sol. Useful for children with canker sores. There is bad breath and profuse salivation (the child may even drool). Canker sores tend to ulcerate, and the entire body smells offensive and per-spiration increases, especially at night. The ulcers are flat and super-ficial and may be accompanied by diarrhea and swollen glands in the neck. The gums are spongy, soft, and swollen.

Natrum mur. Helpful for burning cold sores on the gums. Small vesicles occur on the mouth, lips, and chin. Blisters on the upper lip may be filled with blood.

Nitric acid. Blisters and ulcers on the tongue and the lips can be helped by *Nitric acid.* There may be an unusual pricking sensation as though a splinter is sticking into the mucous membranes. Pro-fuse salivation and a strong, foul mouth odor are present.

Rhus tox. Helpful for blisters on the mouth and chin. The cor-ners of the mouth tend to ulcerate, and the tongue is red on the tip, extremely sore, and cracked.

COLDS AND RHINITIS (INCLUDES RUNNY NOSE)

Colds are caused by several types of viruses. Usually the symptoms are sneezing, a stuffy nose, a sore throat, fatigue, a headache, and a dry cough. The fever is usually low-grade, and the person does not have the severe muscle aching and pains in the joints that accompany the flu. There may also be ear pain or nausea and vomiting along with the cold, especially if the person swallows a lot of mucus.

Natural treatments for colds include getting plenty of rest, drinking lots of fluids, and not overexerting or working too hard. Gargling with salt water or a mixture of one-half warm water and one-half hydrogen peroxide can also soothe sore throats. Using a cool mist humidifier sometimes helps drain stuffy noses. Nasal sprays and decongestants should only be used when there is extreme difficulty in breathing, since they sometimes have a reverse effect, causing the person to get more stuffy after initial improvements. Avoiding caffeine because of the overstimulating effects, dairy products because they thicken the mucus, and alcohol because it generally weakens the immune system is important. Certain vitamins and herbs are known to help colds and rhinitis.

Aconite. Useful for treating colds that come on suddenly after exposure to cold, dry wind. The remedy should be taken as soon as the person begins to feel sick. It can be used frequently (every fifteen to sixty minutes for the first few hours). The body becomes chilly, and a fever may follow. The nose is congested and swollen, but these symptoms may occur without nasal discharge. Nasal stoppage seems to alternate between nostrils. A throbbing frontal headache with sneezing is a possible symptom. The person is hot, thirsty, and restless and generally feels worse in a stuffy atmosphere. Open air improves the symptoms.

Allium cepa. The cold helped by *Allium cepa* occurs with nasal discharge that irritates the nose and the area between the nose and mouth. This type of cold is accompanied by an excessive amount of non-irritating eye drainage (such as the discharge that occurs from peeling an onion). Frequent bouts of sneezing are a common symptom. A peculiar symptom is that nasal discharge stops when the person goes into the open air and returns when the person enters a warm room. Damp, cold weather often triggers a cold. Sneezing occurs when entering a warm room. The person may feel the sensation of a lump at the base of the nose. Nasal discharge may be accompanied by a headache, cough, and hoarseness. A difference between *Allium cepa* and *Arsenicum alb* is that a person with a cold associated with *Arsenicum alb* sneezes in cool air after leaving a warm room. This type of cold also lacks the larynx symptoms commonly seen with an *Allium cepa* cold. These two symptoms can differentiate the remedies, especially when accompanied by a thin, constantly flowing, irritating nasal discharge and excessive sneezing.

Arsenicum alb. Especially useful for treating winter colds that occur with a thin, watery, nasal discharge that irritates the upper lip, causing it to become raw. Although the discharge is constant, the nose still feels stuffed up. A throbbing, frontal headache and excessive sneezing occur, but the sneezing does not relieve the stuffiness. Stuffiness is worse in the open air. The person is quiet and chilly and feels extremely restless, anxious, and weak. There may be fussiness about neatness and a sensitivity to any disorder around the person, especially while feeling ill.

Arsenicum iod. Useful for a cold characterized by thin, watery, nasal discharge that irritates the skin inside and below the nose. Excessive sneezing makes the person feel worse. Nasal discharge may become chronic, leading to a stuffy, swollen nose with profuse, thick, yellow discharge. The symptoms of this type of cold are similar to the symptoms of a cold associated with *Arsenicum alb*, but do not have the characteristic restlessness and anxiety.

Arum triphyllum. Useful for treating a cold characterized by a stuffy nose with excessive, irritating nasal discharge; the discharge will even produce raw sores around the nose. The nose is obstructed, and the person must breathe through the mouth. A very important, peculiar symptom is that the person constantly picks at the nose until it bleeds. Pain in the nose is described as boring.

Calcarea carb. Useful for a person who gets a cold with every change of weather. *Calcarea carb* is often used for chronic rhinitis or acute exacerbations of chronic problems. A peculiar symptom is that nasal discharge may alternate with abdominal pain. The nose is stopped up and a yellowish, odorous discharge may occur. The nostrils can become sore and ulcerated. This type of cold is associated with enlarged lymph glands in the neck. If this remedy is used for recurrent or chronic problems, the person who most often needs *Calcarea carb* tends to gain weight easily and be anxious and fearful about getting other serious diseases.

Calcarea sulph. The type of cold helped by this remedy settles in the head and causes nasal discharge to become thick with pus and often tinged with blood. There may be a yellowish discharge in the back of the nose that drips down the throat. The edges of the nostrils are sore. Discharge often comes from one side of the nose.

Dulcamara. Useful for a cold characterized by either complete nasal blockage or an extremely runny nose. If there is complete nasal stoppage, this occurs especially when there is a cold rain. The person wants to keep the nose warm because cold air stops it up. Symptoms often come on after the person sits on cold and damp ground or on hot days when the nights turn cold toward the end of summer. Possible associated symptoms include diarrhea and joint pain that are relieved by moving about. When the nose is extremely runny, sneezing can be severe and great amounts of watery fluid can stream from the eyes and nose (except when the person is exposed to cold dampness, when the nose gets stuffed up). The person often develops cold sores with the cold and nasal problems.

Euphrasia. Useful for treating colds associated with profuse, thin, non-irritating nasal discharge. Discharge from the eyes irritates the skin below the eyes and eyelids. This type of cold has the opposite symptoms as the cold associated with *Allium cepa,* which has non-irritating eye discharges and irritating nasal discharges. A common associated symptom is a headache and profuse drainage from both the eyes and nose. The nose runs during the day but gets stuffy at night. Nasal problems are improved by being in the outside, open air.

Ferrum phos. Useful for treating the first stages of a cold in the head and nose. There are few mental guiding symptoms. The person often has a predisposition to getting colds. Useful when symptoms of general inflammation and irritation occur early in the illness. A nosebleed is a possible symptom. *Ferrum phos,* a tissue salt, is often used in the 6x potency.

Gelsemium. Useful for a cold accompanied by watery nasal discharge and sneezing. These symptoms can alternate with a fullness at the base of the nose. Common symptoms include a dull headache and fever. The cold symptoms come on slowly in warm, moist weather. The arms and legs ache and feel heavy. The person is usually not thirsty, and a chill seems to run up and down the spine. The person is weak, lethargic, and not very responsive. The eyelids appear heavy. The person is not particularly bothered by the cold or flu-like symptoms and appears tired and weary; the exception to this is that he or she may become worried and agitated when anticipating an upcoming event that will bring particular attention to oneself (such as taking a test, giving a speech, or entertaining guests), or will cause him or her to feel insecure or not in control (such as riding in an airplane).

Hepar sulph. Colds that come on in cold, dry weather may be treated with *Hepar sulph.* The person sneezes often and, at first, there may be an excessive amount of thin, watery nasal discharge that later becomes thick, odorous, and yellow or green in color. The person is chilly, bothered by drafts (especially around the neck), and wears scarves around the neck, even indoors, to provide protection from drafts and cold air. The person is extremely irritable. Anguish and anxiety are common at night. A possible symptom is a sore throat with the unusual feeling that a splinter, needle, or other sharp, pointed object is stuck in the throat.

Hydrastis. Useful for a cold with the symptom of a thick, sticky, discharge dripping down the back of the nose. This type of cold tends to develop into sinusitis after the runny nose slows. The ears tend to be stuffed up. The person feels the sensation that a hair is in the nostrils, and there is the constant desire to blow the nose. The nose feels raw and burning.

Kali bich. This type of cold is associated with tough, sticky, stringy nasal discharge that comes out of the nose, or extends from the back of the nose to the throat, causing the person to choke; sometimes, this sticky discharge completely blocks the nose. *Kali bich* is often useful for chronic nasal congestion. Nasal discharge may be initially runny and irritating, and this type of discharge is relieved by warm air. Then the discharge changes to the typical tough, stringy, tenacious discharge, and the person wants to blow the nose, but nothing comes out. Colds that can be treated with *Kali bich* can be distinguished from those treatable with *Hydrastis*. Although both types of colds have the symptom of a thick, sticky mucus, the mucus associated with *Hydrastis* is more distinctly bright yellow in color.

Kali iod. Helps a cold where pain in the frontal sinus is a major symptom, as well as violent sneezing and excessive thirst. With this type of cold, both the eyes and nose become sore and red from the burning tears and nasal discharge. The person may alternate between feeling cold and hot.

Kali mur. Useful after *Ferrum phos* when the nose stuffs up. Nasal discharge becomes white and relatively thick in consistency. The tongue is white or gray at the base. Usually, few mental symptoms are associated with this remedy. *Kali mur* is often used in the 6x potency.

Lycopodium. Useful for treating a cold characterized by complete stoppage of the nose both day and night, with small amounts of discharge that can sometimes burn and irritate the skin. Sticky crusts and plugs form in the nose. Useful for a child who awakens from sleep needing to rub the nose. An unusual symptom is that the nostrils flare out and move as the person breathes.

Natrum mur. Helpful for a cold with profuse, watery nasal discharge that lasts one to three days before blocking and stopping up the nose, making breathing difficult. Discharge is thin and watery (similar to the raw white of an egg). Excessive sneezing is common. This remedy is helpful in stopping a cold that starts with sneezing. The person may lose the senses of smell and taste.

Natrum sulph. Useful for treating a cold with thick, yellow, salty-tasting nasal discharge.

Nitric acid. Useful for chronic nasal discharge that is yellow, offensive, and irritating to the skin around the nose. A characteristic, peculiar symptom of this type of cold is the sensation that a splinter or stick is poking inside the nose.

Nux vomica. Useful for colds when nasal discharge flows heavily during the day, but the nose stuffs up at night. The nasal discharge is worse inside, but better outside; this characteristic helps distinguish it from the cold treatable with *Dulcamara,* which is worse outside and better inside. *Nux vomica* is often useful in the first stage of a head cold brought on by cold, damp weather or by sitting on cold, damp ground. The nose is dry with little discharge. The person feels a scraping sensation in the throat, and dullness and fullness in the frontal sinuses. This remedy should be given as soon as the dryness and tickling in the nose begins because it is of little use once the cold is established. *Nux vomica* is also useful for colds that begin in a person whose resistance is lowered (by getting little sleep, drinking, smoking, or partying).

Phosphorus. Useful for treating a cold with chronic nasal stuffiness associated with minor, but recurring, nosebleeds. Like the symptoms of a cold treatable with *Lycopodium,* the nostrils move inward and outward when breathing.

Pulsatilla. Useful for a well-established head cold. There is a tendency to cry often and to desire company. The discharges are bland, non-irritating, thick, and yellow in color. There is little sneezing. The person feels chilly, but likes cool air blowing, since it improves the symptoms.

Sabadilla. Helps a cold associated with frequent sneezing and a watery, runny nose. Symptoms include severe frontal head pain and red eyes with excessive watery discharge. The eyelids sometimes burn. There is the sensation that a lump is in the throat and a constant need to swallow. The symptoms are sometimes similar to symptoms associated with allergies and hay fever, which can also be treated with *Sabadilla.*

Sanguinaria. Useful for chronic rhinitis and nasal congestion. Discharges can be offensive and yellow in color. The nasal membranes always feel dry and congested. The person may have nasal polyps. An unusual symptom is that when the nose and cold symptoms stop, diarrhea begins. A possible symptom is a migraine-like headache located on the right side of the head that begins in the back of the head and moves toward the eye.

Sepia. Useful for chronic nasal obstruction and discharge (especially for post-nasal discharge of heavy, lumpy mucus). The discharge must be expectorated through the mouth. The thick, greenish discharge forms a crust and thick plugs. A yellowish discoloration across the nose is sometimes seen. The person often looks sad, with a drawn and droopy facial appearance, and may cry easily when discussing problems and not want comfort and consolation.

Sticta. Helpful for the type of cold associated with a constant desire to blow the nose, but nothing comes out. The person has a stuffed feeling deep inside the nose. A very distressing symptom is dryness of the mucus membranes. When the secretions dry quickly, scabs form and are difficult to dislodge. There is a dull, frontal sinus headache. Often, the person feels as if he or she is floating in the air and may feel a stiffness in the neck. The symptoms seem to come on during sudden temperature changes.

Thuja. Useful for treating chronic nasal discharge with thick, green mucus mixed with blood and pus. When the person blows the nose, there is pain in the teeth.

COLIC OF INFANTS AND CHILDREN

Colic occurs in infants and newborns and is usually associated with the accumulation of gas in the abdomen. The inability to relieve the trapped gas causes pressure and discomfort, and the baby cries, whines, and thrashes about.

Generally babies who have colic have immature and undeveloped digestive systems; it sometimes takes up to six months for the baby's digestive system to fully mature. Placing the baby's abdomen on a person's shoulder or gently massaging the abdomen may help the baby pass gas, relieving the discomfort. Lying the baby on the stomach on the mother's or father's lap with the knee gently pushing against the stomach may also help the baby pass gas.

If the mother is bottle feeding rather than nursing, colic may be due to soy allergies or the inability to digest milk products. Breast-feeding is probably the best way to minimize colic in infants.

Belladonna. Colic that causes a child to cry out suddenly and stop crying just as suddenly can be treated with *Belladonna*. The child tends to bend backward. This type of colic is often associated with a high fever, flushed face, large dilated pupils, and irritability.

Calcarea phos. Useful for older children who develop colicky pains in the abdomen at every attempt to eat. The child may vomit easily and have cold extremities. This remedy is particularly helpful for growing adolescent children. Breastfeeding infants who vomit after nursing may also benefit from this remedy.

Chamomilla. One of the most important remedies for treating the colic of a teething child. The child is very fretful and angry, but calms down for just a few minutes when carried. The child is often thirsty, may be very irritable, and may cry excessively. This type of pain is accompanied by a great deal of gas, but passing the gas does not bring relief. The painful area is distended and sensitive to touch. Warm applications and compresses may bring relief.

Cina. Useful for abdominal pains in children who may also have pinworms. (With pinworms the child will have an itchy anus.) The child will bore and pick at the nose. Sleep is extremely restless. The child only sleeps when rocked.

Colocynth. Useful for the relief of spasms and cramps in the middle of the abdomen. The baby or child twists and doubles over to relieve the pain, and pressing something hard against the abdomen may also bring relief. The child is very restless and moans between the spasms.

Ipecac. Useful for colic characterized by pain in the abdomen and excessive nausea and vomiting.

Magnesia phos. Useful for cramping abdominal pains that are relieved with warmth and gentle pressure.

Nux vomica. Helps abdominal pain associated in babies with constipation and large amounts of gas. The babies are very irritable and seem angry. Colic may occur in children who are overfed.

Pulsatilla. Vomiting, passing great amounts of gas, and foul-smelling stools are associated with the type of pain helped by *Pulsatilla*. The child is weepy, but stops crying when picked up and cuddled. *Pulsatilla* may also help a breastfeeding baby with colic whose mother gets indigestion from meat or fatty foods. The baby suffers along with the mother since the problem is being passed through the breast milk.

Staphysagria. Helps abdominal pain in children who are very peevish and irritable. The child pushes and throws things away. Colic may occur in an infant whose mother suppresses emotions (such as anger).

Veratrum alb. Useful for treating violent colic associated with cold sweat on the forehead. The body is cold, especially the feet. Large amounts of diarrhea often make the child weak.

COLLAPSE AND FAINTING

There are many causes of collapse and fainting. Some people have nervous or cardiovascular systems that are very sensitive to exercise or high levels of heat. These people may suffer from dilation of the blood vessels causing a decrease in the amount of blood flowing to the brain; this causes lightheadedness, darkness of vision, dizziness, and temporary loss of consciousness. Problems may occur when a person exercises heavily and then immediately takes a hot shower (the heat dilates the blood vessels and causes a sudden drop in the blood pressure). The person should cool down ten to twenty minutes before showering. Drinking plenty of fluids during exercise is important. These are not often serious problems and in most cases can be treated by loosening the clothes, keeping the person horizontal, providing fresh air, and keeping the feet elevated above the head.

If a person is feeling faint, have him or her sit in a squatting position with the knees up, either in a chair or lying on the ground. If, however, fainting persists or recurs frequently, the person should consult a doctor. If the person is very ill and loses consciousness, a physician or emergency room should be contacted.

Aconite. Useful for treating fear and sudden shock resulting from an overwhelming experience or from overexposure to the sun (heatstroke). The person fears death. Extreme terror and restlessness with a rapid pulse occur. Severe pain can cause the person to faint. Any situation that involves collapse or fainting should be considered an emergency and should be referred to a qualified medical professional or hospital as soon as possible.

Antimonium tart. Can be helpful for respiratory distress in a newborn where there is great rattling of mucus in the throat and lungs that cannot be expectorated. Any situation that involves collapse or fainting should be considered an emergency and should be referred to a qualified medical professional or hospital as soon as possible.

Arnica. Useful for treating shock or collapse from sudden injury with extensive soft-tissue damage (such as a car accident). Panting is common. The person is pale and pulseless. The person either fears death is imminent, or seems unaffected by the severity of the injury. The person does not want to be touched. Any situation that involves collapse or fainting should be considered an emergency and should be referred to a qualified medical professional or hospital as soon as possible.

Carbo veg. Useful for collapse and shock after prolonged bouts with diarrhea. The person hungers for air and needs to be fanned. The body and breath are extremely cold. Any situation that involves collapse or fainting should be considered an emergency and should be referred to a qualified medical professional or hospital as soon as possible.

China. Can help when collapse and shock occur from loss of bodily fluids (such as from hemorrhaging or diarrhea). The head and carotid arteries in the neck throb intensely. A feeling of shock is associated with a sense of faintness. The person is so weak that walking or standing causes dizziness. Loss of sight and a ringing in the ears may accompany a sense of faintness. Perspiration, accompanied by great sensations of thirst, sometimes occurs. Any situation that involves collapse or fainting should be considered an emergency and should be referred to a qualified medical professional or hospital as soon as possible.

Coffea. The person needing *Coffea* has acute senses, and this remedy is useful when the person faints, especially after being frightened. *Coffea* is often helpful after *Aconite.* Any situation that involves collapse or fainting should be considered an emergency and should be referred to a qualified medical professional or hospital as soon as possible.

Nux vomica. The symptoms associated with *Nux vomica* can be caused from staying up too late or from overworking. Drinking too much coffee or alcohol may precede the feeling of faintness and collapse. Fainting can occur from unpleasant odors. Feelings of faintness get worse in the morning or after a meal. Any situation that involves collapse or fainting should be considered an emergency and should be referred to a qualified medical professional or hospital as soon as possible.

Veratrum alb. Cold perspiration on the forehead is an important symptom. The person feels extremely cold, and the skin is blue. Lips, nails, and fingertips are also blue. The person feels very weak. The pulse is weak and barely perceptible. Saliva often dribbles from the mouth. Violent retching, vomiting, and diarrhea occur. Cramps in the extremities are common. The person may alternate between feelings of extreme melancholy and indifference. The person will lie or sit, noticing nothing. At other times, the person may be almost manic, with a desire to cut and tear things. Delirium drives the person to curse and howl. The person feels as though death is near. Any situation that involves collapse or fainting should be considered an emergency and should be referred to a qualified medical professional or hospital as soon as possible.

CONSTIPATION

Constipation is a common problem for many people. Inactivity, not moving bowels regularly, and improper diets all contribute to constipation. It is important to keep the stool bulky and soft with plenty of fresh fruits, vegetables, and whole grains. Avoiding white flour and white sugar can also be helpful, since these substances pass too slowly in the digestive system, making it difficult to pass the stool. It is often helpful to use bulking agents for a person who has chronic problems with constipation. Using bran is a way to bulk the stool, but unfortunately this often causes gas and can be harsh on the intestines.

Busy routines are another cause of constipation—people are often too busy to sit and relax without straining to have a stool. If the urge to have a stool occurs, the person should not wait. Passing the stool as soon as possible is important.

Regular exercise is another way to avoid constipation. The bowels, like any body tissue, need to be stimulated and activated through exercise. Exercising at least twenty minutes three or four times a week is necessary.

Drinking seven or eight glasses of water each day can also be helpful. Certain herbs are known to help constipation.

The homeopathic remedies listed here are useful for acute or recurrent problems of constipation. From a homeopathic perspective, constipation is just one of many symptoms; the person must describe other symptoms for a clear remedy picture.

Anacardium. Useful if the person feels as if a plug is in the rectum and it cannot be expelled. The bowels are very inactive and the rectum seems powerless to unplug itself. Even soft stools pass with difficulty. Only small quantities of stools are expelled with each attempt.

Antimonium crud. Especially useful for constipation in elderly people. The person alternates between constipation and diarrhea. A white, thickly coated tongue is often associated with this type of constipation.

Bryonia. When constipated, the person helped by *Bryonia* is often irritable and does not like to be bothered or disturbed. *Bryonia* relieves constipation due to dryness. The person does not have an urge for a stool. The intestines just do not seem to have any ability to contract to push the stool out. This remedy can also be used for constipation in young children. *Bryonia* is particularly helpful for a person who has constipation in the summer or who has constipation associated with joint, tendon, and muscle attachment problems. Headaches often accompany this type of constipation. A great thirst for large amounts of cold water at infrequent intervals is common.

Causticum. Useful for relieving constipation when stools are passed easier when standing up. The stools are generally hard, covered with mucus, and expelled with much straining. This type of constipation is due to a feeling of powerlessness or paralysis of the rectum where the rectal tissues are not able to expel the stool.

Graphites. One of the best remedies for constipation. The main symptoms of this type of constipation are mucus in the stool, no urging for a stool, extreme soreness and aching of the anus after a stool, and depression. The person is depressed and overweight. This remedy is helpful for people who wait too long to go to the bathroom after having the urge. The person can go for days without a stool. When a stool does come, it looks like small, round balls, which are connected with tiny shreds of mucus. Passing a stool may cause pain, often because an itchy, burning fissure has developed. The pain from the fissure can last for a long time after a bowel movement.

Lycopodium. Useful for a person with a sensation that a stool was only partially eliminated (like constipation associated with *Nux vomica*). The rectum feels constricted (like constipation associated with *Silica*). The stools are sometimes initially hard and dry, but are softer at the end. A lot of gas is trapped in the lower part of the abdomen and passing gas gives some relief. This type of constipation is also associated with hemorrhoids. The rectum contracts and actually protrudes down with the stool. The typical person affected by this type of constipation is worried, apprehensive, and hardworking. If overstressed or bothered, the person will lose his or her temper. This remedy is often useful for constipated children and pregnant women, especially when the constipation is accompanied by extreme amounts of gas buildup in the intestines. Pregnant women may feel pain in the small of the back as if it would break.

Natrum mur. Useful for a stool that is hard and crumbling, difficult to expel, and causes bleeding and soreness in the rectum. The person has urging to have a stool, but nothing seems to come. A stitching pain may shoot into the rectum. The stool seems to recede into the rectum while the person is trying to pass it. The person must strain to get any stool to come out. Headaches occur during constipation (like constipation associated with *Bryonia*). An unusual symptom is that the person is unable to pass a stool if anyone is present. The person tends to brood, be somewhat of a hypochondriac, and worry and think a lot about the past.

Nux vomica. Probably the most frequently prescribed remedy for constipation. The person has a constant urging for a stool, but nothing seems to come out. When a stool finally occurs, it feels as though a part of the stool was left behind. Absence of the need for defecation contraindicates *Nux vomica*. The affected person generally has sedentary habits, works too hard, or studies too hard at night. The person also tends to be irritable, anger easily, and indulge in stimulants, alcohol, cigarettes, or coffee. Generally, no pain or inflammation is associated with this type of constipation. *Nux vomica* is also a very important remedy for the effects of using too many stool softeners, laxatives, and enemas. This remedy is also useful for constipation from allopathic medicines. *Nux vomica* is one of the most important remedies for constipation in newborn children who are bottle fed with artificial formula; the baby seems to have the desire to pass a stool, but only small amounts of stool come out. Constipation sometimes occurs on alternate days. This remedy is also useful for constipation during the menstrual period and while traveling abroad.

Sepia. Useful for treating constipation characterized by the feeling of a ball in the rectum. Pains shoot upward from the rectum into the abdomen. Stools are large and hard, and attempting to have a stool causes great pain. Constipation is worse during the menstrual period, and during and after pregnancy. The intestines may feel overly relaxed. A bearing-down sensation feels as if the intestines and rectum may actually pass out through the anus. Besides shooting pains up the rectum during a stool, the pains may also shoot up the vagina in women. Note that while homeopathic remedies are safe during pregnancy, labor, and breastfeeding, a pregnant woman should confer with her obstetrician or midwife to coordinate treatment.

Silica. Useful for treating constipation when the stool comes down with difficulty and is partially expelled but recedes again. The person strains excessively for a stool and the rectum stings. The rectum actually closes when the stool comes out. This type of constipation is often associated with rectal fissures. Constipation is related to the menstrual cycle, being worse before and during the menstrual period. This type of constipation is due to inefficient expulsive force of the rectum and also from spasms of the sphincter muscles.

Sulphur. This remedy can help the person who has urges to have a stool, but little comes out. The person feels a sensation of heat and discomfort in the rectum that is relieved by cold compresses or water. Overall, the person is often irritable, lazy, and somewhat disorganized. Useful in children who avoid having a bowel movement because of a memory of painful stools. The stools are hard, dark, and dry. The stools are expelled with great straining; the first effort for a bowel movement is extremely painful. The person may alternate between constipation and diarrhea. *Sulphur* is also a good remedy for irritable bowel syndrome. Due to the sluggishness and internal body heat of the person, the constipation is better with exercise or when it is cold outside. The rectal burning after the stool is better from cold applications.

Veratrum alb. Usually a diarrhea remedy, but it also has important effects in treating constipation. The stools are large, and the person must strain for a stool. This great strain causes exhaustion and is also associated with a cold sweat. This remedy is also useful for relieving the constipation of infants, especially during very cold weather. *Veratrum alb* is often useful after *Nux vomica* has partially treated the person. The intestines are very sluggish, and the feces accumulate in the rectum, causing the person to strain tremendously and break into a sweat. The person may give up the straining and have the feces removed. The person may be faint and lightheaded after the stool.

COUGHS (INCLUDES BRONCHITIS)

Coughing can be a simple and benign symptom, but it can also represent a more serious illness. It can be due to irritation from cigarette smoking or pollution in the inside or outside air. Cigarette smokers often cough in the morning, thinking it is a common and normal problem, not realizing it reflects continual irritation of the respiratory tissue.

Upper respiratory infections caused by viruses can produce a cough that is usually dry and nonproductive. Other forms of nonproductive coughs are post-nasal drip, sinusitis, allergies, side effects from certain medications, especially blood pressure medications, or as the result of acid being regurgitated from the stomach up to the esophagus and irritating the throat and trachea.

A cough that does not go away within a few weeks should always be evaluated by a physician because it may indicate a problem with chronic bronchitis, emphysema, or a tumor. Asthma should always be treated by a professional, especially if it is unable to be controlled and the coughing is extreme. If the mucus becomes thicker and turns yellow or green, it is possible that the bronchitis is more serious or that it is pneumonia. These cases should also be treated by a physician.

If home prescribing does not bring relief, a person should always contact a physician. It may be necessary for the doctor to listen to the lungs or take an X-ray to determine if there is a more serious problem underlying the cough.

Aconite. Useful only during the beginning of an upper respiratory infection and cough. The symptoms often come on after exposure to dry, cold wind. Fever and anxiety are usually present in the beginning, and the person sneezes frequently, has a high fever, is thirsty, and is restless at night. The cough is dry.

Allium cepa. Useful for treating a cough that is triggered by breathing in cold air. A raspy cough does not produce mucus; a tickling in the throat sometimes triggers this cough. An unusual symptom is that the larynx tickles and feels split or torn, and the person may place a hand over the voice box so it will not feel torn apart. While the cough gets worse from breathing in cold air, the person generally feels better in cold or open air and worse in a warm room. Allergy symptoms are often present with this type of cough.

Antimonium tart. Useful for a loose cough when the person is unable to expectorate mucus. Successive coughing is sometimes seen. Symptoms get worse at night and in bed.

Argentum nit. If the person has difficulty breathing once coughing starts, *Argentum nit* may be a useful remedy. There is extreme apprehension and a desire to do things in a hurry. Spasms of the chest muscles make breathing difficult. Laughing and singing high notes can trigger a cough. The person may feel unable to breathe, especially in a crowded room. Symptoms get worse with any type of heat; cold, fresh air makes the symptoms better. Touching the ear canal provokes a cough.

Arnica. Useful for a cough associated with yelling or overuse of the voice. This problem can also occur when the lungs are overworked from too much exercise. The chest wall and ribs are painful. This remedy can be helpful when a person breaks a rib when coughing. A coughing episode can also be brought on after a person cries hard.

Arsenicum alb. Useful for a cough with burning chest pains. The coughing and burning pain are relieved by heat. The cough gets worse when lying down, and the person feels suffocated. The person is irritable, restless, and often wheezes. Symptoms get worse between midnight and 3:00 A.M., and the person often awakens with a cough. Watery, thin nasal discharges burn the skin above the lip and below the nose. The person is thirsty, but only for small amounts of water at a time.

Belladonna. Useful for a cough that comes on quickly and violently after a chill (especially in the head area); it often follows *Aconite* well. Dry skin is an important symptom. The person has a red, hot, flushed face and may have dilated pupils. A dry cough comes in spasms, and the head feels as if it will burst when the person coughs. Often, children cry before the coughing begins.

Bromium. Useful for a dry cough with hoarseness, burning pain behind the sternum, and much rattling of mucus. Chest pain tends to travel upward and causes a cold sensation when the person breathes in. Breathing in also provokes the cough. The bronchial tubes feel full of smoke. Asthma, which may be an associated symptom, is usually better when the person is on the ocean (such as on a cruise, sailboat, or small island) and worse when the person comes inland.

Bryonia. Useful for a cough accompanied by dry mucous membranes. The person is irritable, but if left alone is quiet and does not complain. If bothered, the person reacts angrily. The cough gets worse from any kind of movement and when going from the open air into a warm room. If chest pain accompanies the cough, the person may try to hold the sides of the chest to prevent it from moving or shaking. There are stitching pains in the side, and headaches are often accompanied by a bursting feeling.

Calcarea carb. Useful for a loose cough in the morning that tends to be dry at night. The person feels short of breath. After exertion, there is a feeling of fullness in the chest. An unusual symptom is that the person coughs when playing a piano (as in the original proving) or when eating. With the cough, the person feels suffocated with a tightness, burning, and soreness in the chest. Symptoms are worse going upstairs, causing the person to sit down. The chest is sensitive to any kind of touch. The person desires to be out in the fresh air. When the person is able to bring up expectorant, it tends to taste salty. Useful for children with chronic, recurring coughs.

Calcarea phos. Helpful for suffocating coughs that get better when the person lies down. Pain is felt in the lower part of the left lung with the cough. The nose drains in a cold room, but becomes stuffed up in a warm room or outdoors. The person is fretful. Children who need this remedy tend to whine.

Carbo veg. A helpful remedy for a cough in an elderly person. This remedy is also useful for bronchitis (especially if the person has difficulty breathing and coughs up yellow, foul-smelling expectoration). There is a burning sensation and excessive rattling of mucus in the chest. The cough gets worse in the evening, in the open air, and after eating and talking. The face may have a blue tint, and there may be a desire to be fanned; these symptoms often accompany the cough because the person does not seem to get enough air.

Causticum. Useful for a dry, hollow cough that is relieved by drinking cold water. The person cannot cough deep enough to expectorate the mucus, because it seems to stick in the bronchial tubes. An unusual symptom is pain in the hips (especially in the left hip). During the cough there may be involuntary urination.

Cuprum met. If the cough has a gurgling sound, *Cuprum met* is a useful remedy. This type of cough gets better by drinking cold water. Suffocating coughing attacks get worse at 3:00 A.M. Spasms, cramps, and constrictions in the chest area are important symptoms. Asthma may be associated with this type of constriction and may alternate with vomiting. This remedy is also useful for whooping cough, which has symptoms of vomiting, chest spasms, and a purplish tint to the face. Other symptoms associated with whooping cough or other types of cough may include cramps in the palms of the hands and in the calves and the soles of the feet. A metallic taste in the mouth is a common symptom.

Drosera. Used for whooping cough before the pertussis vaccine was developed. Symptoms include a spasmodic, dry cough that repeats in quick succession. The person can scarcely breathe and feels as if choking. Another type of cough is associated with the sensation of crumbs in the throat or a feather in the larynx. The cough is much better during the day and almost disappears, but as soon as the person lies down in bed at night, it returns (especially in children). Vomiting may occur if the person is unable to expectorate the mucus.

Dulcamara. Helps a cough that occurs after exposure to wet weather or after a person becomes chilled when overheated. The cough becomes worse with sudden temperature changes from warm to cold (often seen in late summer or early fall when hot days and cold nights are common). A person who has been camping or sitting on the cold, damp ground is susceptible to this type of cough. Sneezing and runny eyes and nose are common symptoms. The nose will be stuffy in cold weather and extremely runny in warm weather. The muscles, bones, back, and skin are very sore. The cough is worse at night and better by getting on the hands and knees. Perspiration improves the symptoms (except the headache, which is often in the back of the head). Symptoms get worse when lying down, and there is a sense of weight in the back of the head.

Eupatorium perf. Useful for a cough with extreme soreness in the chest; the chest is so sore that the person must hold it with the hands (similar to *Bryonia*). In coughs associated with *Bryonia,* the lips and tongue are dry, but in *Eupatorium perf* they are not.

Ferrum phos. Useful in the very early stages of an upper respiratory infection. The person has a fever and cough, but few other guiding symptoms. The person is feverish, but the face is pale.

Gelsemium. Useful for coughing with flu-like symptoms. The person feels tired and weak. The eyelids appear heavy, and the person does not want to move. The person is thirstless and has chills moving up and down the spine. The cough is dry and tearing, and the chest is sore.

Hepar sulph. Useful for a loose cough that gets worse in cold air and after drinking cold water. The person is chilly and does not want cold air blowing on the body (especially around the neck and chest area). Yellow or green mucus tends to be easy to expectorate, but causes the person to choke. This remedy can be used for croup in children (especially when the cough is loose).

Hydrastis. Useful for the cough that accompanies bronchitis (especially if the cough lingers). The mucus tends to be thick, yellow, and sticky, and is difficult to expectorate. Sinusitis is an associated symptom with this type of cough. The chest feels raw, sore, and burning.

Ignatia. Useful for a cough associated with stress and worry. One important symptom is a nervous cough when the person has dry coughs in rapid succession (especially common when a person is under stress). Coughing actually increases the desire to cough. This type of cough is also accompanied by sighing (especially when grief, loss, or anxiety accompany the stress). There is little expectoration.

Ipecac. Can help a loose, rattling cough accompanied by asthma, nausea, and vomiting. (Nausea and vomiting are the two most important symptoms.) As with symptoms associated with *Antimonium tart,* the chest is full of mucus that cannot be expectorated.

Kali bich. Useful for a constant, recurring, barking cough with green or yellow, thick, sticky mucus that is difficult to expectorate. Before the measles vaccine, this remedy was often used for coughs following measles (especially a morning cough when mucus is difficult to expectorate). The cough tends to get better at night in bed.

Kali carb. Useful for a cough that accompanies bronchitis and asthma. The cough is usually worse between 2:00 and 4:00 A.M. There is stitching pain in the chest, and the person cannot lie down. The person often buries the face in a pillow while resting on the knees. Mucus is difficult to expectorate. There may be a feeling of anxiety in the pit of the stomach.

Kali mur. Useful for general swelling in the upper respiratory tract. Symptoms include a white tongue, blocked eustachian tubes, and a congested nose. Swollen glands and tonsils are also possible symptoms. The cough is short and spasmodic, and there is light mucus that is difficult to expectorate. Few mental symptoms are associated with this problem.

Lachesis. Useful for a dry cough with a suffocating feeling that gets worse upon awakening. The cough is brought on by putting pressure on the chest or larynx. The cough gets worse in the open air. Mucus is difficult to expectorate because it gets stuck in the lungs and bronchial tubes. When the person falls asleep, breathing almost seems to stop. Touching the ear canal provokes a cough. Mentally, the person may be talkative and easily irritated.

Lycopodium. Useful for relieving a tickling cough accompanied by burning in the chest. The cough is worse when walking downhill, and the expectoration is gray, thick, and tastes salty. Infants who have rattling mucus in the chest may also have increased flatulence. The cough is worse between 4:00 and 8:00 P.M.

Manganum aceticum. Helpful for a cough that always gets better when lying down and worse when sitting up. The cough is also worse in the evening and in damp weather. Mucus is difficult to loosen. The person affected with this type of cough tends to get bronchitis whenever a cold is present. Hoarseness is also a symptom. Touching the ear canal may provoke a cough.

Mercurius sol. A loose cough that comes on in the later stages of an upper respiratory infection can be helped with *Mercurius sol.* The expectoration is green or yellow in color. The cough gets worse when the person lies in a warm bed and at night. Excessive perspiration sometimes awakens the person. Much yellow or green nasal discharge makes the nostrils sore and raw. The entire body smells bad.

Natrum mur. Coughs caused by a tickling in the pit of the stomach can be relieved with *Natrum mur.* The cough occurs with burning pains in the head and shortness of breath (especially when going up stairs). Urine may leak out when the person coughs. Thin, watery mucus from post-nasal drainage triggers a cough. Sneezing, diminished senses of taste and smell, and an alternating runny and stuffy nose are common symptoms. The person is irritable and wants to be left alone.

Nux vomica. Useful for a cough that sometimes begins after exposure to dry, cold air or after the person overindulges in food or alcohol. The person is irritable, angers easily, and is extremely sensitive to noise, bright light, and travel. A person who smokes or has a smoker's cough often needs this remedy. The nose is usually stuffed up at night and runs during the daytime and when the person is in the warm air. The body is very chilled. Often, a bursting headache is brought on by the cough. The person may feel as if something were torn loose in the chest.

Phosphorus. A cough that often arises with irritation in the trachea can be treated with *Phosphorus*. The cough is worse when talking or overusing the voice. Inhaling cold air, reading, laughing, talking, and going from a warm room into cold air also make the cough worse. There is a sweet taste while coughing. The person feels a tightness across the chest and a great weight on the chest. Chest pain is worse when lying on the left side. A nervous cough is often provoked by such things as strong odors and the presence of a stranger. The person tends to be unfocused and has recurring respiratory problems.

Pulsatilla. A cough that comes on in the later stages of respiratory infections can be relieved with *Pulsatilla*. The person is weepy, desires attention, and wants to be held. The nose, throat, eyes, and bronchial tubes discharge a thick, yellow, non-irritating substance. The cough is worse in the morning. There are often chills running up and down the back. Despite a dry mouth, the person is not thirsty. The person feels better in the cold air (which improves the cough).

Rhus tox. Helpful for a dry, teasing cough that is worse from midnight until morning and during a chill, or when putting hands outside of bedcovers. This cough may accompany influenza when the joints ache. The person is restless, agitated, and may need to constantly change position.

Rumex. Useful for a cough brought on by constant tickling at the base of the throat. The cough is worse when touching the throat or voice box and from cold air. When the chest is warmed by covering the body and head with sheets and blankets, the cough stops. The dry, teasing cough prevents sleep. Pressure, talking, and breathing in cool air aggravate the cough. The cough is worse at night. The larynx and trachea are raw. After coughing for a long time, a thin, watery, frothy expectoration is brought up into the mouth. Later, this substance becomes stringy and tough. Intensely itchy skin is a possible associated symptom.

Sanguinaria. A cough accompanied by flushed skin (especially the face) and a dry throat can be relieved with this remedy. This type of cough is relieved by belching. A burning sensation occurs in the right chest through to the right shoulder. An odorous, rust-colored sputum is difficult to bring up. After influenza has improved and a cough remains, this remedy is helpful. The cough tends to return with every new upper respiratory infection and cold. The person must sit up in bed because of the cough.

Sepia. A dry, tiring cough that seems to come from the stomach can be relieved with *Sepia.* An unusual symptom is the taste of a rotten egg when coughing. The person is short of breath. Symptoms get worse after sleeping and are relieved from rapid motion (such as walking quickly, dancing, or playing sports). The cough is worse in the morning, and the expectorant tastes salty.

Spongia. Useful for a dry cough with dryness of the air passages and a burning sensation in the larynx. The cough is better after eating or drinking (especially warm drinks) and is worse in cold air. The person often wakes up feeling suffocated. *Spongia* is useful for a croupy cough, especially in young children when the cough is dry. The cough is dry and barking and gets worse when inspiring and before midnight. There may be the feeling that a plug is in the larynx. Sometimes there is a feeling of an irresistible cough from a spot deep in the chest, as if it is sore and raw. The chest sometimes feels so weak the person can hardly speak.

Sticta. Useful for a dry, hacking nighttime cough. Post-nasal drip, which causes the throat to become raw, initiates the cough. The cough is worse when breathing in, toward evening, when tired, and from sudden temperature changes. Sometimes the person experiences the sensation of floating in the air. There is a tendency to talk excessively. Pain in the right upper extremities (especially the right shoulder, deltoid, and biceps muscles) is a possible symptom. Before measles vaccines, this remedy was used for a cough that occurred after measles.

Sulphur. Seldom useful in the first stages of a cough and instead often helps clear up symptoms that linger (including coughs from simple viruses, bronchitis, and pneumonia). The person is often disheveled, disorganized, messy, and oblivious to surroundings. There is an aversion to bathing and possibly an unpleasant body odor. The person has difficulty breathing and wants the windows open. The cough is loose and gets worse from talking in the morning and from heat. The expectoration tends to be green in color, infected, and sweet-tasting. The chest feels heavy. Shortness of breath in the middle of the night is relieved by sitting up. There may be burning pain in the chest, throat, and lips. The person may be hoarse or lose the voice. Heat flushes are often felt (especially on top of the head), and the feet may burn although they are cold to the touch.

Tabacum. Can relieve a cough brought on by intense hiccoughs. The person must swallow cold water (similar to *Causticum* and *Phosphorus*) to relieve the dry cough. There is shortness of breath and a tingling sensation down the left arm (especially when lying on the left side).

Veratrum alb. The person with this type of cough has excessive mucus in the bronchial tubes that cannot be expectorated easily. *Veratrum alb* is often used for older people with chronic bronchitis. The loud, barking cough is better with belching and worse in a warm room, especially when coming from the cold air (similar to *Bryonia*). Urine escapes when the person coughs.

Verbascum. Useful for a deep, barking, hollow cough. The person coughs while sleeping, but does not awaken. The cough is better from deep breathing.

Zincum met. Useful for a cough that comes on with spasms and causes weakness. The person often has restless legs and moves them constantly. Eating sweet things makes the cough worse. A child who coughs tends to grab the genitals while coughing. Shortness of breath with the cough tends to get better as soon as the expectoration begins. Sleeping is fitful; the body jerks and the person cries out during sleep.

CRACKED SKIN (ALSO CALLED FISSURES)

Fissures, or cracks in the skin, can occur for many reasons. Skin can often have problems in the winter since it loses its normal moisture and begins to crack and bleed. Eczema can also lead to cracking of the skin, especially if there has been a lot of itching. Contact with water, especially washing dishes or clothes by hand, can also create fissures.

Fissures can occur in various parts of the body, including the anus and nose. Anal fissures can be very painful and are often difficult to heal because the tear becomes larger with each new bowel movement. These fissures often bleed and cause pain on defecation. Fissures also form on the side of the nose, especially during dry, cold winter weather when indoor heat is used. Fissures can also form in the corners of the mouth.

Fissures are treated in the same way as eczema. Lotions should be applied to keep the skin moist. Hot baths should be avoided. Fissures on the tips of the fingers can be treated with *Calendula* ointment and covered with a band aid. Gloves should be worn when washing dishes or having one's hands in water. For anal fissures, it is helpful to dab the anal tissues after a bowel movement rather than wiping with harsh toilet paper. Wetting the toilet paper with cool water can often help relieve pain after a bowel movement. Certain vitamins and oils are known to help fissures.

Antimonium crud. Useful for treating cracked fingers (especially around the nails) that are worse from washing.

Calcarea carb. Useful for treating cracks in the hands that are worse in the winter and from getting wet. Cracks in the fingers are also typical.

Graphites. Can be used to treat extremely painful cracks in the hands and fingers (especially in the joints and tips of the fingers). The cracks often ooze a thin, sticky discharge. The cracking is worse in the winter. Cracking is usually associated with eczema, and the person is constipated and tends to be depressed.

Lycopodium. Deep cracks on the heels can be helped by *Lycopodium.*

Manganum aceticum. Helpful for relieving deep cracks in the bends of the elbows. These areas tend to become infected and can turn into ulcers or skin infections.

Mercurius sol. Useful for treating deep, bleeding cracks that emit an extremely foul odor. Cracks that may ulcerate occur on the joints of the fingers.

Natrum mur. Cracks between the toes that itch violently can be relieved with *Natrum mur.* This remedy is also useful for cracks along the fingernails and hangnails that tend to crack along the edges.

Nitric acid. Deep, bleeding cracks that are worse on the hands may be relieved with this remedy.

Petroleum. Burning, deep, bleeding cracks on the hands that are worse during the winter can be relieved by *Petroleum.* The symptoms also affect the fingers (especially the very tips). This remedy is also helpful for cracks that occur on the palms of the hands.

Sarsaparilla. Cracks on the feet (especially between the toes) may be relieved with *Sarsaparilla.* This remedy may also help cracks on the fingers. Symptoms occur in the spring. The affected area tends to burn, and the cracks are often deep and bleeding. Cracks on the thumbs are also seen.

Sepia. Helpful for treating cracks in the skin that occur in the winter and after washing. The cracks often occur on the backs of the hands.

Silica. Useful for treating cracked feet (especially between the toes). Cracks also occur along the sides of the nails. Abscesses and boils that do not heal properly and tend to crack along the sides may also be seen.

Sulphur. Cracks on the hands that occur from getting wet, in the winter, and after washing may be relieved with *Sulphur.* These cracks tend to be deep and bloody. Fingers can crack along the joints. There may be redness, itching, and burning around the cracks. Cracks in the palms of the hands may be present.

CRAMPS

Cramps can occur anywhere in the body, but they are mostly a problem in the calves, soles of the feet, toes, thighs, hands, and forearms.

Leg cramps occur most frequently, and causes and treatments are discussed below.

Leg cramps most commonly occur after exercise when the person has rested a while. Cramps can also occur from wearing shoes that do not fit properly or are uncomfortable; this is especially seen in women who wear high heels. Another cause of leg cramps is from the side effects of medication, such as diuretics, which lower potassium and magnesium in the body. Another common cause of leg cramps is calcium deficiency; this kind of cramping is usually experienced at night, waking the person from sleep. It is particularly troublesome for growing children who have high demands for calcium as their bones grow, strengthen, and harden. It is also troublesome for post-menopausal women, especially those who are trying to lose weight and do not consume enough calcium in their diet. Pregnant women are also susceptible to leg cramps because of their unusually high need for calcium as the baby's bones are being developed.

Treatment of leg cramps includes stretching the leg in the opposite direction that the cramp is occurring. For instance, if the calf muscle is cramping, it is important to stretch the heel out toward the ground and pull the toes back up toward the head. Prevention is also important, making sure that the medication the person is taking does not cause cramping. Making sure to have enough calcium in the diet so calcium deficiency is avoided is important. Avoiding certain types of food that may interfere with the absorption of calcium is essential, especially foods that are high in sugar and caffeine. Certain vitamins and supplements are known to help cramps.

Calcarea carb. Useful for cramps in the calves that occur while the person is sleeping. The cramps tend to get worse when stretching the feet out in bed and when pulling on shoes. Cramping also occurs in the hands in the morning or at night. Cramps in the soles of the feet and in the toes are worse at night and during pregnancy. Note that while homeopathic remedies are safe during pregnancy, labor, and breastfeeding, a pregnant woman should confer with her obstetrician or midwife to coordinate treatment.

Colocynth. Useful for cramps in any part of the lower extremities, as well as in the hands. The person experiences cramps in the thighs that can occur after embarrassment or humiliation. The cramps get better when pressure and warmth are applied.

Cuprum met. Useful for hand or leg cramps that come on after profuse diarrhea (such as after shigella or salmonella infections) or after a severe case of viral gastroenteritis. Cramps may occur in the fingers during childbirth. Note that while homeopathic remedies are safe during pregnancy, labor, and breastfeeding, a pregnant woman should confer with her obstetrician or midwife to coordinate treatment.

Magnesia phos. Associated with cramps in the fingers that result from writing or playing the piano, violin, or any instrument that requires fingering (such as trumpet, saxophone, or cello).

Rhus tox. Useful for cramps in the calves, especially those that occur at night in bed. Also helpful for cramps in the calves that occur while sitting and when sitting down after walking. *Rhus tox* is associated with restless legs.

Sulphur. Useful for cramps in the calves after severe diarrhea. *Sulphur* is also associated with cramps that occur while dancing, at night, while in bed, during a bowel movement, and while stretching out the feet. The person also experiences cramps in the calves while walking. The soles of the feet cramp at night. This remedy is usually associated with hot, sweaty feet that need to remain out of the covers at night.

Veratrum alb. Useful for foot and leg cramps after severe diarrhea. The body feels extremely cold, as do the extremities.

CROUP

Croup is an acute viral infection that primarily affects children six months to three years old; it is less common in children under six months. Many different viruses can cause croup, including the parainfluenza viruses, respiratory syncytial virus (RSV), and influenza. Croup spreads either by airborne viruses or by contact with infected saliva.

Usually croup follows an upper respiratory infection. It occurs at night, waking the child with breathlessness, a barking, metallic cough, and a hoarse voice. A fever occurs in about 50 percent of the cases. The chest wall often retracts in an effort to get enough air into the lungs. Croup can affect the larynx, trachea, bronchia, and lungs. The attack is most intense for one to four hours, especially at night, and often recurs for up to three or four nights. The child often becomes frightened, which aggravates the croup and causes more spasms.

If the respiratory distress continues and there is a rapid pulse, fatigue, blue lips, blue fingertips, or dehydration, seek immediate medical attention.

Resting and drinking plenty of fluids are essential for the body because the respiratory passage can get quite dry from the coughing. Steam often relaxes the respiratory system and eases the spasms. Sitting near a shower with hot water generating steam is helpful. If this is not successful, the child should be wrapped warmly and taken for a drive with the windows open, allowing exposure to cool, moist night air.

While several homeopathic remedies are useful for croup, *Aconite, Hepar sulph,* and *Spongia* are the most commonly used. Repeat remedies hourly for intense cases of croup, and every two to three hours when the cough and breathing problems are less troublesome.

Aconite. Helpful for a dry, barking cough with little or no rattling mucus. It is most useful during the first stages of illness. The attack may come on after being chilled by a cold wind. If the croup occurs at night, the person awakens feeling restless, agitated, and anxious. Fever is often present, and the skin is hot and dry. Often there is no mucus drainage from the nose.

Drosera. Noted for treating whooping cough, *Drosera* is also useful for croup. This remedy is characterized by a deep, barking cough associated with difficulty catching the breath. It is difficult to cough deep enough to get relief and to expel mucus. Generally the symptoms are worse in the early evening and after midnight.

Hepar sulph. The child who needs *Hepar sulph* has a loose, wet-sounding cough. Mucus production is generally associated with this cough. There are often yellow or yellowish-green discharges from the nose, eyes, or lungs. Sometimes there is so much mucus that the croupy cough ends with gagging or vomiting. There may be a general sensitivity to cold drafts, especially around the head and neck. Throat pain may extend to the ears when coughing or swallowing.

Kali bich. Ropy, sticky, thickened mucus is common in coughs associated with *Kali bich.* The mucus is so thick that the person awakens choking and gasping for air. The cough has a metallic sound. Aggravation occurs in the early morning hours, often between 3:00 and 5:00 A.M. Wheezing sounds may accompany the barking cough.

Spongia. Used when croup is characterized by dry air passages. The cough and respiratory membranes are dry. Often there is a feeling of suffocation with this type of croup. Eating warm foods or drinking warm drinks can bring relief of symptoms. *Spongia* is given later in the course of treatment (*Aconite* is usually given in the beginning). When the cough changes from dry to wet, *Hepar sulph* is used (and vice versa).

CUTS AND INCISED WOUNDS
(INCLUDES CLEAN CUTS AND STRAIGHT CUTS)

Incised wounds occur when the skin is cut by a sharp instrument such as a knife, razor, or scalpel during surgery. Both the skin and the underlying tissues may be injured. A physician's attention is often needed to repair the wound, particularly if it is wide and gaping and involves deeper structures. Butterfly strips or stitches are often necessary.

Homeopathy can be helpful, especially when the cut involves only the skin and not deeper structures. Using *Calendula* tincture or lotion on the injured area and thoroughly cleansing the area with water (soapy water if the edges are dirty) are helpful. Once the area is covered with a sterile gauze, *Calendula* ointment can be used to protect and heal the injured site. This dressing should be changed daily to avoid contamination. *Hypericum* ointment or lotion can also be used, especially if there is a lot of pain associated with the injury.

Aconite. Useful for the shock or fear that accompanies a laceration. *Aconite* can be used every five to thirty minutes for the first two hours. The signs of shock include: a rapid, weak pulse; cool, clammy skin; lightheadedness; irregular breathing; confusion; or loss of consciousness. If any of these signs of shock are present, a doctor or person trained in emergency medicine should be contacted.

Arnica. Useful for symptoms of bruising and shock that accompany a laceration. When the person is in shock, *Aconite* is used first and can be given every five to thirty minutes in the first two hours, followed by *Arnica*. The signs of shock include: a rapid, weak pulse; cool, clammy skin; lightheadedness; irregular breathing; confusion; or loss of consciousness. If any of these signs of shock are present, a doctor or person trained in emergency medicine should be contacted.

Calendula. May be used as a lotion, tincture, or ointment. *Calendula* 30c may also be used. This remedy is helpful when bleeding stops because it decreases the possibility of infection. *Calendula* can also be used in combination with *Hypericum*; the two tinctures can be mixed in equal parts, or the ointments of both used together.

Hypericum. Useful if the incised wound is extremely painful (such as a wound over areas rich in nerves, like the fingertips or toes). The pain usually moves up the body from the injury. This remedy can be used alone in tincture, lotion, or ointment form. *Hypericum* tincture can also be mixed with *Calendula* tincture in equal parts, or the ointments of both can be used together.

Staphysagria. Particularly helpful for cuts from sharp instruments (such as knives or scalpels). After surgery, this remedy helps decrease the pain from the scalpel wounds. Often, *Staphysagria* 200c is used once or twice a day for a few days. This remedy can be alternated with *Arnica* 30c or 200c throughout the day at three- to four- hour intervals (so that each remedy is taken twice during the day) until the pain is lessened and healing has progressed (two to ten days). Note that high-potency remedies are not recommended for home prescribing. Consult a physician or skilled homeopathic consultant for potencies above 30c.

DEPRESSION
(INCLUDES SADNESS, GRIEF, CRYING, AND DESPAIR)

Take special care. A health care professional, psychiatrist, or psychologist should be involved with the care of a depressed person or person exhibiting suicidal behavior. Any verbal suicidal threats or acts of self-destruction should be taken seriously. Some clinical features and symptoms associated with suicide are depression; extreme agitation; intense feelings of guilt or remorse; severe hypochondrial preoccupation, having AIDS, cancer, heart disease, or other disease; drug abuse; chronic physical illness; or loss of a loved one or job.

Depression is diagnosed if a person experiences at least five of the following symptoms during a two-week period. These symptoms often represent a change from previous functioning. Always consult a physician if depression is suspected.

Depression symptoms include: (1) sadness (children may be irritable most of the day); (2) diminished interest and pleasure in daily activities almost every day; (3) increased or decreased amount of sleeping, and early morning awakening at least two hours before the usual hour; (4) feelings of restlessness or being slowed down; (5) weight loss or gain when not dieting; (6) loss of energy or fatigue nearly every day; (7) feelings of worthlessness and inappropriate guilt; (8) indecisiveness or inability to think or concentrate clearly; (9) recurrent thoughts of death or suicide; (10) loss of sex drive; (11) worsening of symptoms in the morning or at night; (12) being withdrawn from friends or family; (13) low frustration levels or no motivation; (14) feelings of hopelessness and helplessness; (15) preoccupation with problems and unpleasant events in the past; (16) distractions and complaints of poor memory; and (17) impaired judgment.

Other types of symptoms are also associated with depression. Physical complaints (such as worries or complaints of the heart, gastrointestinal tract, central urinary tract, sexual problems, low back pain, or extremity problems) may mask feelings of depression. A person can also experience different symptoms at different ages. In children, before the onset of puberty, depression may take the form of complaints of body pain, agitation, hearing voices, anxiety, and developing phobias such as to school. During the adolescent period, depression can be manifested by skipping school, restlessness in class, antisocial behavior, substance abuse, promiscuity, or poor hygiene. In the elderly, depression can sometimes take the form of memory loss, disorientation, confusion, apathy, and distractibility.

There are many different forms of depressive disorders. Major depression, also called unipolar depression, is a severe disorder. It is more common in women (two-to-one ratio), with an average onset at forty years of age, although it can occur at any time. There is a severe loss of interest or pleasure in almost all activities, and a lack of ability to react to usually pleasurable stimuli, even when something good happens. It is commonly worse in the morning upon awakening. There may be a family history of depression; however, in at least 25 percent of major depression cases, a direct, precipitating cause, such as job loss or death of a family member, can be determined. These causes are usually seen in people who have major depression followed by complete or nearly complete recovery and usually have good responses to normal antidepressive therapy, such as medication and counseling.

One treatment for depression is medication. Serotonin re-uptake inhibitors (such as Prozac and Zoloft) and tricyclic antidepressants (such as Elavil and Tofranil) are generally prescribed for major depression. Lithium is useful for manic depression. Anti-anxiety medications are useful when there is anxiety associated with depression. Consult a physician, psychiatrist, or psychologist for further information.

Other conventional forms of therapy are psychotherapy with or without antidepressants. This can take the form of psychoanalysis, supportive psychotherapy, group therapy, family therapy, behavioral therapy, or cognitive therapy. Psychotherapy is not used when a person is acutely manic because often medication and hospitalization need to be considered for the safety of the person in this condition. This is also true with depression that is severe and suicidal in nature. Any verbal suicidal threats or acts of self-destruction should be taken seriously. A psychiatrist, psychologist, or social worker should be consulted.

Homeopathy has long been used to treat the effects of depression. Sadness, grief, and mild forms of anxiety are problems that a person can treat at home; however, if any of these problems persist for more than two weeks, professional help is needed. The homeopathic remedies listed here can also be used, but it takes great skill in treating a person who has depression. Homeopathy can be used on its own, in conjunction with psychotherapy, or, in more severe cases, when a person is taking conventional drugs. A health care professional, psychiatrist, or psychologist should be involved with the care of a depressed person.

Aloe. Helpful when the person feels that life is a burden, does not want to work, and becomes lazy. Laziness, however, may alternate with bursts of mental activity followed by tiredness and weakness. The person may tremble and become upset from music or noise. There is a great sense of insecurity and general dissatisfaction and anger, and the person may want to be alone. This is particularly true when there is a problem with the bowels, such as diarrhea, with a sense of insecurity and weakness in the rectal area causing the person to be unsure of whether passing gas or stool. Depression may be associated with symptoms of colitis.

Anacardium. People who need *Anacardium* often have an inferiority complex, lack self-confidence, feel powerless, and feel they must constantly prove themselves. They may feel disliked by others and attempt to attract the attention and affection of others through achievements (such as receiving honors at school, getting good grades, or being promoted at work). If they do not succeed, the lack of self-confidence becomes worse. As depression gets worse, anger turns inward. They may offend easily, swear, and become paranoid, possibly even refusing to eat for fear of being poisoned. There is despair of never getting better, and there may be thoughts of committing suicide by shooting themselves. The memory may fail, and they will suddenly forget names and recent activities. They feel separated from the world and, having lost all self-confidence, believe nothing will ever be accomplished. This remedy is also helpful for depression after childbirth.

Antimonium crud. Helpful for the person who is overly sentimental, especially the person whose love life seems disappointing. The person is weepy, weary, and sleeps too much. There is a curious symptom of being intensely sentimental with this remedy, especially when the person walks in the moonlight, before the menstrual period, and, curiously, when the stools are loose. There may be a suicidal disposition with this remedy, and constant thoughts of committing suicide may sometimes drive the person out of bed with anxiety. Shooting is often the most common form of suicidal thought.

Antimonium tart. Useful when the person feels apathetic, indifferent, and wants to be left alone. If ill, there may be feelings of never being able to recover from the illness, and the person often complains of suffering, even saying that death is welcome. A child who needs this remedy may cry easily, seem sad, tend to whine (especially when sick), and cling to the parents; the child does not even like to be looked at when ill.

Apis. Helpful when the person is weepy and cries all day and night without cause. Apathy, indifference, and fear of death are felt, and the person may be unable to concentrate, especially when reading or writing.

Argentum nit. Useful when the person feels hopeless, neglected, and despised by family. The will to live is lost, and the person may avoid conversation and will often lie down with closed eyes to avoid talking. *Argentum nit* is helpful when the person loses ambition, cries, and is frightened and depressed about having a serious disease and feels no hope of recovery. The person is often tormented, and has strange ideas, feelings, and impulses that cause depression. There may be unusual impulses, such as driving a car into a wall, jumping off a bridge, or sticking the hands into a garbage disposal. Time may seem to pass too slowly, and the memory may weaken. Sadness and loss of hope occur because of phobias and anxieties; impulses become overwhelming and the person feels unable to continue.

Arsenicum alb. May help depression and despair in a person who has a deep sense of insecurity, anxiety, and health worries (see Anxiety). The person becomes obsessed with the need to control and hide insecurities; when attempts fail because the person cannot control everything, he or she becomes anguished. As anger and frustration increase, the person becomes even more angry, which leads to a deeper, darker depression. These feelings may eventually lead to thoughts of suicide (by poison, a knife, hanging, or suffocation). These symptoms may be associated with breathing difficulties and asthma.

Baptisia. Useful when there is a high fever associated with an infection, and the person feels extremely sick. Mentally, the person is dull, confused, unable to think, apathetic, and indifferent. He or she does not want to move or think. The person feels no hope for recovery, is certain of death, may fall asleep while answering questions, and may not complete sentences when talking.

Belladonna. Helpful when the person feels dejected and discouraged. The person may get worse at night and have a throbbing headache, red face, and dilated pupils. There is continuous moaning and sighing, even during sleep. This depression is generally associated with restlessness and anxiety that drive the person out of bed. Bouts of crying may last a long time, and the person is inconsolable while crying. Persistent insomnia is often experienced, leaving the person feeling dull, slow to act, indifferent, and apathetic. This remedy is often used after an acute manic episode has left the person exhausted, tearful, and weak.

Bromium. Helpful when extreme sadness is accompanied by the peculiar symptom of looking constantly in one direction without saying anything. This person may also have the delusion that strange people are looking over his or her shoulder and someone would be there if he or she turned to look.

Causticum. Useful for sadness associated with long, drawn-out grief that may be the result of the death of a friend, relative, or child. This remedy may also be associated with the loss of a close relationship. Anxiety can become extreme, and the person becomes almost paralyzed with worry. This leads to a deep depression accompanied by feelings of helplessness, worthlessness, and despair. The person may cry without cause, and this crying may last day and night. After a while, the person may become extremely depressed and want to die. The person often feels as if he or she committed a horrible crime, which leads to feelings of guilt. *Causticum* helps the person who is obsessed and hopeless about injustices in the world and becomes extremely rebellious, idealistic, and moralistic in response to these feelings.

China. Helpful for sadness and depression that is associated with a loss of bodily fluids (such as after heavy bleeding, diarrhea, or heavy menstrual bleeding). The person may feel unloved and rejected by others who do not provide attention deserved. The person often blames others for problems, and may even be sad enough to lose the desire to live. Suicide may be considered, but the person does not have the courage to follow through with it.

Cimicifuga. Useful when the person is depressed, despondent, and feels as though covered by a black cloud, which leads to feelings of confusion. There is also a feeling that the heart is as heavy as lead, and that impending doom will come at any time. These problems become worse around a woman's menstrual cycle, and particularly during menopause when depression is associated with the fear of going crazy. Ailments from disappointed love are also seen here; the person may become indifferent and uninterested in household affairs, will sigh and moan often, and is suspicious of everyone. Depression is also associated with fear of death and being murdered; these feelings may be particularly noticed during a pregnancy. Note that while homeopathic remedies are safe during pregnancy, labor, and breastfeeding, a pregnant woman should confer with her obstetrician or midwife to coordinate treatment.

Cocculus. Useful for sadness that is a result of being with and caring for sick people. It occurs particularly late at night. *Cocculus* is also helpful when the person experiences extreme sorrow accompanied by the constant inclination to sit in a corner, bury oneself in thought, and take no notice of the surroundings.

Gelsemium. Helpful when the person wants to be quiet and left alone. The mind feels dull and the person is extremely apathetic, especially during an illness (such as influenza or high fever). There is a complete absence of fear. Useful for ailments that come on after grief and disappointment. After a sad event, the person is unable to cry; this is usually associated with aching in the body, a heavy head, absence of thirst, and drooping eyelids, especially when the person is ill. Depression may come on after anxiety attacks, when the person is worried about upcoming events (such as speaking in public or taking an exam). The person feels unable to participate in the event, and often sits and stares, feeling paralyzed.

Graphites. Helpful when the person is shy and unable to make decisions; this often leads to depression, apathy, and laziness. Sensitivity to music is seen and the person may cry as a result of listening to it. There is uneasiness in the stomach, and the person may be overweight, constipated, and have dry, itchy, and cracked skin that oozes a sticky discharge.

Helonias. Useful for the person who is profoundly melancholic but becomes less depressed when busy and the mind is engaged. When not busy, the person may be depressed, irritable, and unable to endure criticism. With this depression, the person may be critical and find fault in others. This remedy is often associated with women who have problems with slow and late menstrual periods. *Helonias* is also useful for women who are tired and aching, often have urinary tract problems, or are worn out from years of hard work.

Ignatia. An important remedy for the effects of sudden shock, loss, disappointment, and grief (such as the loss of a job or a relationship, or the death of a family member or friend). The person tends to hold feelings inside and does not like to cry, especially in public. If feelings are uncontrollable, hysterical crying often results; the person will quickly try to regain control. Sudden shock often causes the person to become speechless. If feelings are not expressed, the person may become hard, cold, critical, and angry. The person may sob and sigh at the same time. Problems such as a lump in the throat, nervous coughing, or diarrhea may develop.

Lachesis. Helps the person who experiences depression upon awakening. The person tends to get better as the day goes on and becomes active at night, even somewhat manic, only to again feel sad and emotionally paralyzed in the morning. Depression and sadness are often experienced during the menstrual period; this is a particular problem for prepubescent girls and during the premenstrual time in women. Generally, these feelings of sadness and aloneness improve once the menstrual period starts. *Lachesis* is also useful for menopausal women who are depressed because the menstrual periods have permanently ended. In general, *Lachesis* helps those who always feel better when discharge of any kind begins to flow (such as the menstrual period, nasal discharge, or a boil that drains).

Lycopodium. Helpful when the person experiences shyness, indecision, and a loss of self-confidence; these symptoms all result in a lack of self-esteem, and they increase depression and promote the fear that the person will break down under stress. The person feels unable to do anything new and, as the depression continues, may want to avoid all people and be alone; the person may even avoid his or her children. *Lycopodium* is generally associated with the person who has digestive problems; he or she becomes depressed and develops indigestion between 4:00 and 8:00 p.m., as well as upon awakening in the morning. The person often cries, especially when criticized, and tends to cry for no reason at all when depressed. There is weeping before the menstrual period as well as before urination, especially if there is a urinary tract infection. The person may have the unusual symptom of crying when being thanked for doing something for others. Generally, crying makes the person feel better, and the person may alternate between crying and laughing.

Mercurius sol. Helpful when the person has poor self-confidence and an inability to make decisions. The person may become easily discouraged, dejected, and disgusted with life. Indifference and suicidal thoughts may be experienced. The person often does not want to eat because of a lack of appetite.

Natrum mur. One of the most important remedies for people who have suffered grief, loss, or disappointment, leading to emotional problems or physical illness. *Natrum mur* helps the person who broods about death or broken relationships that occurred a long time ago; the person may also brood about past insults and other disappointments. Vulnerability and fear of rejection cause the person to become very cautious in relationships; this causes inner tension that often results in emotional outbursts. The person may laugh inappropriately at sad events (such as funerals), or become irritable and angry when someone tries to console him or her. Uncontrollable sobbing may occur after the person holds back tears for a long time, with great shaking and jerking of the body; the person, however, is able to quickly regain control. The person may cry when thinking of sad events, or when spoken to or looked at. The person prefers to cry alone and tends to get aggravated when someone offers consolation.

Natrum sulph. An important remedy for emotional problems resulting from a head injury or fall. Depression becomes worse when the person listens to music of any type (classical music as well as upbeat, lively music). The person may experience the unusual symptom of feeling depressed while sitting near stained glass windows, especially in church. Sensitivity, suspicion, and dislike of speaking or being spoken to may be experienced. *Natrum sulph* is an important remedy for suicidal impulses when the person must use self-control to prevent suicide by shooting. (A physician should be contacted immediately. Criteria for hospitalization rests on the answer to one question: Could the person harm oneself or someone else?) This remedy is also useful for alternating depression and mania (classically called manic depression or bipolar disorder). Physical and mental symptoms get worse in cold, damp weather and become better in warm, dry weather.

Phosphorus. While generally sensitive, friendly, open, and creative, people who need *Phosphorus* become stressed because they overlook their own needs to help others. Fears develop, and they are concerned about the health of others. They become afraid of the dark and being alone at night. They may become self-absorbed, dwell on fantasies, become spacey, and have few emotional defenses. If these vulnerabilities continue, they may feel overwhelmed and break down, become paralyzed with anxiety and fear, and lose the ability to interact with the world, eventually becoming indifferent, unable to function, insensitive, and depressed. Adolescents with depression who need *Phosphorus* tend to grow quickly and fall in love too quickly. They tend to be artistically oriented and intelligent, yet have a hard time maintaining focus. These adolescents are easily hurt by love relationships because they try to care for the needs of others and avoid their own needs; this can lead to depression and withdrawal.

Pulsatilla. Helpful for the depressed person who tends to be kind and easily hurt. The person cries easily and feels better afterward and when being consoled. The person tries to adapt to the environment. As a consequence, there may be an inability to reveal true feelings, and the person suffers in silence and feels self-pity. The person is generally easygoing and giving, but if not in a healthy relationship may be easily embarrassed and afraid of the opposite sex. Feelings of rejection may be easily experienced, especially when the person is separated from loved ones (as when a parent dies or is absent early in childhood). Useful for grieving, especially when the person is unable to express grief. The person likes to be around others, and likes consolation, sympathy, and pity. The person is friendly, yet can be manipulative. The person may form dependent relationships with loved ones and be easily jealous. Children with depression who need *Pulsatilla* are generally bright, bashful, and tend to cling to their parents to feel secure. As these children get older, they tend to be followers rather than leaders, and are easily influenced by strong-willed friends. They may be easily hurt, and keep their feelings to themselves to avoid causing problems.

Rhus tox. Along with apprehension at night, and restlessness with continuous changing of positions, the person may also feel depressed; these symptoms get worse at night. Thoughts of suicide may occur, especially by drowning, and the person may feel sad, helpless, and hopeless. The person may cry and not know why. Generally, the depression is relieved when walking outside in the open air.

Sepia. Helpful when the person is sad, quiet, withdrawn, tends to avoid others, and often lacks the energy to interact with others. The person can sometimes appear hard and stern. There seems to be an absence of any joy. This type of depression is often associated with bouts of crying for no reason; the person may cry all day and night. Physicians can identify those who need *Sepia* because they often cry during the medical interview. The person does not want consolation when feeling sad and becomes irritable if someone attempts to cheer him or her. Desperation and inability to cope may be experienced, and the person may even lose interest in a job or housework. These people often avoid their children and spouse.

Silica. Useful for the person who has low energy and feels depressed. There are problems with endurance and stamina, and the person may have low self-confidence. The person may become easily discouraged and unwilling to take risks because of fear of failure. While the person is capable and conscientious about work, there may be a lack of mental stamina; this leads to an inability to concentrate and the feeling that tasks are too complicated. There is difficulty in initiating new activities, and the person may be shy, reserved, and want to please others. The person likes to avoid conflict and, when stressed, feels unable to cope because of a general lack of stamina; this may lead to an inability to concentrate and express thoughts verbally or in writing.

Staphysagria. The person who needs this remedy suppresses feelings, is shy, likes to please others, avoids conflict, and wants to control the ability to be hurt. The person is often compliant and resigned to fate. However, when hurt in a love relationship or disappointed in another aspect of life, the person tends to suffer in silence; this suppression of feelings creates anger. The person who needs this remedy may feel angry and frustrated despite a pleasant façade. Depression may result when the person has been assaulted in some way (such as a rape or robbery) and does not express the feelings involved; appropriate professional help is needed to help the person communicate these feelings.

Sulphur. The person who needs *Sulphur* is intelligent, enjoys exploring new ideas and deep meanings of things, and may be philosophical about life itself. The person is often a leader, and likes to be the center of attention. If the person feels unappreciated, sulking and depression may be experienced. Self-absorption may cause the person to become mentally overactive, physically lazy, scatter-brained, and disorganized; conversations and tasks are begun but remain uncompleted. The person may withdraw from and lose interest in life. He or she may become disheveled, messy, and inactive. The person may be possessive and collect things; he or she may live in this world of possessions. Personal hygiene may not be maintained.

Veratrum alb. Helpful when depression alternates with restless activity. On one hand, the person can be charming, witty and talkative, and may exaggerate, even to the point of telling lies. On the other hand, depression, solemnity, and indifference may be experienced. The person often hangs the head down or broods in silence and wants to be alone. The person feels despair about self-worth, feels unlucky, and worries about future misfortunes.

Zincum met. Useful for the person who is physically and mentally restless. The person startles easily and constantly moves the legs and feet. Restlessness is often associated with working excessively (at home, school, or work). The person is sensitive to noise and begins to break down mentally because of exhaustion. Depression sets in and the thinking process slows. The person is confused, cries when angry, and feels unable to continue. Peculiar fears may be experienced, such as a fear of being arrested for an imaginary crime. Depression may occur after drinking too much wine.

DIARRHEA

Diarrhea is a common problem that can range from being a sublimated annoyance to severe and life-threatening. Increased stool liquidity, a sense of urgency, increased frequency of bowel movements, and incontinence of stool are different problems of diarrhea. It is important to know the person's normal bowel habits to understand whether diarrhea is a problem.

There are many different causes of diarrhea. Acute diarrhea is defined as loose or frequent stools that persist for less than three weeks. It is usually caused by infections from viruses, bacteria, protozoa, drugs, or bacterial toxins ingested in food. It is important to remember events that may have caused the diarrhea. For example, unpurified water consumed when camping or swimming may often result in an infection with giardia or cryptosporidium. Foreign travel often leads to diarrhea, caused by certain viruses or ameba. Eating foods at a party or in a large group where many people get sick often results in diarrhea related to salmonella or shigella.

Causes of chronic diarrhea include: medications; overuse of laxatives; ulcerative colitis; Crohn's disease; radiation; pancreas disease; irritable bowel syndrome; diabetes; hyperthyroidism; microorganisms such as viruses, bacteria, or protozoa; and intolerance of lactose, magnesium, and antacids.

Diarrhea symptoms can range from loose, watery stools to more serious problems of bloody diarrhea with abdominal cramping, bloating, and nausea and vomiting. It is important, especially when there are bloody or black stools, to have a physician evaluate the diarrhea symptoms thoroughly to determine whether the cause is bacterial or due to problems such as ulcerative colitis or Crohn's disease.

Treatment for diarrhea, especially if it is mild, is to wait it out and drink plenty of fluids. It is important to eat foods that contain carbohydrates. Easily digested foods, such as soups, crackers, and dry toast are also encouraged. It is often recommended to avoid fats, milk products, caffeine, alcohol, and high-fiber foods such as salads and heavy grains. Fruit should also be avoided, except for fruits that tend to bind the stool, such as unripe bananas.

It is very important to watch for signs of dehydration. These include dry mouth, decreased urinary frequency, skin that looks dry and lacks elasticity, rapid heartbeat, lightheadedness, fainting, or problems with concentration. A physician should be contacted if dehydration is suspected.

Severe diarrhea may necessitate the use of intravenous fluids administered by a medical professional. A solution of one teaspoon sugar, a pinch of salt, a pinch of baking soda, and a quart of orange juice or water can also be helpful, and there are products in a pharmacy for oral rehydration. Antidiarrhea agents that slow down the intestinal speed are available over-the-counter in pharmacies. Bismuth (Pepto-Bismol) may reduce symptoms in those experiencing traveler's diarrhea because it is anti-inflammatory and antibacterial. Lactobacilli, the normal inhabitant of the intestinal tract, can be found in yogurt. It is often helpful to replace the normal bacteria that is excreted during diarrhea. Kaolin or pectin (Kaopectate) can also be helpful because of its antidiarrhea action. Antibiotics are sometimes used for severe bacterial infections which lead to diarrhea.

Aconite. Useful at the onset of acute diarrhea (such as diarrhea that comes on after being frightened or after drinking cold drinks). *Aconite* is also useful for treating diarrhea of a child (especially one who is afraid, restless, and extremely anxious). This type of diarrhea may also occur in a person who feels chilled and gets sick quickly when exposed to cold, dry winds. The stool is watery, green, and resembles chopped spinach. The person experiences a cutting pain in the abdomen before and during the stool.

Aloe. Useful for diarrhea with symptoms of a constant bearing-down sensation in the rectum and weak sphincter muscles. The rectum feels insecure, especially when passing gas; the person is uncertain if gas or stool will come. The stool passes without effort, almost unnoticed. Diarrhea in the early morning drives the person out of bed to get to the bathroom. These stools are jelly-like with mucus and cause pain and soreness in the rectum. The abdomen rumbles just before the stool. Eating acidic food or fruit and drinking beer cause diarrhea. Walking and standing tend to aggravate the diarrhea. Passing of stool when urinating is a possible symptom. Hemorrhoids are swollen and sore. Stools are yellow, pasty, lumpy, and watery. Before the stool, gripping pains travel across the lower part of the abdomen. Passage of stool usually relieves pain. Weakness and perspiration follow the stool.

Antimonium crud. Diarrhea that alternates with constipation (especially in the elderly) is relieved by *Antimonium crud.* Diarrhea can occur after consuming acidic foods, sour wine, and too much food. This type of diarrhea can also occur after bathing or swimming, especially when the water is cold. A white, thickly coated tongue is often seen.

Argentum nit. Useful for treating diarrhea brought on by great mental excitement or emotional problems. This remedy is very useful for diarrhea that is associated with the nervous anticipation of an event (such as giving a speech, taking a test, attending an important business meeting, or going to a dinner engagement). This remedy is also useful for a child who gets diarrhea from eating too much candy, especially chocolate. Stools are expelled with much sputtering and noisy passing of gas. The stool looks green and slimy, like chopped spinach, and tends to turn green after remaining in a diaper for too long. The abdomen is enormously distended, and expelled gas has an offensive odor. Diarrhea can be worse after breakfast. An unusual symptom is that diarrhea is made better by belching, which relieves some of the excess gas in the abdomen.

Arsenicum alb. Useful for diarrhea accompanied by a severe burning in the rectum that is relieved by warm baths or compresses. Restlessness, agitation, and anxiety are common mental symptoms. The person often paces the floor or moves from room to room, but feels quite weak. Great prostration and weakness after the stools seem almost out of proportion to the amount of diarrhea. The person is often thirsty for small quantities of liquid. Stools come out in small quantities and are dark and offensive. Diarrhea tends to be worse at night and after eating and drinking (especially after cold food or water, such as ice water or ice cream). *Arsenicum alb* is also useful for treating diarrhea caused by eating spoiled food.

The anus, which is often raw and excoriated, burns painfully. Applications of warm water on the anus sometimes relieve these symptoms. The person can be very sick and weak, even while feeling restless. Bacterial infections such as salmonella or shigella may cause the diarrhea.

Bryonia. This remedy, although more often associated with constipation, is sometimes useful for treating diarrhea. A specific symptom includes the desire to lie down quietly; the least movement causes diarrhea. There is great thirst for large amounts of cold water with a long span of time between feeling thirsty again. The lips are dry and cracked. Diarrhea is worse in the morning, in hot weather, and after drinking cold drinks.

Calcarea carb. Useful for treating diarrhea of children, especially when loose stools of undigested food are experienced. The stools appear white and watery and smell like rotten eggs. Profuse, sour-smelling perspiration on the head (especially during sleep) is a common symptom. Diarrhea is worse in cold and damp weather, during teething, after drinking milk (in a milk-intolerant person), after getting wet, and while walking.

Calcarea phos. Useful for treating diarrhea in children and babies that comes on after anger and frustration. It is also useful for treating diarrhea of girls around the time of their first period. This type of diarrhea comes on after eating fruit or drinking apple cider. Stools tend to be undigested, green, slimy, and hot. They come out with a sputtering sound and a very odorous gas. *Calcarea phos* tends to be helpful for children who are older looking than their age and more wrinkled; *Calcarea carb* is better suited for overweight children with a ravenous appetite.

Carbo veg. Useful for treating a person who has frequent, involuntary stools that smell like rotten meat. The diarrhea occurs after eating spoiled meat (similar to diarrhea associated with *Arsenicum alb*). The rectum discharges an acrid, corrosive moisture, and burns after stools are passed. This remedy is especially useful for older people who tend to be cold, have bluish-colored skin, and are short of breath.

Chamomilla. An important remedy for teething infants who have diarrhea. The diarrhea is worse in the evening, and the infant is often very restless and irritable. The infant wants to be carried. When carried, the infant stops whining and crying for a while, and then starts again. The child wants and demands things, but will throw them away when they are given. The stool is hot, green, watery, odorous (like a rotten egg), and slimy. It resembles chopped eggs and spinach (because of white and yellow mucus in the stool). Great abdominal pain is a characteristic symptom.

China. Very important for the relief of painless diarrhea (similar to the diarrhea associated with *Podophyllum*). An excessive loss of fluids in the stool leads to rapid exhaustion and emaciation. The entire body perspires, and the person has a great thirst. The abdomen is very bloated and rumbles often. One aspect that distinguishes this type of diarrhea from *Arsenicum alb* is that it does not burn. Slimy, black stool contains undigested food. The odor is extremely foul (like rotten meat). Eating fruit either causes the diarrhea or makes it worse. Diarrhea is often worse at night and after eating. The diarrhea tends to be worse during the summer (similar to the diarrhea associated with *Iris*). Often diarrhea occurs in a weakened person after attacks of other acute illnesses. Note that a physician should be contacted for an excessive loss of fluids or black stool.

Cina. Useful for treating diarrhea that occurs in a child who has pinworms. The child will tend to pick and bore at the nose. Stools are often white and look like popcorn. The child may grind the teeth during sleep, wake frequently, and change positions often.

Colchicum. Diarrhea that occurs every autumn may be relieved by *Colchicum*. The stools contain large quantities of white, shredded particles. Pain in the anus feels as if it has been torn apart; the rectum will often be prolapsed. The person may have great prostration and internal coldness and may even collapse or faint from weakness. Diarrhea may also occur after studying hard at night or staying up late caring for a sick person.

Colocynth. Relieves diarrhea that is associated with cramping and extreme pain in the center of the abdomen that is better with pressure and by bending over double. The person feels as if stones were being ground together in the abdomen. Intestines feel bruised. The person is usually irritable and easily angered, especially when questioned or offended. Bouts of anger can cause diarrhea. This type of diarrhea tends to be copious and yellow, and occurs immediately after eating or drinking. Eating fruit results in a loose, jelly-like stool. Cramps in the calves and abdomen often occur while the person has diarrhea.

Croton tig. This type of diarrhea is characterized by a constant urge to have a bowel movement followed by sudden stools. The stool is copious, watery, yellow, and always forcibly shot out. Diarrhea often alternates with skin problems such as eczema. When the diarrhea gets worse, the skin tends to improve (and vice versa). The diarrhea is usually worse in the summertime. Much gurgling in the intestines is a common symptom. The diarrhea and gas buildup are worse while eating or from drinking even a small amount of water. Nausea and vomiting are also associated with this type of diarrhea.

Cuprum met. Useful for treating very loose stools associated with extreme abdominal cramps or cramps in the legs and calves. The stool can be black or bloody and painful. (Note that a physician should evaluate a person who is having black or bloody stools.) The rectum cramps and feels weak after the stool. Useful for treating cholera and other severe types of diarrhea with cramping throughout the body.

Gelsemium. This type of diarrhea is caused by emotional excitement, being frightened, bad news, or anticipation of a future event (such as giving a speech, taking a test, or flying in an airplane). A person with a flu-type illness who is weak, tired, and has heavy eyelids may also benefit from *Gelsemium.* The legs are so weak that the person can hardly move them. A high fever and thirstlessness are also common.

Gratiola. Useful for treating gushing, watery diarrhea (like water from a fire hydrant). Useful for irritable, easily offended people who have large egos and do not like to be contradicted or challenged. *Gratiola* is often useful for treating summer diarrhea caused by drinking too much water or other liquids. The forceful evacuation of the stool is usually painless, but tires the person out. The person feels abdominal relief after passing the stools, but the anus burns. Sometimes the person feels like the tailbone is being torn out. A cold feeling in the abdomen is associated with this type of diarrhea.

The stools are yellowish-green and bubbly. Diarrhea often occurs after dinner.

Ignatia. An important remedy for diarrhea that comes on after grief (such as loss of a loved one). The loss of a job or the fear of losing a close relationship may also cause this diarrhea.

Ipecac. Diarrhea associated with extreme nausea and vomiting may benefit from *Ipecac.* Useful for amebic dysentery, especially when the symptoms include passing a great amount of blood in the diarrhea. Children with diarrhea who tend to be chubby and catch cold in warm, moist weather also respond to this remedy. A cutting, gripping pain is located in the center of the abdomen around the navel. The person passes stool that is either green or very dark (similar to molasses). The person sometimes feels great pain in the rectum while passing the stool. The straining can be so severe that it may actually create nausea. Despite being sick, the tongue stays relatively clean and pink.

Iris. Useful for treating watery diarrhea when the area from the anus through the intestinal tract to the stomach area burns. Vomiting and nausea with increased amounts of saliva in the mouth are common associated symptoms. A migraine headache may be seen along with the diarrhea. This headache tends to settle over the right eye or temple, have blurring of the right eye before the headache begins, and is associated with increased saliva and vomiting.

Magnesia carb. Useful for treating diarrhea in a nursing child where the milk passes undigested through the system. Diarrhea can be green, watery, and bubbly (similar to the green scum that floats on a pond). The diarrhea is most common after dinner.

Mercurius sol. Useful for slimy diarrhea with blood in the stools. The person can appear very sick. This remedy is sometimes used in severe cases of diarrhea (such as in cholera, shigella, or salmonella). Diarrhea is accompanied by chilliness, a sick feeling in the stomach, and increased saliva. An increase in odorous perspiration does not give the person any relief and is worse at night. The person feels great pain and cramping in the anus. The person feels like there is more stool, even after profuse diarrhea.

Natrum sulph. Helps in treating loose morning stools that are worse after a spell of cold, damp weather. Stools are often passed involuntarily. Eating fruit causes diarrhea.

Nux vomica. Typically a remedy for constipation, *Nux vomica* is useful for diarrhea in a few cases. The person is irritable and hypersensitive to noise, sound, and being bothered. *Nux vomica* may be useful after drinking too much alcohol or taking allopathic medicines that have a side effect of diarrhea. Frequent, small amounts of diarrhea with a constant urging are typical. The pain stops after the stool. In the early morning, diarrhea is usually at its worst. The person feels a constant uneasiness in the rectum. This type of diarrhea may also be associated with liver problems such as hepatitis. (Note that a person with hepatitis should be under the care of a physician.)

Petroleum. This type of diarrhea occurs only during the daytime (especially in the early morning). Diarrhea may occur after riding in cars or boats and is associated with seasickness and carsickness. The stools are watery and gushing, and the anus itches. Cabbage causes diarrhea. The stomach often has an empty feeling.

Phosphorus. Helps painless, copious diarrhea that causes weakness and tiredness after a stool. The diarrhea is often associated with great amounts of bleeding from the rectum during the stool, especially when hemorrhoids and rectal fissures are present. Note that profuse bleeding from the rectum should be evaluated by a physician. The stools tend to have an offensive odor and great amounts of gas pass with the stool. Lying on the left side causes a desire for a stool. The person may involuntarily have a stool; this is accompanied by a feeling that the anus remained open too long. The profuse diarrhea is forcibly shot out. Eating warm food aggravates the diarrhea. This type of diarrhea is also associated with vomiting, especially of drinks as soon as they become warm in the stomach. A weak, empty feeling in the stomach and a burning between the shoulders may be associated symptoms.

Podophyllum. Helpful for gurgling in the abdomen that is followed by profuse, watery, odorous stools that gush out of the rectum. The stools are also pasty and undigested. This occurs without pain, but there is weakness in the rectum after the stool. (The rectum is prone to prolapse before, during, and after the diarrhea. Prolapse also occurs from straining, urination, during the menses, from overlifting, and during pregnancy. Note that while homeopathic remedies are safe during pregnancy, labor, and breastfeeding, a pregnant woman should confer with her obstetrician or midwife to coordinate treatment.) Diarrhea tends to be more severe in the morning (between 3:00 and 9:00 A.M.) and is often followed by a normal stool later in the day. Diarrhea is worse after eating and in hot weather. Abdominal cramping is relieved by firm pressure and heat (as with *Colocynth*). Headaches either alternate or are relieved by diarrhea. Sometimes diarrhea may alternate with constipation. Diarrhea is seen in infants during teething. The cheeks tend to be hot with a glowing red color. The diarrhea may be worse from being bathed or eating acidic fruits. The baby's cramping seems better when lying on the stomach.

Pulsatilla. Used when no two stools are alike. The stool alternates between being soft, liquid, and hard. The person is usually weepy, wants consolation and comfort, and is generally thirstless. The problem often occurs after eating excessive amounts of fruit, fat, or overly rich food (such as pastry and ice cream). Certain meats also cause diarrhea (especially pork products). Warm rooms aggravate the diarrhea and cold air makes the person feel better.

Rhus tox. Useful for treating diarrhea associated with a person who is very restless and changes positions often. The person moves from place to place and cannot remain in bed. Diarrhea is often associated with dysentery from ameba and other types of bacteria and protozoa. There may be a high fever and the person may appear very ill and dehydrated. The stool, which smells like decaying flesh, is accompanied by tearing pains down the thighs. Note that a person with these symptoms should be under a physician's care.

Rumex. Useful for treating diarrhea that occurs in the early morning, especially with a cough that drives the person out of bed. The stool tends to be brown and watery.

Sulphur. Useful for morning diarrhea (especially around 5:00 A.M.) that drives the person out of bed to go to the bathroom. The diarrhea is generally painless; however, the area around the anus is sore and red. Severe itching and burning in this area is relieved by cool compresses. Alternating diarrhea and constipation are typical. The stools are offensive; the odor of the stool follows the person.

This type of diarrhea may be associated with hemorrhoids that tend to burn after a stool.

Veratrum alb. Useful for treating a profuse, watery stool that is forcefully evacuated. An important symptom is great prostration and weakness following the stool. Other very important symptoms include cold perspiration and coldness and blueness of the body after the stool. Pain in the abdomen precedes the stool. Severe nausea, vomiting, and sometimes cramps in the feet and legs accompany the stool. The watery stools contain small flakes and are commonly called rice water discharges. This type of diarrhea is different from the diarrhea associated with *Arsenicum alb* because the stools are profuse. Also, the person affected with the diarrhea helped by *Veratrum alb* is not restless, anguished, or overreactive to the pain. Another difference is that a person with diarrhea associated with *Veratrum alb* has great thirst for large amounts of cold water; *Arsenicum alb* has great thirst, but only for small quantities of warm water.

DRUG SENSITIVITY (INCLUDES REMEDY SENSITIVITY)

Some people react very strongly to almost any drug they take, whether it is aspirin, antibiotics, or cold medicine. These same people are often sensitive to homeopathic remedies. The homeopathic remedies listed here can actually help the person become less hypersensitive to either allopathic or homeopathic medication. (See also Antibiotic Side Effects, Chemical Hypersensitivity, and Chemotherapy Side Effects.)

Chamomilla. Particularly helps the person who abuses narcotics (such as morphine, opium, or cocaine). Daily use of this remedy can help kick the habit or decrease the effects of quitting addictive drugs. This remedy is associated with the typical *Chamomilla* symptom picture of oversensitivity, thirstiness, whining, restlessness, impatience, and intolerance to being spoken to or interrupted. While similar to *Nux vomica* in many ways, *Chamomilla* is not associated with overindulgence in other areas (such as smoking, drinking alcohol and coffee, and overworking). The person who needs *Chamomilla* is sensitive to medications and drugs and reacts quickly to any of them. This is even true of homeopathic remedies, in that the person overreacts to the remedies and has a more significant aggravation or proving.

Nux vomica. Very important remedy to help the side effects of drugs. This remedy is associated with addiction or dependence to medication (even herbal medication) and drugs. There may be an hypersensitivity to medications, with side effects being produced quickly. Narcotics, herbal medicines, and homeopathic remedies all can cause greater-than-typical reactions in a person who needs *Nux vomica.* The person who needs this remedy is the most susceptible to drug abuse. Often, drugs create a situation that aggravates the already hypersensitive, overreactive *Nux vomica* temperament.

Phosphorus. Associated with people who are very sensitive to medications and drugs because the reaction to any drug occurs quickly. Illegal drugs or prescribed medications may cause the person to become spacey, overly theatrical, or flamboyant. The person also fears taking too much and may ask the doctor to prescribe the bare minimum. This is even true of homeopathic remedies where the person will overreact to the remedies and have a more significant aggravation or proving.

Pulsatilla. The person taking *Pulsatilla* may be very sensitive and weepy, and seek consolation. Generally the person is not irritable but likes a lot of fuss and caring. The person may be susceptible to taking drugs because of feeling very vulnerable and insecure. These people may take illegal drugs due to peer pressure and often feel guilty and remorseful after indulging in drugs. If they have a bad reaction to drugs, they get very weepy and need people around them.

Sulphur. Useful for the person who develops rashes, diarrhea, and redness of the skin after taking drugs. There is often itching and the person has trouble keeping organized and maintaining good hygiene.

EARACHE

Earaches are caused by inflammation or infections of the eardrum or ear canal, which may be the result of viruses, bacteria, allergies, and trauma. Symptoms include a painful ear, loss of hearing, ringing in the ear, dizziness, or fever. The eustachian tube, which normally adjusts the pressure in the middle ear and drains fluid from it, is often blocked. The ear is usually red and inflamed (supportive otitis media) or dull with fluid behind the eardrum (serous otitis media).

Earaches are especially a problem for young children. Their eustachian tubes are narrower, shorter, and lie more horizontal than in adults. When their tubes become swollen due to the effects of upper respiratory infections or allergies, the flow of fluid is obstructed. This problem is compounded at night because the horizontal position of the tube allows fluid from the mouth and throat to flow back into the middle ear. This fluid sits in back of the eardrum and becomes thick or infected, leading to a painful ear infection. Children often awaken at night because of this great discomfort. To treat this condition, homeopathic remedies may be used to help the pain and reduce inflammation and infection. Acetaminophen (Tylenol) can be used if pain is not controlled by homeopathic remedies. Warm compresses placed on the ear can help in some cases. Elevating the head in bed may help facilitate draining of the eustachian tube and relieve pressure. Drinking lots of fluid can help keep the mucus thin. Swallowing helps open up the tubes and encourages them to drain. Using a clean, cool mist vaporizer in the bedroom at night sometimes helps the child sleep better. To help slow the development of allergies in babies, breastfeeding should be continued as long as possible. Babies should not be encouraged to drink from a bottle while lying down, especially if they have a tendency toward ear infections, since fluids can collect in the middle ear.

Eliminating foods that cause allergies and swelling of the mucous membranes can be helpful for earaches. Allergies commonly come from foods such as dairy products (which have an enzyme that can thicken mucus), eggs, corn, citrus, wheat, and nuts. Avoiding foods that are high in carbohydrates such as sugar, candy, honey, or ice cream and drinks such as fruit juices is also important.

If the pain continues or a discharge appears in the ear canal, indicating a rupture of the eardrum, a physician should be contacted immediately. High fever associated with an earache is also reason to contact a doctor. If the mucus in the nose is green or yellow or if a cough is producing discolored phlegm, it is a sign of a bacterial infection and a doctor should be contacted.

Aconite. Useful for a sudden onset of violent pain in the ear, especially after exposure to a cold wind or draft. The external part of the ear is red, hot, and swollen. Ear pain is worse at night and gets better when heat is applied. The ear is sensitive to noise, and there may be the sensation that a drop of water is in the left ear.

Arsenicum alb. Useful for burning ear pain, especially if a thin, offensive, irritating discharge causes the skin around the ear to become raw and burning. The person may hear roaring noises with the ear pain.

Arundo. Useful for burning and itching in the ear canals. Ear pain is often associated with allergies when there is a stuffed-up sensation in the ear. There is annoying itching in the nostrils and roof of the mouth.

Baryta carb. Useful for painful, swollen glands around the ears. Ear pain is due to a sore throat in which the tonsils are swollen and block off the flow of fluid from the middle ear to the throat. Crackling noises in the ear are worse when swallowing and walking and cause a decrease in hearing.

Belladonna. Useful for an acute ear infection in which tearing pains suddenly occur. The eardrum is covered with swollen blood vessels. Pain comes on suddenly, and all symptoms are worse at night. Application of warmth provides relief. Thirst is often absent, even with the fever. *Belladonna* can be associated with sore throats and swollen glands and the typical red and flushed face, dilated pupils, and mental agitation.

Calcarea carb. Associated with chronic ear trouble (such as a ruptured eardrum that does not heal and causes a decrease in hearing and humming and roaring in the ears). Ear discharges look infected, and the glands around the ears are swollen. The ears are sensitive to cold, and there is often a pulsating pain in the ears as if something could pass out of them. With any sign of rupture, such as intense pain suddenly relieved and followed by yellowish discharge from the ear, a qualified health care provider should be contacted.

Calcarea sulph. Will help heal a ruptured eardrum. Useful for discharge from the middle ear that is yellowish, thick, often lumpy, and mixed with blood; these symptoms may cause loss of hearing. Any sign of rupture should be evaluated by a qualified health care provider.

Chamomilla. Useful for infants and young children with earaches. *Chamomilla* can be associated with earaches that occur during teething. The person is in great pain, has red cheeks, is restless and fretful, and seems to be suffering greatly. The pain gets worse at night and when warmth is applied. A child is fretful, demands things, and refuses them when they are offered. A child feels better when held and often cries out in pain.

Ferrum phos. Useful for earaches that occur after exposure to cold. *Ferrum phos* is often used after *Aconite* (*Aconite* is generally useful only during the first few hours after exposure to a cold wind or draft), especially if there are not many guiding symptoms other than fever and earache. The ear tends to burn and throb, and there is pulsation in the ear and head. The eardrum looks red. *Ferrum phos* is often useful for earaches that result from exposure to cold or wet conditions.

Hepar sulph. The person is irritable and senses the slightest draft of air. Useful when pus behind the eardrum causes sensitivity and soreness with the slightest touch. There may be thick, creamy, offensive discharge if the eardrum ruptures. Sensitive to the least draft of air, the person may want to have the ear warmly wrapped by scarves. There may be stitching pains traveling from the throat to the ear during swallowing. Note that any sign of rupture, such as intense pain suddenly relieved and followed by yellowish discharge from the ear, should be evaluated by a qualified health care provider.

Kali mur. Useful when the person experiences an earache accompanied by swollen glands, a sore throat, and a white coated tongue. The person hears a crackling noise when blowing the nose and swallowing. The nose is often congested.

Mercurius sol. Useful for middle ear infections when pus forms behind the eardrum. *Mercurius sol* is usually associated with offensive breath and excessive perspiration. The pain is worse at night. The tonsils may be swollen. A raw feeling and an internal sensation of soreness are present in the throat, eustachian tube, and ear area. If there is a discharge from the ear, it is often thin and corrosive. The ears, teeth, and face often ache.

Pulsatilla. One of the most important ear remedies along with *Aconite, Belladonna,* and *Hepar sulph.* The person has the characteristic *Pulsatilla* picture of weepiness, chilliness, and a desire for company and consolation. *Pulsatilla* is also associated with a lack of thirst. *Pulsatilla* is useful for ear infections in the ear canal in which the ear is red, hot, and swollen, and severe pulsating pains get worse at night. This remedy is also useful for middle ear infections and a ruptured eardrum in which the discharge is thick, yellow, and non-irritating. The person feels as if the ears are stuffed up. Note that any sign of rupture, such as intense pain suddenly relieved and followed by yellowish discharge from the ear, should be evaluated by a qualified health care provider.

Silica. Useful to help ear drainage, restore healing, and help heal a ruptured eardrum. A peculiar symptom is itching and tingling in the area of the eustachian tube. The person experiences shooting pains through the ear and perspires profusely. *Silica* is the most common remedy associated with persistent, chronic ear drainage from ruptured eardrums that have not healed, especially when the person is hypersensitive to sound. *Silica* may also be given to prevent the eardrum from rupturing when it is red, swollen, and has pus behind it, especially when given in higher potencies. The signs of rupture include intense pain suddenly relieved and followed by a yellowish discharge from the ear. Any evidence of rupture or threatened rupture should be evaluated by a physician or health care provider and only knowledgeable professionals should prescribe higher potencies.

Verbascum. Useful for ear pain associated with facial aching below the eyes and near the nose. The left side of the face seems to be more sensitive, and the pain is worse when the temperature changes, especially from warm to cold. The pain is often worse at night. *Verbascum* can be given in 30c potency or can be used as a tincture mixed one-to-one with warm (not hot) olive oil, dropped directly into the ear. Cotton can be used to keep this warm fluid in the ear canal.

ECZEMA

Eczema is an allergy of the skin and is more common with people who have respiratory allergies, asthma, or a tendency toward hives. It is a superficial inflammation of the skin characterized by redness, swelling, crusting, scaling, and oozing of fluid. Often appearing on the elbows, wrists, face, and inside the knees, eczema is very itchy, and causes the person to scratch and rub the skin. Infants and babies are common sufferers of eczema, but the disorder can continue into childhood and adulthood.

There are several types of eczema. One type is called contact dermatitis, which is either an acute or chronic inflammation produced by substances that come in contact with the skin. The most common irritants include topical antibiotics; plants such as poison ivy, ragweed, or primrose; sensitizers in the manufacture of shoes and clothing; metal compounds such as nickel or chrome; dyes; cosmetics; and industrial agents. Sunlight can also cause an allergic reaction to the skin in some people.

Another type of eczema is called atopic dermatitis. This is a chronic, itching, superficial inflammation of the skin. It usually occurs in individuals who have a family history of allergies, such as hay fever or asthma. It is usually seen in the first few months of life and generally subsides by the age of three or four, although exacerbation and remission occur during childhood, adolescence, and adulthood.

Other types of eczema include seborrheic dermatitis, nummular dermatitis, stasis dermatitis, and neurodermatitis. Seborrhea dermatitis is an inflammatory scaling of the scalp and face. It is called dandruff in adults and cradle cap in infants. Nummular dermatitis has red or coin-shaped lesions that are itchy and inflamed. Stasis dermatitis is a persistent inflammation of the skin on the lower legs with a tendency toward increased pigmentation. It is commonly associated with leg swelling and vein problems, such as varicose veins. Neurodermatitis is a chronic and superficial itching and inflammation of the skin characterized by dry, scaling, hyperpigmented spots that are oval or angular. This disorder has a strong psychological component, and the allergy appears to play no role. Itching usually occurs because of stress and tension.

Treatment of eczema is complicated and very interesting from a homeopathic point of view. Homeopaths believe that eczema in any form should not be suppressed or treated with medicated creams. It is believed that production of skin lesions or eruptions represents the body trying to heal itself and externalize internal illnesses. Suppressing eruptions is similar to a person suppressing emotions. By stopping the healing, or in this case, stopping the itch and eruption, the problem is driven in deeper to create more serious problems. People who suppress their feelings sometimes find themselves depressed or angry at the wrong people or at inappropriate times. In a similar way, people who suppress their eczema find that they may have increased problems with asthma, allergies, or emotions.

Practical steps to relieve symptoms include using warm (not hot) water for bathing. An unscented bath oil should be used to soften the skin in baths. A person needs to be cautious about lanolin in skin lotions since it sometimes causes the body to react. It is important to avoid temperature extremes and to wear cotton or other natural fibers next to the skin. Wool is often a problem in people who have eczema. Exercising can be helpful in decreasing stress and helping the skin sweat. It is important to take a shower after exercise to wash away any irritants in the sweat. It is also important to practice stress-reduction techniques, since stress often increases the amount of eczema and itching.

Identifying food allergies and eliminating foods that may cause eruptions can be very important. Foods that may cause eczema are eggs, milk, chocolate, peanuts, soy, and wheat. Breastfeeding infants for as long as possible can be helpful because breast milk helps the baby's immune system. While the mother is breastfeeding, she should avoid foods that cause the baby's skin to get worse. Certain vitamins and oils are known to help eczema.

Homeopathic remedies are very helpful for not only keeping the eruptions on the surface, but also for increasing the body's ability to heal itself.

Anacardium. Intense, itchy eczema with mental irritability can be treated with *Anacardium*. This type of eczema sometimes forms small blisters filled with a clear liquid. The skin feels worse with applications of hot water and better from eating and from rubbing the affected area gently.

Antimonium crud. Useful for treating dry, itchy skin that cracks easily and forms thick, horny calluses. The symptoms are worse from the heat of a bed and from cold bathing. The eczema may form thick, hard, honey-colored scabs (especially around the face) and is often associated with stomach problems (such as excessive belching, heartburn, and nausea). The tongue has a thick, white coating. The person is very irritable (especially a child, who cannot bear to be looked at or touched). Angry feelings may be evident. Often, eczema is located on the hands, with cracking around the nails. Cracking in the nostrils and the corners of the mouth are also common.

Arsenicum alb. Useful for dry, scaly eczema that resembles fish scales. The affected area itches excessively and burns. The burning is relieved with the application of hot water or warm cloths. Discharge from this type of eczema is often putrid. Great mental restlessness is a common symptom, and the person is most irritated by the skin late at night (midnight to 3:00 A.M.).

Calcarea carb. Eczema of newborn infants that occurs on the scalp and sometimes extends to the face can sometimes be treated with *Calcarea carb.* The crust can be white and tends to itch, especially in the morning after waking up. The child scratches vigorously. The skin is not healthy; the eczema may ulcerate and does not heal well. Glands may swell because the eczema can get infected.

Dulcamara. Useful for treating eczema characterized by a thick, brownish-yellow crust that bleeds when scratched. The itching is always worse in cold, wet weather. Eruptions tend to occur on the face (usually on the forehead, nose, chin, and cheeks).

Graphites. One of the most important remedies for eczema. The skin tends to be dry and rough and secretes a very thin, sticky, gluey substance. Cracks that bleed easily may be seen. This remedy is especially helpful for eczema on the eyelids, behind the ears, around the mouth and chin, in the bends of the elbows, and behind the knees. This eczema oozes a fluid that is usually watery, transparent, and sticky, but can be dry, thick, and honey-like. The skin is always very dry, and the person seldom perspires. Constipation is usually a symptom.

Hepar sulph. Useful for eczema that becomes infected, especially if the lymph glands swell around the infected area. Eczema associated with deep cracks on the hands and feet can be helped by *Hepar sulph.* The eczema tends to spread from new eruptions that appear underneath the originally affected area. Itching and a sticky or prickly pain characterize this type of eczema. The person is also sensitive to touch.

Hydrastis. Eczema that tends to dry into a crust and burn excessively (often like fire) can be helped by *Hydrastis.* This eczema may ooze a thick, yellowish, milky secretion. The eczema is worse from warmth and from washing.

Kali mur. Helpful for chronic eczema of the scalp, especially when the eczema is moist and wet and tends to be difficult to treat. The tongue tends to be white.

Lycopodium. Useful for treating chronic eczema that is associated with urinary tract infections, gastric problems, and abdominal distention. The skin forms very thick patches that bleed easily when scratched. Symptoms are worse from warm applications and better from cold applications.

Manganum aceticum. Useful for eczema that is accompanied by amenorrhea (abnormal loss or absence of periods). This type of eczema can also be worse during menstrual periods or menopause. It is also worse in cold, wet weather or during weather changes.

Mezereum. Eczema characterized by intolerable itching, great chilliness, and a sensitivity to cold air may be helped by *Mezereum.* Itching with this type of eczema is worse in bed. This remedy is also useful for treating itchy eczema that occurs at the spot of a vaccination. Eczema on the head is covered with a thick, leathery crust. Pus collects under this crust. This remedy is also useful for children who have cradle cap (especially when the child scratches the head or face furiously). Scabs form on the face or head. The child constantly tears scabs off, leaving raw spots.

Natrum mur. Useful for red, raw, inflamed eczema that is particularly bad around the hairline. This type of eczema tends to be worse from eating too much salt or from being near salty water (such as an ocean). The affected person often craves salt. Hangnails with cracks along the edges of the nail bleed. Crusty eruptions may form at the bends of the elbows, behind the knees, and behind the ears. Small vesicles may also be seen.

Petroleum. Useful for treating dry, constricted, sensitive, rough, and cracked skin. Eczema forms a thick, greenish crust that burns and itches. This area becomes raw and red, and cracks and bleeds easily. The eczema and cracking are worse in the winter. The itching is intolerable at night. The fingertips crack and the hands chap, particularly in cold weather. This remedy is also helpful for eczema of the face, scrotum, genitals, and bends of the skin (such as the elbows and behind the knees), as well as behind the ears. After scratching, the eczema becomes moist and oozes.

Rhus tox. Useful for acute outbreaks of eczema (especially if the entire body is affected). The eczema has small, fluid-filled eruptions. All symptoms are worse at night, in cold, damp weather, and in the winter. Scratching causes an even greater need to scratch. The eczema tends to burn and can form a thick crust that oozes an offensive substance. The person is restless, especially at night, and often paces.

Staphysagria. Useful for eczema located on the head, ears, face, and fingers. This type of eczema forms thick, dry scabs that itch violently. Scratching changes the location of the itch.

Sulphur. A very important remedy for eczema that feels extremely good from scratching. After scratching, however, the skin becomes sore and there is more burning. The eczema tends to ooze if scratched too much; otherwise, the skin tends to be dry, red, and rough-looking. Contact with water (such as washing the hands or face, taking a shower, or swimming) aggravates the eczema and causes great burning. The person is often sensitive to heat, tends to look or be dirty, and has many skin problems. Discharges from this type of eczema are offensive. The face flushes easily and the lips are very red.

ELECTRICAL SHOCK (INCLUDES LIGHTNING)

Electrical shock is the passage of electrical current through the body. It can be caused by contact with lightning, high-voltage electrical lines, or low-voltage lines in the home or business. Factors that determine the severity of the injury, ranging from minor burns to death, include the type and magnitude of the current, resistance of the body at the point of contact, the current pathway, and duration of the current flow.

Electrical shock can startle the person, causing him or her to fall down or drop objects, or have severe spastic stimulation and contraction of the muscles. Unconsciousness can occur, either from respiratory shock or fibrillation of the heart ventricles. Treatment consists of separating the person from the electrical source and re-establishing the vital functions of the body immediately. Breaking contact can be done by either shutting off the current or removing the person from contact with it. Shutting off the current is done by disconnecting the device from its electrical outlet, throwing a circuitbreaker or switch, or cutting the wires using an insulated tool such as an ax with a wooden handle. While removing a person from the source of the electrical current, rescuers must be well insulated from the ground and use an insulated material (such as cloth, rubber, dry wood, or a leather belt) to pull the victim free. The rescuers should then quickly determine whether the vital systems of the victim are functioning. A physician or emergency room should always be contacted immediately. In the meantime, mouth-to-mouth resuscitation may be necessary if heart or lung problems are present.

Prevention of electrical injury includes proper design and installation of all electrical devices, especially circuits that contain failsafe equipment.

The homeopathic remedies listed here have been helpful immediately after electrical shock and for long-term problems associated with electrical shock.

Arnica. Often the first remedy to give after a person is struck by lightning. The body feels sore and bruised, and the person may be in shock.

Nux vomica. Used after a person is struck by lightning or electrically shocked. This remedy can also be used for the effects of electroshock therapy for depression. Important symptoms are irritability and agitation.

Phosphorus. Given after a person is struck by lightning. The person is confused and unable to concentrate, feeling unable to remember facts or events. Blindness sometimes follows the strike of lightning.

EYE INFECTIONS

One type of eye infection is conjunctivitis, which is the swelling of the conjunctival membrane including the white of the eye and the underside of the eyelid. In this condition, the white of the eye looks red due to the swelling or dilation of the small blood vessels. There may be clear discharge or thick pus, and the eye feels irritated with the sensation of grit in it; the eyes are often stuck together in the morning. If the condition is caused by a virus, the discharge is usually thin and watery. If caused by bacterial infections, the discharge tends to be thick, sticky, and white, yellow, or green. Allergies from wind, dust, smoke, or air pollution may also cause this condition. Irritation can occur from intense light, sunlamps, or reflections from snow. When the condition is infectious, it can spread to the other eye or to other people. If the pain gets worse and the discharge lasts more than a couple of days, a physician should be contacted.

Another type of eye infection is blepharitis, an inflammation of the eyelid. The eyelid is often red, scaly, and thickened, and there may be scale-like dandruff. Bacteria may grow on the eyelids, causing them to discharge, swell, and possibly develop small ulcers. In this condition, the eyes should be washed three or four times a day either with warm soap and water or salt water. If the condition is due to seborrhea or eczema, using a shampoo that has selenium in it may be helpful. It is also important to keep the hands clean.

Dry eyes can lead to conjunctivitis or blepharitis if there is constant irritation. It is helpful to use artificial tears, which are available in most pharmacies. A humidifier during the winter, when the air is dry and indoor heating is used, may also be helpful. It is important to wear sunglasses in bright, sunny weather. It is important not to share towels or washcloths and to change the linens on the bed, especially the pillowcase. Certain herbal solutions are known to help eye infections.

Aconite. Useful in the first stages of conjunctivitis or blepharitis. Eyelid irritation may occur after an injury or after exposure to dust and cold, dry wind. The eyelid feels dry and heavy, is red and swollen, and often waters profusely. *Aconite* is useful for irritation from snow reflection and after cinders or other foreign objects are extracted from the eye.

Allium cepa. Useful for profuse, non-irritating discharge and watering of the eye (similar to the experience of chopping an onion). The eyes burn and are red, but the discharge does not irritate the tissue under the eyes. The eyes are sensitive to light and feel better in the open air. *Allium cepa* is often useful for allergies that affect the eyes and cause excessive discharge.

Apis. Useful for swollen, red, and puffy eyelids. The eyes sting and burn and are relieved by cold water.

Argentum nit. Helpful for swelling of the conjunctiva. Discharge is abundant and full of pus. The eyes ache and feel tired, and the eyelids are sore, swollen, and thickened. For many years, silver nitrate *(Argentum nit)* was used in allopathic dosages as drops to help prevent gonorrhea in newborns. This caused the eyes to swell and secrete pus. Homeopathically, *Argentum nit* is useful to treat these types of symptoms.

Arsenicum alb. Useful for swelling of the eyelids that may completely close the eye. The tears tend to be corrosive and burning, which makes the eyelids and cheeks sore. The burning is relieved by heat. *Arsenicum alb* is often associated with allergies when the tears burn.

Belladonna. Useful for hot, red eyelids that burn. The pupils are dilated, and the eyes are sensitive to light. *Belladonna* is associated with a red face, dry mouth, and high fever.

Calcarea sulph. Associated with inflamed eyes that discharge thick, yellow mucus and pus. Useful for bacterial eye infections, especially when discharge flows freely, since this remedy helps keep the infectious material flowing out of the eyes.

Calendula. Helps soothe infected eyes. It also is useful after a foreign object is removed from the eye. This remedy is used as a tincture by diluting the mother tincture with water in a one-to-twenty ratio.

Dulcamara. Useful when a cold or upper respiratory infection has settled in the eyes. A profuse, watery discharge is worse in the open air. There can also be a thick, yellow discharge. *Dulcamara* is useful for allergies that affect the eyes, especially those that cause excessive tearing.

Euphrasia. Useful for eyes that water profusely. The eye discharge is acrid and irritating, while the nasal discharge is bland and non-irritating (this is the opposite of *Allium cepa*). *Euphrasia* helps eye infections where the discharge is thick, burning, and irritating to the skin under the eye. (With *Mercurius sol,* the discharge is thin and burning.) There is great inclination to blink, and mucus seems to stick to the cornea. The eyes are sensitive to light, and eye problems are often associated with colds and headaches.

Gelsemium. Useful for eyelids that feel heavy and are difficult to open. *Gelsemium* is often associated with flu-like symptoms. The person experiences blurred and smoky vision and extreme pain around the eye.

Graphites. Helps dry, cracked, and bleeding eyelids. *Graphites* is often associated with eczema, especially on the eyelids, head, and behind the ears. The discharge is sticky and has a honey-like consistency.

Hepar sulph. Useful for profuse, pussy discharge that irritates the eyelids and conjunctiva. Eye discomfort gets worse from touch and exposure to cold air. The eyes and eyelids are red and inflamed, and the eyeballs are sore to the touch. These symptoms can often be the early stages of ulceration of the cornea. If pain occurs in the eyes, seek medical advice at once.

Kali bich. Helps burning, swollen, and puffy eyelids. The mucus is sticky, thick, and difficult to rub off and comes from the corner of the eyes and the conjunctiva. *Kali bich* is often associated with sinusitis.

Mercurius sol. Useful for thin, burning, yellowish-green eye discharges. The eyelids are red, thick, and swollen. There may be excessive perspiration, increased salivation, and nighttime aggravation of the eyes.

Pulsatilla. Useful for profuse, white or yellow discharge from the eyelids and conjunctiva. The discharge does not irritate the tissue below. The eyelids are inflamed and sticky. They feel worse inside in the warmth and better when outside in the cool air. *Pulsatilla* is often associated with upper respiratory infections and colds in which the person is chilly, weepy, and likes to have consolation and sympathy.

Sulphur. Useful when the person experiences burning and heat in the eyes (similar to *Arsenicum alb* and *Belladonna*). The eyelids tend to ulcerate, and the eyes itch and feel worse when washed or rinsed with water.

EYE INJURIES

Take special care. Eye injuries can be serious and result in a loss of vision. An ophthalmologist, advanced medical care facility, or emergency room should always be contacted when there is trauma to the eye or the surrounding area, a foreign object embedded in the eye, a scratched cornea, or intense eye pain. Intense eye pain should be evaluated by a physician, since this can represent a more serious eye condition.

Foreign objects such as cinders, sand, or eyelashes can be washed out of the eye using large amounts of tap water. If there is a sensation that a foreign object remains in the eye, a person can invert the lid to try to remove it. Inverting the lid is done by placing a thin object, such as a matchstick, above the eye but below the eyebrow and bony orbit of the forehead. The eyelashes are then grasped and pulled first downward and then upward over the object, while the person is looking down. If the foreign object can be seen, it can be removed by moistening the end of a tissue and gently brushing the object away from the lining of the eye. Irrigation with large amounts of plain water will also help removal.

If there is blunt trauma to the eye, such as being hit by a snowball or fist, the eye should be covered with a clean, moist cloth.

For chemical spills in the eye, the best treatment is rinsing with water constantly for at least fifteen minutes. This is especially true if the substance that is irritating the eye is basic or alkaline, such as lye. A *Hypericum* tincture may be helpful. Note that a physician should be contacted in this situation.

An injury to the area around the eye, such as the eye socket or cheekbone, may have discoloration and swelling. This often results in a black eye in any shade of black, blue, green, or purple. It is always best to check with a physician to make sure there has been no fracture in the orbit around the eye or in the skull.

Aconite. When fear and anxiety are associated with an eye injury, *Aconite* is the best remedy. The eye becomes inflamed after the injury.

Arnica. Often the first remedy given after any eye injury. The eye area is extremely sore.

Calendula. Can be used as a tincture for inflammation that occurs after an eye injury. This remedy can be used as an eyewash (especially for splinters in the eye or wounds from cuts or surgery). To prepare an eyewash, mix one part *Calendula* tincture with five parts boiled and cooled water. For a scratched cornea, mix one part *Calendula* tincture and one part *Hypericum* tincture with five parts boiled and cooled water.

Euphrasia. This remedy can be used after an eye injury if the eye waters all the time and there is an excessive amount of irritating, burning discharge. The eyelids burn and swell, and the person always wants to blink. Often, there is a sticky mucus on the cornea, and the person must blink to remove it.

Hypericum. Used along with *Calendula* as an eyewash, especially for a scratched cornea, a cut or surgical wound, or a splinter in the eye. There is often extreme pain with this type of eye problem because it affects the nerve endings. To prepare an eyewash, mix one part *Calendula* tincture and one part *Hypericum* tincture with five parts boiled and cooled water.

Ledum. Useful when the eye has been hit by a blunt object, causing aching and bleeding. *Ledum* may be helpful for an injury to the deeper structures of the eye, the conjunctiva, or the iris. A doctor should be contacted in this situation.

Silica. An important remedy when splinters or sharp objects in the eye cannot be removed. This remedy helps the object to come out on its own. This remedy is also used to help soften scars on the cornea.

Staphysagria. Useful after a sharp incision to the eyeball (such as from a surgical procedure). *Staphysagria* is useful after cataract surgery when an incision causes great pain.

Symphytum. An important remedy for a blunt trauma to the eye (such as being hit by a snowball, baseball, elbow, or fist). The eyeball itself is usually not damaged, but the area around the eye has the appearance of a black eye because of the damage and pain around the supporting structure of the eye (such as the bones of the forehead, eye socket, and cheekbone). With this kind of injury, a break in the cheekbone or eye socket is possible, and *Symphytum* may help to heal it more quickly. A physician should always be contacted if vision is affected or a break is possible as a result of an eye injury.

FALSE LABOR

Take special care. While homeopathic remedies are safe during pregnancy, labor, and breastfeeding, a pregnant woman should confer with her obstetrician or midwife to coordinate treatment.

When a woman goes into labor, it is important that a health care professional, such as a doctor or nurse midwife, be managing the care. Natural childbirth is a wonderful way to have a baby if the mother's health is good and there are no complications.

Homeopathic remedies should only be used by qualified people who have delivered many babies as an adjunct to normal medical intervention. The homeopathic remedies listed here can be used in conjunction with medical care to both prepare the uterus for labor and relax and stimulate the uterus during labor.

Belladonna. Useful for pains that come and go suddenly. There is a feeling that the uterus will fall out of the vagina. *Belladonna* is often useful for older women in their first delivery when muscles are rigid (not stretched by a previous pregnancy) and there are contractions of the cervical opening. The person is restless, hot, flushed, and sensitive to noise, light, and especially jarring of the bed. The carotid arteries seem to throb.

Calcarea carb. Useful for false labor that occurs in heavy women who have had many babies and tend to be flabby, weary, and weak. The uterine muscles seem unable to contract. The head and feet perspire, and the person is cold, fearful, and apprehensive of going crazy and having other people observe this.

Caulophyllum. Useful for false labor pain that feels like spasms and moves quickly from one part of the body to another. *Caulophyllum* helps extreme exhaustion and weakness that accompanies false labor.

Cimicifuga. Helps false labor when pain shoots across the abdomen, causing the person to double up in agony.

Gelsemium. Useful when the cervix and uterus are soft and flabby. Labor pains seem to stop, and the uterus does not contract at all. The person is drowsy and dull, the face is flushed, the eyelids are heavy, and there is a lack of thirst.

Pulsatilla. Useful for labor pains that start too early and are slow, weak, and ineffectual. The person may feel faint and wants the doors and windows open because of a suffocated feeling. The person likes cold air blowing despite being chilly. The person is often tearful and wants consolation and comfort. Another important use for *Pulsatilla* is when the baby is lying across the uterus or is breech. *Pulsatilla* 30x or 30c three times a day during this pre-labor stage may be helpful in turning the baby.

FEVER

Human body temperature is around 98.6°F measured under the tongue. When measured under the armpit, it is usually one degree lower than the temperature under the tongue; when measured rectally, it is one degree higher. The temperature in the ear is similar to the temperature under the tongue.

It is wise to take the temperature frequently when a person feels hot to the touch or complains about feeling warm or cold. A fever is an indication that the body has been challenged by a virus, bacteria, or inflammation. The fever represents part of the healing process and the body trying to eliminate foreign substances or microorganisms. Homeopaths believe that the fever process should usually not be suppressed because it represents the body trying to heal itself. Homeopathic remedies are used to enhance this immune response. At the same time, remedies should help decrease the symptoms and the pain that accompanies the fever and its associated illness.

It is only when fevers are very high, generally over 103.5°F, or when the fever goes up or down rapidly, that intervening with other forms of therapies or medicines should be considered. One easy and useful method is a lukewarm sponge bath, which may help bring down the fever one or more degrees and give comfort. If the person is hallucinating, in great pain with the fever, or the temperature seems to be rising or falling rapidly, it may be helpful to consider using acetaminophen (Tylenol) to gently bring down the fever. This will not interfere with the homeopathic remedy; however, if it is needed, it may cause a confusion of symptoms and the true remedy picture will not be seen.

In the case of a very high temperature, such as 105°F, a cool sponge bath can be used along with acetaminophen (Tylenol). A health care provider should be contacted if the high fever persists or if the person has great pain or appears very ill.

Homeopathic remedies can be useful for a fever. The symptoms must match the entire picture to be useful, since a fever is just one of many symptoms that a person has when ill.

Aconite. This remedy is given in the first stages of fever before the nose begins to run or other symptoms appear. *Aconite* is especially helpful for fever brought on by exposure to cold, dry wind. Fever can also be brought on by overheating (such as when a person is exposed to the sun for a long period of time). The mental symptoms are extremely important and include anxiety, restlessness, and fear. There is frequent chilliness, a hot, red face and head, and a headache with a sensation that something is pressing outward. Dry skin, excessive thirst, and a pounding pulse are experienced. Perspiring relieves these symptoms.

Apis. Useful for fever that is often preceded by a chill. The chill is accompanied by thirst, and the fever accompanied by a lack of thirst. The fever often begins around 3:00 p.m., progressing into the evening and night. The person often perspires after the fever breaks, but this does not relieve the symptoms. There is usually a part of the body that has stinging pains associated with this fever (such as the throat); there may also be some swelling.

Arsenicum alb. Useful for fever that begins at midnight, is worse around 2:00 A.M., and gets better around 3:00 A.M. There is restlessness, but the person feels weak from any exertion.

Baptisia. Useful for fever accompanied by weakness and a bruised feeling throughout the body. While the body feels fatigued, the mind is quite restless, especially when the fever is high. *Baptisia* is useful for people who are very sick. The mind wanders and cannot remain on a subject for any length of time. After being restless, the person finds it difficult to stay awake and can fall asleep even while talking to somebody. The head feels dull, heavy, and hard to hold up. The eyes are sensitive to light and the eyeballs are sore, making it painful to read and difficult to move them. The face is flushed, hot, and often dark red. The person cannot find a comfortable position in bed. The back, arms, and legs feel chilly, especially when exposed to open air.

Belladonna. Useful for fever accompanied by burning, hot skin. The face is red, hot, and flushed. The eyes bulge and the pupils are dilated. The fever may be so high that the person is delirious and hallucinates. The head and neck often throb. Perspiration will occur, but does not provide relief. Fever is generally accompanied by a lack of thirst. *Belladonna* is usually used relatively early in illnesses before discharges from mucous membranes occur.

Bryonia. Useful for fever where the person is irritable when disturbed and likes to be alone. The person feels better when lying very still; any kind of movement increases the intensity of the headache and the general ill feeling. An intense headache is accompanied by a sensation that the head could burst. The person thirsts for large amounts of water at infrequent intervals. Along with thirst, the person has a dry mouth and a thickly coated, white tongue. Fever is accompanied by chilliness and the sensation of internal cold. If a cough accompanies the fever, it is hard and dry with little or no expectoration.

Eupatorium perf. Useful for fever that comes on during illnesses like influenza. There are terrible aching pains in the bones, especially in the back and extremities. A morning chill between 7:00 and 9:00 A.M. is preceded by thirst. Perspiration relieves all the symptoms, except for headaches. The person knows a chill is coming because he or she gets very thirsty and cannot drink enough water or other fluids.

Ferrum phos. This remedy has some similarities to the fevers of *Aconite* and *Gelsemium*. This type of fever, however, lacks the mental symptoms of *Aconite* (which is marked by anxiety) and *Gelsemium* (marked by drowsiness and mental dullness). With

Ferrum phos, few emotional symptoms exist. The person has a fever accompanied by a pale face.

Gelsemium. Useful for fever accompanied by drowsiness. The person cannot open the eyes because the eyelids feel so heavy. He or she wants to lie still and does not want to talk or have anybody nearby. The pulse is weak, and the person is not thirsty. There is great muscular weakness and aching in the extremities. This type of fever is often brought on by warm weather, especially in the summer and in areas where the climate is usually warm all year.

Ipecac. Useful for fever accompanied by excessive nausea and vomiting.

Mercurius sol. This remedy is usually associated with fever when the person has bacterial infections and when there is pus and yellow-green discharges. All discharges are foul smelling, including perspiration, breath, and skin discharges. The person perspires excessively, especially at night, yet this does not bring down the fever. There is increased saliva and excessive thirst, especially for cold water. Useful for chills that start slowly, especially in the evening. Fever alternates with chills. The tongue is soft, flabby looking, and thickly coated yellow.

Nux vomica. Useful when the body is burning hot, yet the person cannot move or uncover because the least movement makes him or her feel chilly. The person is irritable, angers easily, and is bothered by noise, touch, and light. Gastrointestinal problems are often present, including indigestion and constipation.

Phosphorus. Useful when the person has the peculiar symptom of increased hunger with fever.

Pulsatilla. Useful for a fever accompanied by a lack of thirst. The person is weepy, sad, and wants comfort and consolation. The head is hot, and the lips are dry. The person has the chills, yet wants to be fanned with cool air. The person feels worse in the evening.

Pyrogenium. Helps fever that is accompanied by extreme sickness, especially when there is an infection (such as a spreading boil). The perspiration has the odor of dead animals. The person shivers excessively and has a desire to move about.

Rhus tox. Useful for fever accompanied by achy limbs and joints.

The person is restless and feels better when constantly changing position, especially at night. This type of fever often comes on after exposure to cold, rainy weather, especially when the person gets wet.

Veratrum viride. Useful for fever symptoms similar to *Aconite* (sudden high fever with dry, burning heat of eyes, mouth, throat, and palms, causing the person to uncover); however, the person needing *Veratrum viride* has less anxiety and more facial flushing than the person needing *Aconite.* The head feels full, and the arteries throb in the neck and head. *Veratrum viride* is useful for the fever that comes on after exposure to the sun. The eyes are bloodshot. This remedy can be helpful for fevers accompanied by respiratory problems (such as bronchitis). The fever rises in the evening and lowers in the morning.

FINGER INJURIES

The first thing a person should do after an injury is make sure there is no damage to deeper tissues such as blood vessels, nerves, tendons, bones, or organs. If not certain as to the extent of the injury, it is best to consult a physician or go to an emergency room. Bleeding should be controlled as quickly as possible by applying direct pressure to the site with a clean, moist cloth. For control of pain and swelling, a cold, moist application can be used, although ice should not be applied directly against the skin. When transporting a person who is injured, it is important not to aggravate the injury. Consulting a Red Cross first aid manual or taking a first aid course can be helpful.

When fingers are hit with a hammer, slammed in doors, crushed by heavy objects, or fallen upon, especially in a work environment with heavy machinery, the homeopathic remedies listed here can help. Because movement of the fingers is so important for normal hand manipulations, they should always be evaluated by a hand specialist or orthopedic surgeon if there is any deformity or chronic pain.

Arnica. Useful for a sprain of the finger joint (especially when a ball hits the end of a finger and stretches it backward). The finger becomes black and blue, swollen, and very sore. *Arnica* 30c or 200c may be used two to four times daily. *Arnica* ointment can be used on any soft tissue or muscle that is bruised or sore, but should never be used when the skin is broken. Note that high-potency remedies are not recommended for home prescribing. Consult a physician or skilled homeopathic consultant for potencies above 30c.

Calendula. Useful as a wash for cuts to the finger. This remedy can also be taken internally to help reduce the possibility of infection.

Hypericum. An important remedy for the extreme pain of a crushed finger (especially when a finger is stepped on or caught in a car door). *Hypericum* can be useful for a cut to the finger (such as a paper cut). This is also an important remedy after a partial or full amputation of a finger to help relieve the extreme pain in the stump.

Lachesis. Useful for a crushed, bruised, or injured finger if the wound becomes infected. The affected part is blue and cold, as if the circulation is compromised. The person worries that gangrene will set in. A physician should be consulted for this condition.

Pyrogenium. Helpful for an infected finger injury. Extreme body aching, coldness, and an offensive, painful discharge from the infected finger are symptoms. The bed often feels too hard when the person sleeps. The finger is better with motion.

Rhus tox. A dislocated or sprained finger may be helped with *Rhus tox.* The pain gets worse from cold applications and initial motion, but seems better from warm applications and sustained motion. The person is restless. A physician should be consulted for this condition.

Ruta. Helpful when the tendon of the finger is stretched. This is an important remedy when the finger is hit by a basketball, baseball, or football.

Silica. An important remedy for removing slivers from the finger or fingertips (especially if the sliver cannot be removed through a minor surgical procedure). *Silica* helps to gently promote the expulsion of the splinter. This remedy is also useful for abscesses under the fingernails (especially when a splinter has been under the nail for a long time).

FLATULENCE (ALSO CALLED GAS)

Producing intestinal gas is a normal process. Each person produces more than a quart of gas every day, and most of it needs to be released at some time. Gas problems occur when gas becomes excessive, odorous, or there is a lack of control when passing it.

Gas is produced in the large intestine by normally occurring bacteria acting on food that has not been totally digested in the stomach or small intestine. Beans, bananas, onions, broccoli, brussels sprouts, and cabbage are more gas productive than other foods.

Some people have difficulties digesting milk because they lack the enzyme lactase. People with an intolerance to milk will develop much intestinal gas. The use of Lactaid, an enzyme bought in pharmacies, can often help milk intolerance.

Other ways to minimize gas are to avoid gas-forming foods and to use activated charcoal tablets to absorb the gas. Soaking beans overnight and then rinsing them before they are cooked helps diminish the gas-forming qualities. A substance called Beano can be sprinkled on food to help decrease the amount of gas formation. It is also important to avoid smoking, chewing gum, and drinking carbonated beverages since these substances bring air into the body, causing gas.

Aloe. Abdominal distention and diarrhea are common symptoms associated with *Aloe.* The person is uncertain whether gas or stool will pass. The gas tends to be hot, loud, and sputtering. An important symptom is that the person has an urging for a stool, but only passes gas.

Antimonium crud. A characteristic symptom with this type of gas is belching that tastes like the ingested food. Often, regurgitated fluid tastes sweet. The person bloats after eating. The tongue often has a thick, white coating.

Argentum nit. The abdomen is greatly distended from gas buildup and can reach an enormous size, causing pain. Gas is extremely offensive when it is passed. Passing of gas is very loud and is worse after eating sweets and sugar. Symptoms are worse after dinner.

Carbo veg. The abdomen (especially the upper portion) is greatly distended. Symptoms are better after passing gas or belching. Gas seems to develop about half an hour after eating. Digestion is slow and food seems to putrefy before it is digested. Gas passes during diarrhea and is hot and very offensive. Sometimes the person feels an urging for a stool, but only passes gas. Symptoms of belching, heaviness, fullness, and sleepiness occur together. Abdominal gas seems to increase when lying down.

Chamomilla. A good remedy for babies and children with abdominal distention from too much gas. Gas buildup occurs after angry outbursts; red cheeks and hot perspiration are often associated symptoms. Gas often smells like rotten eggs.

China. Useful for treating gas that causes abdominal pain. Bending over double relieves this pain. Belching of bitter fluid or regurgitating food does not provide relief. Movement does not make the bloating feel better. Hiccups with sour belching and gas are sometimes experienced. Eating fruit aggravates the gas buildup.

Cocculus. Helpful when there is gas buildup after staying up late at night, especially with the stress of caring for a sick person. Riding in a car or boat may cause a sick feeling and a sensation of abdominal fullness. The abdomen is distended with gas. When moving about, the person feels as if the abdomen is full of sharp stones. Lying on one side or the other brings relief.

Graphites. Helps the type of gas that is almost always associated with constipation. The abdomen is full and hard from increased gas buildup that seems to be trapped. The person must loosen the clothing. Gas pain occurs on the opposite side the person lies on.

Lachesis. The most useful remedy when a person cannot bear anything tight around the waist because of great abdominal distention. This remedy is especially useful for people who drink too much alcohol. Gas is often worse upon waking.

Lycopodium. One of the most important remedies for excess bloating and gas buildup. Immediately after a light meal, the abdomen is bloated and full. There is a constant sense of fermentation in the abdomen (like yeast working); this feeling is worse on the upper left side. Pain shoots across the lower abdomen, from the right side to the left side. Gas rolls in the stomach. Foods such as yeast, breads, cabbage, and beans cause gas buildup. Sweet things are craved. Gas is often worse between 4:00 and 8:00 P.M.

Magnesia phos. Useful for gas buildup in the abdomen that forces a person to bend over double. Pain and discomfort from this excess gas is relieved by rubbing, warmth, and pressure. Belching does not give relief. The person must loosen the clothes, walk about, and constantly pass gas to feel any relief. This remedy is often useful in the 6x potency. Dissolve twenty tablets in one cup of warm water and sip.

Natrum sulph. Useful for treating abdominal distention that is worse in the ascending colon. Symptoms are worse before breakfast. When passing gas, stool sometimes passes involuntarily. The gas that is passed is loud and sputtering.

Nux vomica. Helps gas and flatulence that comes on after eating spoiled food, as a side effect of taking medication, or after drinking too much alcohol or coffee. Irritability and oversensitivity are common. The person desires to pass gas, but only a small amount is passed at a time. A stool is passed in a similar manner. When the gas is passed the person feels better. There may be a bruised sensation of the abdominal wall and muscles.

Sepia. Useful for treating increased gas buildup that is accompanied by a headache. The gas pains tend to shoot up the rectum and into the intestines.

Staphysagria. This remedy may also be used for gas buildup and pain after suppressed emotions (such as anger and frustration). *Staphysagria* is useful after abdominal operations when a person has trapped gas that cannot be passed. Useful for treating children with swollen abdomens due to excess gas.

Sulphur. Useful for treating gas buildup that causes the abdomen to be very sensitive to pressure. The person feels as if something alive is moving in the abdomen (similar to the problems associated with *Thuja*). The gas that passes is hot and is either odorless or smells like spoiled eggs. Gas tends to be passed at night and is usually associated with a burning rectum that is relieved with cold applications.

Thuja. Gas buildup causes the abdomen to protrude in different spots. These protrusions move around from place to place and feel like something is alive in the abdomen. Eating fatty foods or onions causes gas.

FOOD POISONING

Food poisoning can be caused by many different viruses, bacteria, parasites, and toxins. The type of food poisoning is determined by the length of incubation period between eating the food and developing the symptoms; this period can be from thirty minutes to as long as a few weeks. Single cases of food illnesses are difficult to identify unless there is a distinct clinical syndrome, such as botulism.

Most gastrointestinal illnesses caused by food poisoning are relatively simple to treat. The most important aspect of working with food-borne illness is prevention. The World Health Organization has developed the ten golden rules for safe food preparation to help decrease the incidence of food poisoning: (1) choose safely processed foods; (2) cook foods thoroughly; (3) eat cooked foods immediately; (4) store cooked foods carefully; (5) reheat cooked foods thoroughly; (6) avoid contact between raw food and cooked food; (7) wash hands repeatedly; (8) keep all kitchen surfaces clean; (9) protect food from insects, rodents, and other animals; and (10) use safe water. Safe water can be water that has been boiled, distilled, purified, or filtered; water from wells or springs needs to be tested before selling or consuming.

Other treatments for food poisoning include bedrest and the occasional use of antibiotics. Medical professionals may administer fluids intravenously if there is much fluid loss from diarrhea or vomiting. A doctor should be consulted if the symptoms seem to be extreme or the person is very weak from fluid loss. Otherwise, homeopathic remedies can be used to treat the symptoms of food poisoning.

Arsenicum alb. Especially useful for treating the effects of drinking bad water and eating spoiled meat. A characteristic symptom is severe diarrhea and vomiting that burns the rectal tissue or throat. There is extreme exhaustion and restlessness. The person thirsts for warm drinks that relieve the burning in the throat. These drinks are sipped rather than gulped.

Carbo veg. Particularly useful for symptoms of food poisoning from spoiled fish or meat and oily, fatty, and rich foods. Great belching and distention of the stomach are key symptoms. Belching helps temporarily, but the abdominal pain and distention resume quickly. Burning pains are also common. A person feels that there is not enough air in the lungs and wishes to be fanned or have the windows open, despite being chilly.

Colocynth. Severe abdominal cramping and diarrhea are key symptoms of this type of food poisoning. The person is irritable and restless. Symptoms are better from warmth, bending over, and heavy pressure applied to the abdomen.

Ipecac. Can be used to treat food poisoning associated with extreme nausea and vomiting. This type of food poisoning has more vomiting than any other type. The tongue is often clean. Very sour fruits and rich pastry that have been made with rancid oils often lead to this remedy.

Lycopodium. Useful in treating the side effects of shellfish food poisoning. There is a tremendous sense of fullness in the abdomen with great flatulence and abdominal distention. Burning eructations arise in the throat causing it to burn for hours. The symptoms are often worse between 4:00 and 8:00 P.M.

Natrum phos. Useful for stomach discomfort from eating sour, green fruit. Great flatulence, sour belching, and vomiting are key symptoms. The mouth has a sour taste. There is a creamy, yellow coating on the tongue and on the back of the roof of the mouth.

Nux vomica. Useful for digestive problems caused by overeating or from spicy or rich foods. *Nux vomica* is also useful after drinking too much. The symptoms will sometimes occur an hour or two after eating. Irritability, impatience, and anger are common. The person is oversensitive and easily offended. Any kind of stimulation, including noise, touch, and strong odors, cause irritation. While at times there is diarrhea, the person often has an urge to pass a stool, but nothing comes. There is also a feeling that there is still stool left inside, even after extensive diarrhea. Often a weight in the stomach feels like a stone.

Podophyllum. This remedy can be used for food poisoning from shellfish. The most important symptom is that the large amount of diarrhea is often painless and non-irritating.

Pulsatilla. Sometimes helpful in easing the symptoms of food poisoning from spoiled meat. It is also useful after overeating rich food, such as cakes, creams, and pastries. Moods and symptoms seem to change frequently. The person often feels weepy and wants company and attention. Diarrhea that varies with each stool is common. The person feels chilly yet wants to be outside walking slowly in the cool air. Contradictory symptoms are common, and the person may even want to eat the same foods that caused the sickness. The person is thirstless, even though there is a dry mouth.

Pyrogenium. Useful for treating food poisoning from spoiled fish or meat. All discharges (including vomit, sweat, and stools) have a very strong, offensive smell. The breath is often putrid and offensive. The person is restless, and the bones ache. The pulse can seem abnormally rapid, and there is great awareness of the heart beating. Hot drinks and bathing make the person feel better. Aching is temporarily improved by motion.

Urtica urens. An important antidote for the bad effects of eating shellfish. Hives that burn and itch intensely come and go. The hives can occur in small blotches or in large patches that sting and burn. Cold air and touch aggravate the hives.

Veratrum alb. Severe retching and vomiting with diarrhea characterize this remedy. The person feels extremely cold, and there is cold perspiration on the forehead. The skin has a bluish color. Cramping in the extremities is common. The person has a weak, shaky feeling. The person is thirsty for cold water, but vomits as soon as the water is swallowed. A craving for ice or cold drinks such as fruit juice is sometimes experienced.

FOREIGN OBJECTS (INCLUDES SPLINTERS)

When a splinter, thorn, or other small object gets stuck underneath the skin, it is often very painful. Trying to remove it with a pin or needle is helpful, especially if it is close to the surface. If the object is deeper within the skin and cannot be retrieved, homeopathic remedies may help promote expulsion of the object.

Cantharis. Can be used for burning pain from a puncture or when a nettle is stuck in the skin. A physician should be contacted regarding a tetanus shot for puncture wounds, especially if caused by a dirty or rusty object or an object contaminated by animal feces.

Hepar sulph. Useful for pus and infection that form around a foreign object that cannot be removed easily. Fish bones, needles, splinters, and glass can cause infection if lodged in the body, and *Hepar sulph* can help decrease the infection.

Silica. The main remedy for expulsion of foreign objects (such as needles, glass, fish bones, or splinters) from the body. This remedy has an amazing ability to push the foreign object out of the skin surface. *Silica* should be used in the low potency (such as 6x four times a day) along with a *Calendula* or *Hypericum* ointment.

FROSTBITE (INCLUDES IMMERSION FOOT)

The different degrees of frostbite depend on the length of time an extremity has been exposed to cold, the temperature of the air or water, and how the affected area has been treated.

One type of frostbite, immersion foot, is observed in shipwreck survivors or in soldiers whose feet have been wet, but not exposed to freezing temperatures, for long periods of time. Primary injury occurs in nerve and muscle tissue, but there is no damage to the blood vessels or skin. The problems that occur usually result from lack of oxygen, which causes paleness followed by pulsating red, swollen feet. It is important to treat immersion foot frostbite by warming the areas slowly because overheating can lead to gangrene. Long-term problems can occur, including sensitivity to cold and pain in weight-bearing parts of the feet.

Frostbite has similar symptoms as immersion foot, but can be a more serious condition if the blood vessels are severely damaged. When the circulation of blood stops, the frozen tissue is blocked by red blood cells and platelets, which form clots. Early on, this clumping is reversible, but as time passes, the clots cause severe damage to the tissues. It is important not to walk, bear weight, or put pressure on any thawed frostbite areas. Thawing followed by refreezing is especially harmful. Frostbite that has caused irreversible damage or was not treated properly can continue to cause long-term problems including increased sweating, pain, cold insensitivity, numbness, abnormal color, cracking skin, deformed nails, and joint pain. Frostbite can be a very serious problem. A physician or emergency room should be contacted immediately.

When treating frostbite, it is important to warm the core temperature of the body first, followed by warming the frostbitten limb in water that is between 50°F and 59°F and increasing 9°F every five minutes to a maximum of 104°F. Once the frostbitten area has been warmed, the treatment should be conservative and consist of bedrest, elevation of the injured area, tetanus vaccine, and the use of antibiotics.

It is important to wear warm, multi-layered clothing, eat good meals, and keep the hands or feet protected. Avoiding constricting wristbands and tight socks or shoes is important. Wearing warm headgear is important since most heat is lost from the top of the head. It is very important not to be exposed to cold after drinking alcohol, and older adults and young people who are susceptible to stress should avoid long exposure to cold.

The homeopathic remedies listed here can be helpful in treating mild to moderate frostbite.

Agaricus muscarius. *Agaricus* is made from a mushroom that has muscarium in it. Burning, itching, redness, and swelling are typical characteristics of this type of frostbite. Fingers or affected parts of the body feel like they are pierced by needles of ice. Skin is sensitive to pressure and cold air.

Arsenicum alb. Helpful for treating frostbite that has a tendency toward gangrene. The affected area burns. Hot applications bring relief.

Calcarea carb. Fingers tend to ulcerate easily. The affected area gets worse from washing with water.

Petroleum. Cracking and bleeding of the skin, especially at the fingertips, occurs with frostbite. Great itching and pain may be associated with this type of frostbite. Often this itching affects the heel. The affected area becomes painful, swollen, and red. Inflammation sets in when the weather turns cold.

Pulsatilla. The person is weepy, frightened, and seeks comfort and consolation. Affected areas turn a deep red or bluish color. The area burns and itches intensely with throbbing pains. Soles of the feet are particularly affected. Generally, affected areas feel worse by warm applications and in a warm room. Cold applications bring relief.

Rhus tox. Helps itching and burning pains that are intolerable at night. Symptoms feel worse from rest.

Sulphur. The affected area itches and burns intensely with this type of frostbite. The skin may crack and ooze and fingers turn quite red. Symptoms feel worse at night.

GUM DISEASE (INCLUDES GINGIVITIS OR PYORRHEA)

Gum disease, also called periodontal disease, usually involves one of two conditions: severe tooth decay or gingivitis. Gingivitis is an inflammation of the gums around the tooth; pyorrhea is a purulent inflammation of the tooth sockets, usually leading to loosening of the affected teeth. In all instances, the gums become red, swollen, and bleed easily, especially when teeth are brushed or after flossing. Gingivitis and pyorrhea are usually caused by an accumulation of plaque, which attracts bacteria that causes the inflammation of the tissues and gums. Lack of proper nutrition and eating foods that are high in sugar, especially ones that stick to the teeth, can cause gum disease. Some people are more prone to this problem.

Several natural methods can be used to prevent and treat gum disease. Brushing the teeth at least two times a day and after meals, and flossing the teeth properly between each tooth are extremely important. Brushing the teeth at the gum line where plaque is located is essential. Massaging the gum with the index finger after brushing and flossing will help loosen plaque. Brushing the teeth with a solution of hydrogen peroxide, water, and baking soda can also remove plaque and clean the teeth. Regular visits to a dental hygienist or dentist should be made every four to six months. Certain vitamins and supplements are known to help gum disease.

Antimonium crud. The gums bleed easily and seem to separate from the teeth. The tongue has a thick, white coating. Cracks in the corners of the mouth, salty saliva, and canker sores are common characteristics.

Carbo veg. The gums retract and bleed easily, especially when cleaning the teeth. The teeth are very sensitive, especially when eating. The person may be cold, suffer from shortness of breath, and have excessive flatulence.

Hepar sulph. Useful when the mouth and gums are very painful to touch and the gums bleed easily. The gums are infected and often ooze bloody pus. Cold air bothers the gums and teeth.

Kreosote. This type of gum disease is characterized by spongy, bleeding gums and rapid tooth decay. The teeth become dark and crumble. The lips are red and bleeding. A putrid odor comes from the mouth. Dull, throbbing pains in the gums are worse from cold, open air and better from warmth. Ulcerations occur on the gums and inner surface of the mouth. The corners of the mouth burn.

Lachesis. Helpful when the gums are spongy, swollen, and bleed easily. A toothache radiates to the ears. There may be a sensation of constriction around the neck. People who need this remedy often wake up from a nap or sleep and have more pain than before.

Mercurius sol. The gums recede and bleed easily. A putrid odor comes from the mouth and from the body in general. Increased saliva and perspiration are common. The person has much tooth decay and teeth become loose and tender.

Phosphorus. Swollen gums bleed very easily, even from light brushing or flossing. Ulcers, which also bleed easily, may form on the gums.

Silica. Useful for sore, swollen gums that have a tendency to form abscesses and boils. *Silica* helps ripen the abscesses.

Staphysagria. Often useful for people who have smoked too many cigarettes and have other excessive habits. The gums become spongy and bleed easily. The teeth actually turn black and begin to crumble.

HEAD INJURIES

The first thing a person should do after an injury is make sure there is no damage to deeper tissues such as blood vessels, nerves, tendons, bones, or organs. If not certain as to the extent of the injury, it is best to consult a physician or go to an emergency room. Bleeding should be controlled as quickly as possible by applying direct pressure to the site with a clean, moist cloth. For control of pain and swelling, a cold, moist application can be used, although ice should not be applied directly against the skin. When transporting a person who is injured, it is important not to aggravate the injury. Consulting a Red Cross first aid manual or taking a first aid course can be helpful.

Head injuries cause many deaths and much disability. Traumatic damage can result from the penetration of objects into the skull. Rapid acceleration or deceleration of the brain, which damages the tissue at the point of impact and on the opposite side, can also be harmful. There can be damage to the nerves, blood vessels, and lining of the brain. Swelling and bleeding can cause increased pressure. Skull fractures can sever important arteries in the brain. Infections can result when the lining of the brain has been damaged.

A common form of head injury is a concussion or closed head injury. There can be a dazed feeling or a temporary loss of consciousness, but there is no structural damage to the brain. If there has been any kind of head injury, it is important to watch for and report any of the following signs: changes in consciousness, changes in emotions, confusion, dilation of the pupils, nausea, seizure, or vomiting. The person should be watched for twenty-four hours; sometimes it is necessary to wake the person at night to make sure that he or she is not having problems with consciousness.

Minor head trauma can be treated at home with rest and observation. If more serious injuries occur, a physician should be contacted immediately or the person should be taken to the nearest emergency room.

The homeopathic remedies listed here should be used only when there are no signs of internal structural damage. Other homeopathic remedies can be used when there are emotional problems (fear, anxiety, sustained concentration) as a result of head trauma.

Arnica. The first remedy for any head injury (especially for a concussion or laceration). The head feels sore and bruised and may be black and blue. Useful for blunt trauma to the head and when the scalp is bleeding. *Arnica* is also useful when seizures occur after a head injury.

Calendula. Useful for a scalp injury that may become infected. This remedy can be used as a tincture or an ointment.

Glonoine. Useful when the person suffers from migraine headaches after a head injury.

Hypericum. Helpful for a head laceration with extreme pain because of injury to the nerve endings. This remedy can be used internally, or as a tincture or ointment.

Natrum sulph. Useful after a head injury when the mental state is altered. The person may cry excessively or be confused, or possibly even suffer from memory loss. *Natrum sulph* is also helpful for vertigo or dizziness after a head injury. Symptoms tend to get worse during hot, damp weather. This remedy is also useful when seizures occur after a head injury.

Symphytum. Useful for a fractured skull, *Symphytum* helps the bones heal together more quickly. *Symphytum* 30c three times daily can be helpful.

HEADACHES

Different forms of headache include tension, migraine, and cluster headaches. Some headaches are associated with influenza, sinus infections, or other viral illnesses. Other headaches result from the contraction of the neck and forehead muscles. These stress headaches are often due to emotional distress or the physical distress of working too hard or sitting in an awkward position too long. Natural methods to help these types of headaches are relaxation techniques, heat, massage, acupuncture, and rest.

Certain types of headache may be serious. One serious type of headache is meningitis, with the symptoms of a stiff neck, high fever, and a severe and incapacitating headache. These symptoms may also be associated with aneurysms of the brain. Long-standing headaches are associated with a sense of confusion, and changes in behavior may be caused by a brain tumor. Trauma or head injury may also result in a potentially serious form of headache, indicated by any change in consciousness or pupil size, nausea, or vomiting. Meningitis, long-standing headaches, and head trauma are all serious conditions; therefore, a physician should be contacted immediately.

Headaches caused by sinus inflammation are treated the same way as sinusitis. This includes thinning the mucus and eliminating bacteria from the sinuses, drinking plenty of fluids, and steaming the face.

Migraine headaches are caused by an initial constriction of the blood vessels in the temples of the head, which may lead to a sensation of aura because of the lack of blood flow. Symptoms may include a feeling that something is wrong, seeing spots in front of the eyes, losing vision, or getting confused. Following this initial constriction, the blood vessels actually dilate, letting too much blood flow into these arteries and causing great pain characterized by throbbing, blinding headaches with nausea, vomiting, and great weakness. Changes in climate, high winds, loud noises, sunlight, excessive staring at computer screens, high levels of stress, and food allergies can all initiate a migraine headache in a susceptible person. A person is most often susceptible due to heredity.

Learning biofeedback techniques to control blood flow into the temple arteries can be helpful in controlling migraines. There are also allopathic medicines that help prevent migraines just as they are starting or treat them once they have started. Consult a physician or pharmacist for further information. The homeopathis treatment of migraine headaches is complex and should be handled by a homeopathic physician. Headaches caused by trauma can also be treated naturally as long as the trauma has been relatively minor.

Homeopathic remedies can be used to treat all types of headaches. For example, certain remedies are associated with migraines, others with the effects of food or alcohol, and others with trauma. Homeopathic remedies can also be used to treat recurrent or chronic headaches. By carefully analyzing each remedy, a person can choose which one best matches the symptoms, no matter what type of headache it is. Certain vitamins, supplements, herbs, and oils are known to help headaches.

Aconite. Helpful for the treatment of a sudden, intense headache that often comes on after exposure to cold, dry winds or hot sun. The person may feel fear and apprehension. Either the skull feels like it will be forced out of the forehead, or the head feels constricted by a tight band. The head feels full, heavy, pulsating, hot, bursting, and burning. The person also feels as if the brain was moved by boiling water.

Anacardium. Helpful when a person feels like there is a plug in the forehead, the back of the head, or the temples. The person is extremely irritable and may have a tendency to swear and curse.

The head pain is worse from coughing, deep breathing, and mental stress. The headache seems better during a meal and after falling asleep.

Antimonium crud. Helpful when a headache is associated with indigestion (especially after drinking wine or eating candy, fruits, or fats). It is also useful for treating a headache that comes on after bathing or swimming in cold water. The pain is often worse on the top of the head, and it can increase by ascending stairs or while in high places. This type of headache may be associated with a very thick, white coating on the tongue.

Apis. A true migraine remedy, especially useful for treating swelled blood vessels in the head. The head throbs and feels hot. Stinging pains like a bee sting are common. The person may bore the head into a pillow and scream out. The headache feels better from pressure and cold wraps and worse from heat and motion.

Argentum nit. Useful when emotional disturbances (such as the stress of worrying about an upcoming test or job interview) cause headaches. These headaches often occur on one side of the head and are accompanied by coldness and trembling of the body. The person may feel a sense of expansion in the head and an aching in the right frontal area around the eye. The head pain can extend into the teeth. This type of headache may be associated with nausea and vomiting of sour-tasting bile. Although the person may generally feel better with fresh air, the headache may be aggravated by it. Boring head pains feel better with tight bandaging and pressure.

Arnica. Useful for treating headaches associated with a sore, bruised head after an injury. A physician should be contacted if a person changes or loses consciousness, experiences any nausea or vomiting, or shows changes in the eye pupils.

Belladonna. One of the most important remedies for headaches. This remedy is often useful for headaches that occur from overexposure to sun or heatstroke. Symptoms associated with this type of headache are clearly defined; throbbing pain that can drive the person almost wild is the most important symptom. The location of the pain is usually in the right frontal area and is associated with a flushed face and dilated pupils. The person cannot lie down or bear any light, direct air, noise, or jarring. Sometimes sitting up makes the headache feel better. Headaches are often better with warm wraps around the head or firm pressure (as with *Bryonia*).

Bryonia. Useful for treating headaches that have a bursting or splitting pain. The person is very irritable and wants to be left alone. This pain can begin in the front of the head, move over the head to the neck, and continue down the shoulders or back. The headache is worse from any touch except when a hard pressure is applied to the painful area, or when lying, unmoving, or on the painful side. When attempting to sit up, the person feels nauseated and faint. A great thirst for large amounts of cold water is often present. The lips are parched and the tongue may be dry and white. The hair can be very greasy. The head pain is often worse in the morning. Any movement, even movement of the eyes, makes the pain feel worse. Lying perfectly motionless makes the person feel better.

Calcarea carb. Helpful for headaches caused by stress or over-lifting, and associated with cold hands and feet and nausea. It is also often associated with the menstrual period. When the pain is severe, it makes the person feel crazy. The person has a feeling of coldness in the head. When sleeping or lying down, great amounts of perspiration sometimes wet the pillow. This type of headache is worse from weather changes, with any type of motion, or by bending over. The pain is worse in the morning upon wakening. The person feels better when completely still.

Calcarea phos. Useful for treating headaches of children or adolescents who grow quickly; their headaches are often located on top of the head. This remedy is also useful for headaches of young girls when they first get their menstrual period and who may become anemic due to the loss of blood. The person can be thin, have a lack of appetite, and become tired quickly. The growth of the body seems to tire the person out more than schoolwork or other activities.

Chamomilla. This type of headache can be associated with young children who seem almost furious with pain. The child is often very thirsty, restless, and irritable. The headache may be associated with the cutting of teeth. The child may have one red cheek and one pale cheek. Vomiting of bitter bile is a common symptom.

China. Often useful for pain that seems to travel along the nerves. This pain is especially worse after blood loss due to nosebleeds or heavy menstrual periods. The person feels as if the skull will burst open. The head and carotid arteries throb intensely due to anemia. This intense throbbing is unlike the throbbing of *Belladonna*, which is associated with too much blood flow through the blood vessels in the head (*China* is associated with too little blood flow). The headache is worse when sitting or lying; the person must stand or walk.

Cimicifuga. These headaches are typical of high school or college students who are fatigued from overwork and overstress. *Cimicifuga* is especially useful if the person feels crazy from the pain. One type of headache feels as though the top of the head will fly off. Sharp pains in and around the eyes shoot up to the top of the head. Another type of headache is when the head feels like a nail is being driven straight through the head, from the back to the front. Another type of pain may also begin in the occiput and shoot down the spine. This pain is relieved by bending the head forward. An unusual sensation in the head is an opening-and-shutting feeling in the brain, as well as an outward pressure.

Cocculus. This type of headache is triggered by riding in cars or boats and is almost always associated with vertigo and nausea. The headache is generally worse from any kind of emotional or mental stress. The pain is usually located in the occiput and the nape of the neck. The back of the head feels like it is opening and closing; the person cannot lie on the back of the head because of this pain. The person may tend to stretch the head backward. The headache is better when indoors and with rest.

Coffea. A headache associated with insomnia may benefit from *Coffea.* The head pain is intolerable, driving the person to weep and feel despair. The person feels as if a nail has been driven into the brain.

Ferrum phos. Helps headaches that are caused by either an upper respiratory infection or the heat of the sun. Symptoms can include having an earache, sore throat, and fever. This type of headache often pulsates and the person may feel a rush of blood to the head. The scalp and hair are very sensitive to touch. Bending over and any kind of movement cause the headache to get worse. The pain is improved by pressing a cold object against the painful area.

Gelsemium. This type of headache is often accompanied by a fever and flu-like symptoms. The person is generally very weak and apathetic and the entire body aches. The eyelids and limbs feel very heavy, and the eyeballs feel bruised. These congested headaches are often preceded by visual disorders such as double vision or blurred vision. Generally, the head pain is concentrated in the nape of the neck and the occiput. The pain may extend over the head and settle over the eyes. The person feels as if a tight band is wrapped around the head just above the ears. The headache is often worse in the morning and can be relieved by urinating. Any kind of mental effort, the heat of the sun, or tobacco smoke makes the headache worse.

Glonoine. Associated with overexposure to the sun, such as sunstroke, this headache increases and decreases with the rising and setting of the sun. Sometimes the headache can occur from incandescent or florescent light. This type of headache is characterized by an extreme throbbing of the arteries, similar to headaches associated with *Belladonna*; however, unlike *Belladonna,* symptoms are somewhat relieved by motion and the face is not as deeply flushed. Bending the head backward aggravates the headache. The head feels enlarged and distended. The person may feel like a tight band is wrapped across the forehead. The person is very sensitive to the slightest jarring.

Ignatia. This type of headache is often triggered by great mental stress, such as the breakup of a relationship or the death of a loved one. The person feels great grief and loss. The head feels as though a nail was driven into the side of the head. Pains can either come on gradually and stop suddenly, or they come and go suddenly. The head feels heavy. The head pain is better from warmth and lying on the painful side. The person feels relief from the profuse flow of urine, like headaches that are helped by *Gelsemium.* The pain is worse from stooping, but better when bending forward.

Ipecac. Extreme and constant nausea and vomiting occur with this type of headache. The pain in the head extends downward toward the teeth. Consult a physician if symptoms persist.

Iris. An important remedy for headaches that occur on the weekends, especially for working people such as teachers or business people. These headaches commence after a period of prolonged stress like a long work week followed by a let-down. These headaches are also produced by eating sweet things. The headache begins with partial blindness or blurred vision (similar to *Gelsemium* and *Kali bich*). Blurred vision is often preceded by drowsiness. As soon as the blurring disappears, the headache begins. Sharp or throbbing pains are generally located over the eyes (especially the right eye). Excessive, bitter vomiting often occurs when the headache is at its most severe. The vomiting is so sour that the teeth are sensitized. This headache is aggravated by motion, cold air, and coughing; however, moderate exercise in the open air often relieves the pain.

Kali bich. A headache helped by *Kali bich* begins with dimness of vision, but is different from a headache helped by *Iris* or *Gelsemium*. In headaches associated with *Kali bich,* intense pain seems to settle in a small spot. When this happens, the loss of vision disappears. The area of pain can actually be located with a finger. The pains often shift from one place to another and can appear and disappear suddenly. Another important type of headache relieved by this remedy is a sinus headache. This head pain is located above the eyes on the frontal sinus or below the eyes in the maxillary sinus. A thick, greenish-yellow, stringy, sticky mucus drains from the sinus to the nose. This type of sinus headache is often relieved with pressure. If a fever and yellow or green discharge continues after a few days, a physician should be contacted.

Lachesis. Helpful in treating left-sided headaches that are worse in and over the left eye. This type of head pain can be brought on from the heat of the sun, such as in sunstroke. The pain can start on the left side of the head and move to the right side. Changing position makes the head throb. Headaches are worse upon waking up from a nap or in the morning. An important characteristic is that the headaches are better with the appearance of discharges such as menstrual flow or nasal mucus.

Ledum. This type of headache is sometimes caused by a blow to the eye. The head pain worsens from any type of warmth; even a hat creates too much heat for the head. Lying down in bed causes pain because it creates friction and heat. The person feels great relief from bathing the head with very cold water.

Lycopodium. This type of headache can occur if meals are eaten later than usual. Excessive flatulence and gas buildup can also bring on this headache. The headache can begin on the right side of the head and move to the left side. With severe colds, headaches often occur over the eyes. Sometimes the person can only see the left side of objects. The symptoms seem worse between 4:00 and 8:00 P.M. Headaches are worse with heat, although the rest of the body feels better by being warm. The headaches are improved by cool air.

Magnesia carb. A headache treatable by *Magnesia carb* is brought on by emotional stress. The headache is characterized by pain in the side of the head on which the person lies. This pain feels as if the hair is being pulled and the entire body feels tired and exhausted. Excessive worry and sensitivity to touch are common problems. The person moves around and wraps up the head for relief.

Magnesia phos. This type of headache often occurs after spending long hours reading or studying. Shooting pains move around and come on suddenly. The pain is generally located in the occiput and nape of the neck. The person feels exhausted. The headaches are better with warmth and pressure. Often dissolving twenty tablets of the 6x potency in one cup of warm water and sipping the mixture slowly is helpful.

Natrum mur. Useful for headaches that are chronic. Not often used for acute problems, *Natrum mur* is effective between headaches as a preventive. This type of headache is associated with young girls who recently started their menstrual periods (similar to headaches associated with *Calcarea phos*). The headache can also be caused by eye strain (similar to headaches associated with *Ruta*). This remedy is especially useful in children or adolescents who become exhausted from studies because they stay up too late or worry too much. The person may be sad or feel hurt but does not like to be consoled; the person likes to be alone. The person is often sad and likes to dwell on problems. Often, a person who needs this remedy is thin, loses weight easily despite a normal appetite, and tends to crave salt. The pain is usually one-sided, especially over the right eye. Often the headache begins with partial blindness, similar to headaches helped by *Iris* and *Kali bich*. Prior to the headache, the person may experience a temporary numbness and tingling of the lips, tongue, and nose. The person feels like the head is being beaten by a thousand little hammers. A throbbing, blinding headache often begins around 10:00 A.M. and tends to throb all day. The headache is accompanied by dizziness. The person may see zigzags and be very thirsty. The head pain can begin when near the ocean. The headache is worse after menstruation and from sunrise to sunset. A type of headache that is more of an acute headache relieved by *Natrum mur* is associated with colds and sinus problems. Sneezing and excessive amounts of nasal discharge are common. A runny nose changes into nasal stuffiness, making breathing difficult and causing the frontal sinuses over the eyes to hurt.

Nux vomica. The most important remedy for a headache that occurs from excessive alcohol or coffee intake, or other kinds of overindulgence. This headache is referred to as the typical hangover headache. The person feels dull but at the same time is hyperexcited and sensitive to noise and touch. This type of headache is also brought on by sunshine (similar to headaches associated with *Glonoine*). A splitting headache occurs in the morning upon waking. The person feels as if a nail is being driven into the skull at the top of the head. The pain envelops the entire head. The pain can also occur in the front of the head. The person wants to press the head against something to relieve the pain. Hemorrhoids sometimes occur. Nausea and vomiting are common symptoms. The headache is generally worse from coughing, stooping, eating, and moving the eyes or body. Not much seems to relieve this headache; however, the pain seems to improve when rising in the morning and being up and about for a few hours.

Petroleum. This type of occipital headache can be brought on by the motion of cars or boats. The back of the head feels numb and heavy, as if it were made of lead or wood. Pain in the temples is better by holding the temples tightly. Shaking while coughing makes this pain worse. The person often experiences vertigo in the occiput upon rising. The person feels intoxicated. The head feels as if a cold breeze was blowing on it.

Pulsatilla. This type of headache is brought on by overwork and overindulgence, especially by eating rich, fatty foods such as ice cream. The person often wants tender loving care and consolation, which generally helps. *Pulsatilla* is especially useful for women who have late and light periods and tend to cry easily. The head pain seems to shift from one place to another very rapidly, and extends to the ears or teeth. The person may have pain in the right temporal area with profuse eye drainage from the right eye. *Pulsatilla* may also be useful in treating sinus headaches. The person is very sensitive, weeping at the slightest cause. This type of sinus headache is associated with a bland, yellow discharge from the mucous membranes. The person is chilly, but wants to be near cool breezes. The head pain is worse from any kind of warmth and in the evening. Being in the open air and bandaging the head tightly seem to help relieve the pain.

Rhus tox. The head feels heavy, as though a board was strapped to the forehead. The person is extremely restless and changes positions continually. The brain feels loose inside the head. The pain in the forehead often proceeds backward. Sitting without movement seems to make the head pain worse, and warmth and gentle motion make the pain better. Joint pains, especially when the joints are hot and red, sometimes occur.

Ruta. Especially useful in treating headaches that occur after long periods of eye strain, such as from reading small print, sewing, or working with a computer screen. The eyes are tired, hot, and red.

Sanguinaria. Used for treating migraine-type headaches including periodic migraines, especially ones that occur every seven days or even monthly. The pain is felt on the right side, beginning in the occiput, spreading upward, and settling over the right eye. The pain increases in severity until vomiting of food and bile sometimes brings relief. The pain can become so intense that the person will bore the head into a pillow for relief. A bursting pain feels as if the eyes will be pressed out from their sockets. Noise and light are unbearable, and sleep brings some relief. The symptoms increase and decrease with the course of the sun, reaching a climax at the middle of the day. Headaches are generally always better when lying down in the dark, sleeping, belching, or passing gas.

Sepia. Generally a remedy for women. The migraine headache occurs in relation to the menstrual period (often as a premenstrual syndrome headache). Melancholy, sadness, and a desire to be left alone are all common symptoms. The pain is usually associated with the left eye and the left temple, and the pains tend to extend backward. The throbbing over the left eye is often accompanied by hot flashes that are made worse from motion, light, and noise. These headaches tend to occur in women who have profuse leukorrhea and chronic vaginitis.

Silica. Useful for treating a headache caused by nervousness and emotional stress. The person wants to tie the head up with a towel or handkerchief to keep it warm, which brings relief. (People with headaches helped by *Argentum nit* also want to tie the head up tightly, but it is to create pressure rather than warmth.) The pains tend to come up from the back of the head and settle above one eye or the other. The face is often pale at the beginning of the headache. As the pain becomes more intense, the face gets flushed, even though the body remains chilly. Noise, motion, and jarring make the pain worse, and warmth brings relief. This type of headache can be accompanied with profuse sweat on the head. Like headaches helped by *Ignatia* and *Gelsemium,* this headache is often relieved by urination.

Spigelia. The pain rises from the nape of the neck and occiput, over the head, and settles over the left eye. (Headaches helped by *Silica* have the same kind of pain, but the pain settles over both eyes; headaches helped by *Sanguinaria* have pain that settles over the right eye.) The pain can feel like a band around the head. The head is very sensitive to touch. The pain tends to start in the morning, intensify at the middle of the day, and go away in the early evening.

Staphysagria. This type of headache can come on after a person suppresses angry feelings. The headache increases in proportion to the inner feelings of anger. The brain feels compressed and the forehead feels like a ball of lead is inside. The head may also feel compressed, numb, hollow, and wooden.

Sticta. Useful for dull frontal sinus pain located over the eyes. There is dull, heavy pressure in the forehead and root of the nose. The headaches are worse when the nose is stuffy; they are relieved when the nasal discharge begins.

Thuja. The head feels as if it has been pierced by a nail. The pain, usually located on the left side, can be unbearable, causing the person to almost lose consciousness. The headache is worse from 3:00 to 4:00 A.M. Drinking too much tea can make the headache worse.

Veratrum viride. Useful for congestive headaches, such as those corresponding to high blood pressure or severe heatstroke. These conditions should be under the treatment of a physician. The person is irritable and may be delirious. The person tries to initiate fights and arguments. This headache sufferer has a red face with bloodshot eyes and dilated pupils. The head is heavy and hot. The head pain may rise from the back of the head.

Zincum met. Headaches of overtaxed and overstressed school children may be relieved by *Zincum met.* The headache is brought on and aggravated by any type of intellectual effort. This type of headache is also caused from drinking a small amount of wine. The person is restless and constantly moves the feet and legs. The person tends to bore the head into the pillow and roll from side to side. The forehead may feel cool to the touch, but the base of the skull feels hot.

HEATSTROKE (INCLUDES SUNSTROKE)

Heatstroke occurs when there is disruption in the temperature-regulating mechanism of the body. It can be due to overexposure to heat sources such as the sun, a fireplace, or a stove. An increase in the body temperature and a decrease in the amount of sweat are often experienced. Heat exhaustion with headaches, nausea and vomiting, fatigue, vertigo, muscle cramps, and a sensation of clamminess of the skin are also common.

While the sun is generally helpful for the skin, too much exposure to the sun can lead to several problems. One problem in recent years, especially with the depletion of the ozone layer in the atmosphere, is the tendency to form skin cancers, such as basal cell carcinoma or melanoma. More immediate problems are sunburns and headaches caused by exposure to bright sunshine.

Heatstroke, or sunstroke, is a medical emergency; the person should be transported to the nearest hospital as soon as possible. The pulse becomes rapid, resulting in confusion, and there might be loss of consciousness and convulsions. On the way to the emergency room, homeopathic remedies can be given.

Aconite. Symptoms occur suddenly after sun exposure. The person is restless, worried, and thinks of the possibility of death. The skin gets red and dry but does not perspire. There is an intense thirst for large quantities of cold water. The person feels better as soon as sweating occurs. *Aconite* can be used every ten to fifteen minutes if needed.

Antimonium crud. Especially useful when a person is overheated from being too close to a fire or stove. Head pain is common. The person is excessively irritable and is unable to bear the heat of the sun. The person cannot work outside in the sun and cannot bear to be looked at or touched.

Belladonna. Often useful after *Aconite.* The face is very hot, red, and swollen looking, and there is sweating. The person has a throbbing headache, and the pupils are dilated. The person is often fearful and is hypersensitive to light, noise, and touch. This type of sunstroke can lead to convulsions, especially in infants and children.

Bryonia. Sun or heat exposure causes the person to have a severe headache that is worse on any attempt to move or sit up. The person is irritable and does not like to be talked to or interrupted. A great thirst for cold water is common.

Cuprum met. Especially useful for sun and heat exposure. Severe muscle cramping, especially of the calves and legs, is a typical symptom.

Gelsemium. An important symptom is an intense headache that radiates to the neck and shoulders. The person is trembling, weak, and dazed. Sometimes the person complains of double vision. Often the person feels better after urinating. This remedy can be repeated every ten to fifteen minutes.

Glonoine. A throbbing headache comes on when being overheated by a fire or stove. Violent throbbing in the arteries of the head and neck is a common symptom. The face is hot and red with generalized sweating. The eyes are red and bloodshot. Blood pressure may rise, and there will be waves of hot flashes. Cool temperatures and compresses improve the redness. This remedy is similar to *Belladonna* for heat-related problems, but it has less facial flushing and agitation. This remedy can be repeated every ten to fifteen minutes.

Lachesis. The person reacts to the heat by becoming talkative, changing subjects quickly. Being unable to tolerate the extremes of weather, the person often trembles when overheated. The person sticks the tongue out. The throat and abdomen feel constricted. Often the person feels worse after waking up from a nap.

Natrum mur. This remedy is not used for sudden and extreme reactions to the sun; it is used more between bouts of sun reactions as a preventive. Coldness in the legs and numbness and tingles in the fingers are unique symptoms. Mucous membranes are dry. Eye muscles feel weak and stiff. Hot weather fatigues the person, causing the person to feel dizzy, faint, dull, sleepy, and unable to work. Symptoms can be worse in the morning from 9:00 to 11:00 A.M. Generally the person feels better from cool bathing and being in an open area with a breeze. Sweating also makes the person feel better.

HEMORRHOIDS

Hemorrhoids occur when varicose veins in the anus are stretched, weakened, and dilated. They are a common problem in approximately 75 percent of the U.S. adult population.

There are many causes of hemorrhoids. The most prevalent cause is from standing, which places tremendous pressure on the lower veins. This pressure can be aggravated by heavy lifting, pregnancy, childbirth, or sitting for long hours. Coughing, sneezing, and constipation also make hemorrhoids worse.

Hemorrhoid symptoms include bright red bleeding, seen on the surface of the stool or toilet paper. Often large and tender protrusions of blood vessels are felt along the anal or rectal area. Some hemorrhoids are minor and cause small problems such as itching and formation of tags, the remaining piece of tissue after the vein shrinks. Other hemorrhoids are very large, can bleed extensively, and cause a great amount of pain. Hemorrhoids are especially painful when a blood clot develops inside.

Hemorrhoids are often both internal and external. Preventing or reducing the recurrence of hemorrhoids involves eating unrefined whole grain carbohydrates and high-fiber foods. Developing countries, in contrast to industrialized countries, generally have a lower incidence of hemorrhoids because of high-fiber diets full of vegetables, fruits, legumes, and grains. Grains promote peristalsis; fibers attract water, which forms a lattice mass that keeps the feces bulky, soft, and easier to pass. White flour in low-fiber diets causes stools to be hard, lumpy, and difficult to pass; this contributes to increased straining and irritation of the hemorrhoids.

To diminish discomfort with hemorrhoids and hasten their healing, it is often helpful to sit in a warm bath, especially with the knees raised. This helps shrink and soften the hemorrhoids. Exercise is extremely important because it circulates the blood from the lower extremities and the anal or rectal area back to the heart. Avoiding lifting heavy objects is also important. If hemorrhoids are particularly painful or troublesome, it may be helpful to buy a cushion with a hole in the center to relieve the pressure of sitting. It is important not to strain when having a bowel movement, and move the bowels only when there is an urge. A person should never sit on the toilet for long periods of time. Using soft toilet paper is necessary to decrease the friction and irritation. It is often helpful to saturate the toilet paper with cold water and dab the rectum after a stool to help constrict the blood vessels and decrease the burning and discomfort. During pregnancy, it is generally helpful to lie down as much as possible with the feet elevated. (Note that while homeopathic remedies are safe during pregnancy, labor, and breastfeeding, a pregnant woman should confer with her obstetrician or midwife to coordinate treatment.) Certain vitamins, herbs, and supplements are known to help hemorrhoids.

Aesculus hippocastanum. Useful for treating a person with hemorrhoids who has pains that feel like splinters or sticks in the rectum. These hemorrhoids are associated with severe pains in the back, especially in the sacroiliac joint.

Aloe. Helps protruding hemorrhoids that tend to be large and look like a bunch of blue grapes. They bleed often and profusely and are tender, sore, and hot. The application of cold water brings relief. The anus burns intensely, and the person may have diarrhea with the important symptom of insecurity of the rectum (the person does not know if a stool or gas will pass). Hemorrhoids are aggravated by the menstrual period, childbirth, and a stool. Note that while homeopathic remedies are safe during pregnancy, labor, and breastfeeding, a pregnant woman should confer with her obstetrician or midwife to coordinate treatment.

Arsenicum alb. Useful for hemorrhoids that tend to be blue and burn as if on fire. The burning sensation is worse at night and after midnight. Worry, fear, and a fixation on neatness may also be evident.

Collinsonia canadensis. Useful for treating hemorrhoids that bleed almost constantly. *Collinsonia canadensis* is helpful for treating pregnant women who suffer from hemorrhoids with itching. The person has a sensation of sticks in the rectum. A person who is susceptible to chest pains will sometimes develop chest discomfort when the hemorrhoids stop.

Graphites. Painful hemorrhoids associated with itching fissures and constipation may be relieved by *Graphites.* The hemorrhoids ooze a thick, sticky, stringy, honey-yellow colored substance. These hemorrhoids are almost always associated with constipation when there is no urge for a stool.

Hamamelis. Very sore hemorrhoids that bleed excessively (the blood is dark-colored rather than bright red) are sometimes treated by *Hamamelis.* The back feels as if it will break. This remedy can be used in potency, as an ointment applied directly to the hemorrhoid, or as a tincture applied directly to the hemorrhoid. The symptoms are aggravated by heat and the slightest touch.

Ignatia. Useful for treating hemorrhoids associated with sharp, stitching pains that shoot up the rectum. These hemorrhoids are often brought on by stress, grief, or the loss of a job or close friend.

Kali carb. Useful for large, swollen, and painful hemorrhoids. The pain is worse when coughing. These hemorrhoids often occur in heavy people, especially in women with backaches whose legs seem to give out on them when they walk, and who feel weak and sweaty. The affected person generally has a great intolerance of cold weather. Hemorrhoids are aggravated from childbirth and from any kind of touch, but seem to improve when riding in a car. The hemorrhoids are prolapsed, cause stabbing pains, and bleed excessively. They are improved by exposure to cold or sitting on a hard surface.

Lachesis. Useful for treating hemorrhoids that are prolapsed, violet colored, and very sensitive to touch. Throbbing pain and a constriction of the anus are typical symptoms. The pains are actually relieved by bleeding and aggravated by exposure to heat. Hemorrhoids can be worse during pregnancy and especially aggravated by menopause. They tend to be aggravated on waking in the morning or after a nap.

Muriaticum acidum. Helpful for the person who has an extremely sensitive anus. The slightest touch (even the softest toilet paper) is unbearable. Useful for hemorrhoids in the elderly.

Nux vomica. Hemorrhoids relieved by *Nux vomica* are associated with people who have sedentary habits, work too long, or study too hard. These hemorrhoids are also associated with people who abuse stimulants (such as alcohol, coffee, or cigarettes). The itchy hemorrhoids keep the person awake at night and are relieved by cold water. The person feels a constant urging to have a bowel movement and a feeling as though the bowel cannot empty itself completely. Hemorrhoids burn and bleed, and the anus feels constricted. The person is chilly, irritable, and hypersensitive to noise and touch. Hemorrhoids are relieved by cold compresses or ice packs, even though the person is usually hypersensitive to anything cold.

Phosphorus. Useful for treating hemorrhoids that bleed excessively with severe, sharp pains. Blood seems to flow in small streams with each stool.

Sulphur. Useful for treating hemorrhoid problems after the hemorrhoids have stopped bleeding. Associated symptoms include headaches, a feeling of fullness in the head, and a possible discomfort in the liver area. Mental symptoms include being irritable, being disorganized, and having a hot temper. The person usually dislikes heat and feels better in cool temperatures. Constipation is common with these hemorrhoids. The rectum burns and the anus itches, and they are relieved by cold water. The discomfort of the hemorrhoids is generally worse at night. These hemorrhoids sometimes occur in people who drink too much alcohol (especially beer). After childbirth and during the menstrual period are particular times of aggravation. *Sulphur* is also helpful when the menstrual period has been suppressed by medication and stress. Hemorrhoids tend to be worse when standing, being touched, or walking. Wiping after a stool also aggravates the hemorrhoids.

HERPES

The herpes infection has reached epidemic proportions in the United States and throughout the world. Twenty to thirty million Americans are infected today. There are two types of herpes infections that are troublesome: type 1 is associated with cold sores around the mouth; type 2 is generally associated with eruptions on the genitalia, thighs, and buttocks. In both cases, the painful sores that occur are small fluid-filled blisters with a red base. Oral herpes can be transmitted to the genitalia through oral sex, and genital herpes can be transmitted to the mouth.

After the initial eruption and subsequent healing, the herpes virus lives in the nerves in a dormant state. It erupts again when there is stress or minor infection such as sun exposure, respiratory infections, trauma to the area, overheating, or emotional stress.

The main symptoms of herpes are pain, irritation, tingling, burning, and itching in the area one to four days before the eruption occurs. It can be a very serious disease in people who have immune system problems, such as those infected with HIV, or people undergoing chemotherapy treatment for cancer. In these cases, herpes can become systemic and cause such problems as encephalitis. Herpes is also a very serious disease in newborn babies who have acquired the infection from an infected mother. This can lead to blindness or mental retardation.

The area that is infected should always be kept dry. For genital herpes, a person should wear cotton underwear and clothes that are loose fitting. Warm baths with epsom salt can help to relieve a breakout. Using ice on the infected area can help diminish pain. It is important not to share towels, washcloths, or toothbrushes when a person has a herpes breakout. Avoid touching the area since it can spread to the eyes, face, mouth, and genitals. Stress reduction techniques and avoiding excessive sun exposure, especially to the mouth and lips, is necessary.

Prevention is the best way to counteract the herpes infection. Avoiding sex with a person who is infected is extremely important. Using latex condoms will help diminish the contagiousness of the herpes infection if the person is not 100 percent positive of having no eruptions. It is possible to have an eruption and not have symptoms. It is also possible that a person does not have an eruption but has the early warning symptoms of itching, tingling, or burning, which enables the herpes infection to be transmitted.

Foods that are high in arginine, an amino acid, should be avoided; this includes chocolate, oatmeal, nuts, raisins, seeds, and peanuts. Acyclovir, an anti-viral allopathic medication, can be used topically or orally to help diminish the intensity of the initial breakout and increase the length of time between breakouts. However, this medication should only be prescribed by a physician. Certain vitamins and supplements are known to help herpes.

Arsenicum alb. Ueful for herpes of the face and chin. Eruptions tend to burn. Warm applications relieve the burning, and cold applications make it worse. The person is restless, very agitated, and anxious about having herpes. This type of herpes is not usually located on the genitals; it is more often located around the lips.

Croton tig. Herpes of the face and genitals is sometimes helped by *Croton tig.* The eruptions itch intensely, but scratching is painful. The skin feels tight. This type of herpes is often accompanied by diarrhea (especially in the summer).

Dulcamara. Useful for herpes eruptions that tend to bleed easily. These herpes eruptions can occur in clusters all over the body and are aggravated by cold water. The eruptions can open up and form a yellowish crust. Useful for genital herpes, especially when the person develops a cold. *Dulcamara* is also useful when a woman has outbreaks of herpes during the menstrual period. Sometimes the herpes eruptions are actually seen in the hair follicles of the pubic hair.

Graphites. Useful for herpes of the thighs, face, and chin. The herpes eruptions may ooze a sticky, thin discharge.

Natrum mur. Herpes at the corners of the mouth and the lips can sometimes be treated with *Natrum mur.* Blisters that form are more irritating during the menstrual period.

Petroleum. An important remedy for genital herpes. Herpes eruptions can occur on the penis, vagina, or perineum. The affected area tends to be dry, cracked, constricted, and very sensitive. If the herpes eruptions ooze, a thick, greenish crust that itches and burns may form.

Sepia. Useful for treating genital herpes as well as herpes of the hair follicles. This type of herpes seems to occur during pregnancy. The herpes often break out in the spring.

Thuja. Useful for chronic genital herpes that seems to last for a very long time. This type of herpes is often accompanied by chronic vaginal infections (in women) or urethra infections (in men).

HIVES (ALSO CALLED URTICARIA)

Hives represent an allergic reaction of the skin when histamine and other chemicals are released. This causes light red patches, called wheels, to form on the skin. Hives itch and burn but rarely are dangerous, unless they occur in the larynx or voice box, which can cause breathing problems. In people who are very allergic and very sensitive, hives can develop from exposure to cold water, sunlight, being overheated, and emotional stress.

There are many causes of hives, including medications such as penicillin or aspirin and many types of foods and food additives. The most common types of foods that cause hives are shellfish, strawberries, fish, nuts, beans, and dairy products. The types of food additives that cause hives are BHT, food stabilizers (such as those in ice cream), salicylate (found in many over-the-counter medications), and food coloring (such as yellow dye found in some ice creams, jellies, baked goods, candy, hot dogs, toothpaste, bologna, and salami). Artificially colored drinks, soft drinks, some types of beer, and cider vinegar also contain dyes that can cause hives. Certain vitamins and supplements are known to help hives.

Apis. Can be used to relieve hives with great swelling. The pains sting, itch, and burn. The symptoms are worse from any heat and covering. These hives may occur with asthma (especially during a change of weather). Insect bites cause hives. A fever may also cause hives. The hives are worse from any kind of perspiration (especially when exercising). Useful for swelling and hives that occur after eating strawberries or fish. Hives occur more often on uncovered parts of the body.

Arsenicum alb. Hives that cause great anxiety, restlessness, and anguish may be relieved by *Arsenicum alb.* An unusual symptom is that the hives alternate with other health problems (such as asthma, leg cramps, abdominal cramps, or croup). When the hives get better, the other problems get worse (and vice versa). *Arsenicum alb* is useful for hives that occur around salt water (such as when at the seashore or traveling by boat on the ocean). Warm applications relieve the itching and irritation of the hives, and cold ones make them worse.

Calcarea carb. Useful for treating chronic hives that are worse from drinking milk.

Dulcamara. Useful for hives that occur with the common cold (especially when profuse nasal discharge is a symptom). The hives tend to be better in the cold, dry, open air and with the application of water. The hives are worse from warmth, exercise, damp weather, and before and during the menstrual period. The red spots that occur tend to look like flea bites. The affected area does not radiate heat.

Kali iod. An excellent remedy for hives, especially when few other guiding symptoms are present. The hives tend to burn and itch. Both exercise and warmth tend to make the hives worse.

Natrum mur. Useful for hives that are greatly aggravated by warmth and exercising. Hives that occur during a chill or after eating too much salt may also be relieved with this remedy.

Pulsatilla. Useful for hives that are accompanied by stomach problems (such as indigestion and heartburn) and possibly diarrhea. Symptoms are worse from warmth and exercise. Hives can occur after eating fruit, pork, or buckwheat. The person is thirstless, weepy, and chilly, but wants to be in the cold air, which improves the hives.

Rhus tox. Useful for hives that occur after the skin gets wet (such as from bathing or perspiring). Hives also occur after scratching.

Arthritis and other types of rheumatic conditions sometimes occur with the hives. The itching is worse in cold air, during a chill, and with a high fever. The hives are improved by warmth. Useful for people who get hives annually during the same season. In general, the person is very restless and feels better when moving around.

Sepia. Useful for chronic hives that occur when a person goes out in the cold air and disappear whenever entering a warm room. The eruptions sometimes resemble a mark that a whip or small rod would make if hit on the skin.

Urtica. One of the most important remedies for hives that occur with joint pain. These hives occur after bathing and after excessive exercise, especially when the person is overheated. Swelling around the affected area is a common symptom. Many foods bring on this type of hives, including strawberries, shellfish, and some types of vegetables. This remedy is also useful for recurring hives in children, especially when the hives recur at the same time every year.

IMPETIGO

Impetigo is a skin infection seen mostly in children. The infection is caused by the streptococcus bacteria, the staphylococcus bacteria, or both. It is characterized by small blisters and pustules that form on the skin, especially around the face, arms, legs, and genitals. These blisters eventually form yellowish scabs, and they may form shallow ulcers that are covered with a crust. Impetigo is quite infectious; in schools or daycare centers, several children may have impetigo at the same time. Neglected infections can lead to infection of the lymph gland or cellulitis.

Antibiotics are often used either topically or orally for impetigo. Untreated infections can persist for months, and scarring can result if untreated. One of the most worrisome side effects is the streptococcus bacteria invading the bloodstream and settling in the kidney, causing glomerulonephritis in children. A physician should always be contacted in the case of impetigo. Good hygiene is a helpful way to prevent and treat impetigo.

The homeopathic remedies listed here can be useful for superficial and mild cases, or they may actually help the antibiotics work more effectively in more serious cases.

Antimonium crud. Useful for impetigo that has thick, hard, honey-colored scabs on the face, head, and lips. This remedy is one of the most commonly used remedies for impetigo.

Antimonium tart. Useful for treating eruptions on the face that leave a bluish-red mark. Impetigo of the scrotum can be relieved with this remedy.

Arsenicum alb. This particular type of impetigo is characterized by crusty eruptions with infected pustules that ooze an offensive, burning discharge. This burning is relieved by warm applications and made worse from cold applications. The person is restless, agitated, and apprehensive. *Arsenicum alb* is useful when a person is sicker than what is normally seen with a typical impetigo problem.

Dulcamara. Useful for impetigo characterized by a thick, brownish-yellow crust that bleeds when scratched. This remedy may be used more in the late summer or early fall when there are hot days and cold nights. The impetigo may arise as a result of getting chilled, especially in the cold, damp weather.

Graphites. Useful for treating impetigo when there is a thin, sticky, fluid discharge coming out of the eruptions. The person tends to be constipated, chilly, apprehensive, despondent, and indecisive. Cracks, fissures, and eczema may accompany this type of impetigo.

Kali bich. Useful for treating impetigo with a very sticky, thick discharge that is often yellowish or greenish. Ulcers with punched-out edges may form. The eruptions feel better from hot applications.

Mercurius sol. Useful for impetigo with a yellowish-brown crust that often itches and is worse from the warmth of the bed at night. These eruptions become infected easily and have a putrid odor. The affected person salivates excessively and has offensive perspiration. The person is sensitive to both hot and cold temperatures.

Mezereum. The type of impetigo has ulcerated eruptions that form thick scabs. Pus oozes from under these scabs. Eczema with intolerable itching is sometimes an associated symptom with this type of impetigo. The person is extremely sensitive to cold air and feels chilly all the time.

Rhus tox. Impetigo that becomes red, swollen, and itchy may be relieved by *Rhus tox*. This type of impetigo has less crust formation and instead a more red, inflamed, swollen look (similar to a skin infection). The person is restless and agitated. The symptoms are worse at night, and the person cannot remain in bed. The symptoms feel better with gentle rubbing and warm applications and worse from cold applications.

Sulphur. Useful for recurring impetigo. The skin is generally dry, scaly, and unhealthy. Every injury seems to form another impetigo outbreak. The skin itches and burns and is worse from scratching. All water (such as a bath or perspiration) irritates the skin. This remedy is especially useful when impetigo is repeatedly treated and suppressed with ointments and salves. The irritation from inflammation and itching is worse from warmth in the evening. The impetigo generally recurs in the spring (especially when it is damp outside).

INDIGESTION

Indigestion is a common problem, and there are many other problems characterized as indigestion: heartburn, excessive belching, esophagitis, gastritis, diseased gallbladder, food allergies, intestinal or stomach yeast infection, milk intolerance, and ulcers. A hiatal hernia, which is a structural problem where the stomach contents regurgitate into the esophagus, causing a burning sensation, can also be mistaken for indigestion. Acids normally do not burn the stomach because of its protective coating of mucus; however, they cause burning in the esophagus because it does not have a coated surface. Stress is another factor that can lead to indigestion. Strong emotions can result in secretion of certain hormones and enzymes that may cause distress in the stomach.

For treating dairy and milk intolerance, using Lactaid or avoiding dairy products completely is important. Medications can also produce too much acid, leading to indigestion; therefore, a person has to be careful with pain medications such as aspirin and ibuprofen. A person who has a deficiency of pancreatic enzymes will have trouble digesting fatty foods. Certain supplements are known to help indigestion.

The homeopathic remedies listed here can help treat indigestion. Because of the many different types of indigestion, it is important to read each remedy carefully, since some are more associated with heartburn, some with gastritis, and others with flatulence.

Anacardium. Most useful when indigestion is relieved after eating, although symptoms then tend to return with increased intensity and force the person to eat again (similar to *Petroleum* and *Graphites*). An empty, sinking feeling in the stomach comes on about two hours after eating. The person may choke when eating or drinking, and may swallow food and drink hastily. The person is hungry most of the time, and eating temporarily relieves the hunger. This remedy is also helpful for dull stomach pain that extends to the spine and is accompanied by fullness and abdominal distention. For the gas buildup, the person must pound the back to relieve the gas. There is great urging to have a stool, but the desire disappears when the person tries to move the bowels. Symptoms generally get worse at night. There may be hypochondriacal symptoms and, emotionally, the person may experience confusion, loss of memory, absentmindedness, and a lack of self-confidence. There can be outbursts of anger and swearing, especially when the person is offended. Indigestion and gastric symptoms are often caused by excessive studying or worrying.

Antimonium crud. Useful when the person has eaten too much and overloaded the stomach, especially with foods such as bread, pastry, acidic foods, and sour wine. There is constant belching and bloating after eating. Eructations taste like the food that was eaten. A considerable amount of heartburn, nausea, and vomiting are experienced, especially after eating pickles and sour foods, which, ironically, are the things the person craves. *Antimonium crud* is generally associated with a white, thickly coated tongue. This is an important remedy when newborns and infants vomit up breast milk in curds and refuse to nurse afterward and are irritable. Older children or adults with this type of indigestion are often irritable, contradictory, sulky, and cannot bear to be looked at or touched. They are angry at every attention given to them, preferring to be alone and not bothered.

Antimonium tart. Helpful for excessive nausea, retching, and vomiting experienced after eating; these symptoms are followed by faintness. Nausea produces anxiety and fear, causing pressure in the chest area. This is followed by a headache with yawning, watery eyes, and vomiting. The person tends to vomit, and the only position that provides relief is lying on the right side. There is often a thirst for cold water, but the person drinks only a little. There is also a desire for apples, other fruits, and acidic foods. There is a pasty, thick, white-coated tongue. Children who need this remedy are often whiny, especially when picked up or touched. *Antimonium tart* may be associated with a rattling cough and an inability to expectorate the mucus.

Argentum nit. Helpful for stomach pain that gets worse after eating. Stomach pain gnaws and burns the pit of the stomach and radiates in every direction. Applying light pressure causes stomach pain to get worse, as does eating; this pain may be relieved by applying hard pressure and bending over double. The pain increases and decreases gradually, and there may be the sensation of a lump in the stomach and spasmodic muscles in the lower chest around the stomach. There is often a craving for sugar and sweets, although sweets tend to aggravate the condition and may increase the pain. The person desires cheese and salty foods. Stomach pain is often experienced from loss of sleep and worry (such as anticipating taking a test or giving a speech) and by women with menstrual problems. The other important symptom with *Argentum nit* is excessive flatulence, which sometimes causes the stomach to reach an enormous size. Because the person may be unable to belch for a long time, belches are violent and extreme but tend to provide relief.

Arsenicum alb. Useful for burning pain in the pit of the stomach soon after eating; this pain is relieved by warm drinks. Anxiety is felt in the pit of the stomach and is accompanied by pacing and agitation. The person experiences nausea, retching, and vomiting after eating or drinking. Dyspepsia is caused by many foods, such as vinegar, acidic foods, ice cream, ice water, vegetables, watery fruits, melons, and tobacco. The person may crave milk, which helps relieve the burning in the stomach. Excessive heartburn makes the throat raw and is relieved by warm drinks. *Arsenicum alb* is associated with extreme thirst, and the person drinks often but only a little at a time. There also may be an intolerance to the sight or smell of food when nausea is great. In general, the *Arsenicum alb* person is fearful, anxious, often short of breath when having stomach problems, faint, cold, and exhausted and restless at the same time.

Bryonia. Useful for pain and pressure in the pit of the stomach. Pain is sharp and cutting and extends to the shoulders and back. Stomach pain comes on soon after eating food, which seems to lie like a stone in the stomach. The person vomits bile and water immediately after eating. Stomach discomfort gets worse from the least pressure and movement, and the person feels better while lying still. There is nausea and faintness when sitting up. Vomiting occurs immediately after eating or drinking, and a burning sensation in the stomach extends to the throat, especially when the person belches. The lips are dry and parched, and there is excessive thirst for large amounts of water, yet the person drinks infrequently. Cold drinks are preferred because warm drinks are often vomited. These gastric symptoms often get worse during the summer heat. The person is irritable and often wants to be left alone.

Calcarea carb. Helpful for pain in the middle abdomen and the pit of the stomach. *Calcarea carb* is associated with sour belching and sour-tasting vomit. There is also a sense of pressure as of a weight in the stomach. The person experiences a loss of appetite but enjoys eating, and there can be ravenous hunger in the morning. Tight clothing around the waist is not tolerated. There is craving for eggs, salt, sweets, and sometimes indigestible nonfoods such as chalk, coal, or pencils (this is often seen in children and babies). There is usually an aversion to meat and boiled foods. Milk and fatty foods cause discomfort.

Carbo veg. Helpful for extreme abdominal distention, especially in the upper abdomen. The person feels the sensation when eating or drinking that the stomach and abdomen will burst; belching temporarily relieves this distention and discomfort. The gas presses upward. Belching and eructations are rancid, sour, and putrid tasting. There may be burning in the stomach that extends to the back and along the spine. Abdominal distress comes on about thirty minutes after eating, and cramping pains force the person to double over. Digestion is slow, and food seems to putrefy before it digests; the simplest foods, especially meat and fat, cause discomfort. This is an important remedy, along with *Arsenicum alb,* for the ill effects of eating tainted or bad meat. There is an aversion to milk, meat, and fatty foods. Abdominal distention is so extreme that it sometimes causes asthma because of pressure on the lungs; the asthma gets worse from motion, when sitting up, and from 4:00 to 6:00 P.M. *Carbo veg* is useful for elderly people who are tired, weak, cold, and have a blue tint to the skin. Despite feeling cold, they want to be fanned because they feel they do not get enough oxygen. Stomach pain is burning, and flatulence is located in the upper abdominal area (compared to *Lycopodium*, where extreme flatulence is located in the lower intestinal area). There is heaviness, fullness, and sleepiness after eating (similar to *Lycopodium*). Flatulence and indigestion get worse from fat, fish, oysters, ice cream, vinegar, or cabbage. Coffee causes discomfort, and milk increases flatulence. Another difference between *Carbo veg* and *Lycopodium* is that in *Carbo veg* there is a tendency toward diarrhea, while in *Lycopodium* there is usually constipation. Compared with *Nux vomica*, *Carbo veg* has a more upward pressure of gas, while *Nux vomica* has a more downward pressure of gas on the intestines.

Causticum. Useful when acid regurgitates from the stomach into the throat. The person feels as though a caustic material (such as lime) is burning the stomach; this sensation gets worse after eating fresh meat (although smoked meat agrees with the person). There may be an aversion to sweets and a greasy taste in the mouth.

Chamomilla. Useful for abdominal cramping and increased gas buildup in the abdomen; these symptoms come on after anger. *Chamomilla* is useful for babies who are teething. Eructations are irritating, acidic, and taste bitter. Stomach pain feels as though stones are lying in the stomach. In adults, there is nausea after coffee, sweating after eating or drinking, and an aversion to warm drinks. Babies have red cheeks, increased perspiration, irritability, and act angry.

China. Helpful for extreme abdominal distention. There is a sensation of fullness after eating only a few mouthfuls of food. The distention is painful, and belching does not provide relief. The person has sour or bitter eructations, and may also pass offensive-smelling gas. There is a sensation that food is lodged in the back of the esophagus, behind the sternum. Digestion is extremely slow, and food remains in the stomach for a long time; this symptom is particularly worse after eating a meal at night. Abdominal pain and distention occur from drinking tea to excess; milk is also disagreeable. While there is no appetite, the person often feels hungry. After eating, food remains undigested for a long time and causes eructations until the undigested food is vomited. There is very little burning with the rancid belching, which distinguishes this remedy from *Carbo veg.*

Colchicum. Useful when the smell or thought of food causes nausea, even to the point of fainting. The person craves various foods, but the smell of food is nauseating. Stomach pain, flatulence, and vomiting of mucus, bile, and food are experienced. These symptoms get worse with any motion.

Graphites. Helpful when burning, cramping pains in the stomach and upper intestines are relieved by eating (similar to *Anacardium* and *Petroleum*). The stomach and bowels are distended, causing the person to loosen the clothing (similar to *Lycopodium, Carbo veg, Nux vomica,* and *China*). There is a burning sensation in the stomach area and putrid eructations (similar to *Carbo veg*). Hot drinks cause discomfort, and sweets cause nausea and disgust. There may be a rush of blood to the head after eating and a disagreeable taste in the morning as though the person has eaten rotten eggs. There is an aversion to meat (similar to *China*). The gas that the *Graphites* person passes smells rancid or putrid, which distinguishes this remedy from *Lycopodium,* which has odorless gas. People who need *Graphites* are almost always constipated, and may be chilly, overweight, have flabby muscles, and have rashes (such as eczema) that ooze a sticky substance.

Hydrastis. Helpful for gastric uneasiness and dull, aching stomach pain. The person has a loss of appetite, constipation, and depression. The tongue is clean at the sides and tip, but is coated yellow down the center. Digestion is weak, and there may be a bitter taste in the mouth. The person cannot eat bread or vegetables without experiencing stomach distress. Often, there is thick, yellow, sticky mucus that the person has swallowed, which causes nausea and vomiting.

Ignatia. Useful for stomach problems that come on after grief or other stressful occurrences. A sinking feeling in the stomach is relieved by taking a deep breath. Sighing seems to help the person feel better. There are sour eructations and a feeling of emptiness in the stomach. The person may crave acidic foods. Useful for those who overreact to daily circumstances and experience stomach pain that comes on at night or after eating. This pain gets worse from motion or pressure.

Ipecac. Helpful for extreme nausea and for when constant vomiting does not relieve the nausea. The stomach feels too relaxed, as though it were hanging down in the abdominal cavity. Gastric discomfort arises from eating fatty foods, pork, or pastry (similar to *Pulsatilla*). The person vomits all stomach contents, including food, bile, and mucus; the vomit is often bloody. (Note that if there is red or dark blood or black material in the vomit, a physician should be contacted.) The tongue is usually clean and pink, and there is excessive saliva in the mouth.

Iris. Helpful when the entire intestinal tract burns. There is vomiting of sour, bloody stomach contents. (Note that if there is red or dark blood or black material in the vomit, a physician should be contacted.) Indigestion is often accompanied by frontal headaches on the right side that begin with a blur before the eyes or after relaxing from stressful events. Nausea accompanies these headaches, which are often migraine-like. There is profuse saliva in the mouth, similar to *Mercurius sol* and *Ipecac*. (The person who needs *Mercurius sol* smells worse than someone needing *Iris,* and *Ipecac* has more extreme vomiting.)

Kali bich. Helps the person who experiences indigestion after drinking beer. The person feels as if digestion has stopped after eating, and the food feels as if it is lying there like a heavy load.

Kali carb. Useful for indigestion in elderly or weakened people who tend to be exhausted and have backaches and weak legs. *Kali carb* is useful when there has been a long illness (similar to *China* or *Carbo veg*). Anxiety is felt in the pit of the stomach, and there is often a feeling of a lump in the pit of the stomach. Before eating there is a faint, sinking feeling in the middle of the stomach, which is related less to the sensation of hunger and more to nervousness. Sleepiness while eating is common, and after eating the abdomen becomes distended. Everything eaten seems to turn to gas (similar to *Argentum nit*). Putrid belches relieve abdominal discomfort (similar to *Carbo veg*). Most stomach problems are aggravated by coffee or warm soup. The person may desire sugar and sweets. Nausea gets better when the person lies down. There may be a constant feeling that the stomach is full of water. There are sour eructations and vomiting. Ice water can also cause gastric problems.

Kreosote. Useful for stomach distress that comes on three to four hours after eating and results in vomiting. There is a feeling that ice water is in the stomach.

Lycopodium. Helps the person who experiences indigestion that occurs while eating, especially from starchy or fermentable foods (such as cabbage, beans, and certain breads). There is extreme abdominal distention, especially in the lower abdomen. Belching and eructations rise to the back of the throat, causing burning that remains for hours at a time. The abdomen is swollen and distended and is relieved by passing gas, which is generally odorless. The person cannot bear the pressure of clothing around the abdomen when it is bloated (this distinguishes it from *Lachesis,* which does not like tight clothing around the abdomen at any time). Digestion is slow and difficult, and the person is usually sleepy after eating. The accumulation of gas in the intestines is generally lower down, but there is an upward pressure that causes difficulty in breathing (similar to *Carbo veg*). Indigestion and abdominal distention get worse in the late afternoon or evening, especially between 4:00 and 8:00 p.m.; this causes restlessness and insomnia if the gas is not passed before bedtime. Sour belching and sour vomiting are present, and the person is constipated and feels the urge to have a bowel movement, but is unable to (similar to *Nux vomica*). *Lycopodium* may be a good remedy when there are peculiar effects on the appetite. The person is hungry upon eating, but gets full after a few mouthfuls. Extreme hunger is felt immediately after eating a heavy meal, or the person may have no desire for food, but the appetite returns upon eating. There also may be an aversion to solid foods and a desire for liquids. The person may be hungry at night with an empty, sinking feeling.

Magnesia carb. Useful for worn out, tired women with uterine problems, especially those in menopause. Eructations are sour and there is vomiting of bitter water. The person craves meat, fruit, acidic foods, and vegetables.

Natrum mur. Helpful for heartburn accompanied by acid rising from the stomach that occurs after eating, especially during pregnancy. Heartburn is accompanied by heart palpitations, unquenchable thirst, sweating while eating, and a craving for salt. There is an aversion to eating bread, oysters, and fatty foods. These people may brood and hide their feelings, which leads to stomach distress.

Natrum phos. As in all ailments with this remedy, there is an excess of acidity. Sour and acidic fluids rise to the throat from the stomach, and vomiting is sour. The back of the tongue and roof of the mouth have a creamy yellow coating.

*Nux vomica.*One of the most important remedies for indigestion. This type of indigestion is caused by mental overwork, sedentary occupations, and overuse and abuse of stimulants and harmful substances (such as alcohol, coffee, and cigarettes). *Nux vomica* is also useful for those who stay up too late and work too hard. All of these conditions cause crankiness and irritability. The person feels drowsy in the evening and miserable in the morning upon awakening. A dull, frontal headache is a constant symptom in the *Nux vomica* person. When eating (especially dinner), food tastes normal, and the symptoms of indigestion come on about thirty minutes after eating. At this point, there is nausea, vomiting of sour and bitter fluids, and possible dizziness. The stomach region is sensitive to pressure (similar to *Bryonia* and *Arsenicum alb*), and there is the sensation that a stone is lying in the stomach several hours after eating. Indigestion occurs after drinking strong coffee and especially from drinking too much coffee. This is an important remedy for headaches, indigestion, and hangovers. The person tends to desire fatty foods and tolerates them well (*Pulsatilla* is the opposite). As with all *Nux vomica* symptoms, the person feels the urge to pass gas or stool, but is often unsuccessful; this is also true of the urge to belch or vomit.

Petroleum. Helpful for stomach pain and ravenous hunger that is immediately relieved by eating (similar to *Anacardium, Graphites,* and *Sepia*). Indigestion accompanied by diarrhea sometimes indicates this remedy. Cabbage aggravates the indigestion, and there is a strong aversion to fatty foods and meat. The person may feel hungry immediately after a bowel movement. There may be a feeling of great emptiness in the stomach area, and the person is often hungry and sometimes rises from sleep at night to eat.

Phosphorus. Helpful when the stomach is inflamed, with a burning sensation that extends up the throat and down to the bowels. Stomach pain and indigestion are relieved by eating cold foods, but these are vomited up as soon as the food or liquid becomes warm in the stomach. The area where the esophagus empties into the stomach feels contracted and too narrow, and food that is swallowed comes up again. There is sour belching of excessive amounts of gas after eating. Useful when the stomach region is painful to touch and when walking. There is a weak feeling in the stomach around 11:00 A.M. (similar to *Sulphur*), and burning between the shoulder blades. Even small amounts of vomiting can cause bleeding in the stomach. (Note that if there is red or dark blood or black material in the vomit, a physician should be contacted.) The person is hungry at night and often rises from sleep to eat (similar to *Sulphur*).

Pulsatilla. Symptoms helped by this remedy are a putrid taste in the morning upon awakening, a dry mouth without thirst, and the sensation that food is lodged under the sternum. Eructations taste like food the person has eaten; this is particularly true after eating cold foods, fruits, and pastries. There is a feeling of fullness and weight in the stomach one or two hours after eating; this is relieved for a short time by eating again (similar to *Anacardium*). Almost always with indigestion, there are headaches around the eyes that get worse in the evening and from warmth, and are relieved from cool air. The tongue is coated with a thick white or yellow coating, and there is excessive heartburn. The person is sad, weepy, likes consolation, and is apprehensive. While sharing many similarities, the person needing *Pulsatilla* is distinguished from the person needing *Nux vomica* by being worse in the evening, having excessive heartburn, and being weepy and sad; the person needing *Nux vomica* is worse in the morning and after dinner, has less heartburn, and is irritable and domineering. *Pulsatilla* is distinguished from *Ipecac* because it does not have the clean tongue and the intense nausea of that remedy.

Sepia. This remedy is helpful when the person experiences a feeling of emptiness in the pit of the stomach, which is not relieved by eating (this is different from *Anacardium, Phosphorus,* and *Sulphur,* in which the person experiences an empty sensation that always gets better after meals). Nausea is felt from the sight or smell of food. Abdominal pain and increased gas in the liver area are relieved by lying on the right side. There may be nausea in the morning before eating. Burning pain is felt in the pit of the stomach, and acid regurgitates into the mouth. *Sepia* may be useful for indigestion that comes on from too much smoking. There is a craving for vinegar, acidic foods, and pickles, and an aversion and strong dislike of fatty foods. Indigestion gets worse from drinking milk, especially boiled milk.

Sulphur. Helpful for excessive acidity, sour belching, and burning in the stomach. There is weight and pressure in the stomach. Weakness and faintness are experienced around 11:00 A.M., at which time the person must eat. There can be a complete loss of, or an excessive, appetite. The person is often more interested in drinking than eating. There may be a desire for sweets, which cause indigestion, a sour stomach, and heartburn (*Argentum nit* also has cravings for sweets, which cause diarrhea). The person who needs *Sulphur* also craves alcohol and milk; ironically, milk increases stomach acidity and causes vomiting rather than eases the burning, as dairy products usually do for gastritis and indigestion. There is a dislike of meat, and food sometimes tastes too salty. When hunger increases, the person can hardly wait for meals and gets up during the night to eat (similar to *Phosphorus*), but does not feel well and becomes bloated after eating. The general *Sulphur* characteristics are usually present with this type of indigestion, which may include hot flashes, cold feet with a hot head, early morning diarrhea, itching, an aversion to washing and bathing, irritability, and an unkempt appearance.

Tabacum. Useful for incessant nausea that gets worse from the smell of tobacco smoke (similar to *Phosphorus*). The least movement causes vomiting. Seasickness causes faintness and a sinking feeling in the pit of the stomach; this is followed by vomiting. The person feels wretched, despondent, depressed because of extreme nausea and vomiting, is pale and icy cold with sweats, and has an irregular pulse. There is vomiting during pregnancy with excessive spitting. Symptoms get worse when riding in a car, airplane, or boat. Stomach pain extends up to the left arm, and there is also a sense of relaxation of the stomach with nausea (similar to *Ipecac*).

Thuja. Helpful for loss of appetite and an inability to digest certain foods. Rancid eructations are experienced after eating fatty foods, and the person feels sick after eating onions. There is often indigestion from drinking tea and a dislike of meat and potatoes. There is the sensation that something is alive in the abdomen, but there is no pain with this feeling. Flatulence and distention cause the abdomen to protrude in different parts of the abdomen, and this seems to move to different areas, causing the sensation that something is alive in the intestinal area.

INFLUENZA (ALSO CALLED FLU)

Influenza has caused many serious epidemics worldwide. Vaccines are typically 70 percent effective each season, and are recommended for people who are older than 65 or who have a chronic illness, such as diabetes, respiratory problems, or cancer. Influenza is generally most severe in the elderly; however, in 1918, during a major epidemic, the highest fatality rate was among young adults. Reye's syndrome is a complication of influenza, especially in children who take aspirin for the fever.

The symptoms of this viral illness are generally in the respiratory tract and are characterized by a fever, headache, nasal discharge, sore throat, cough, muscle pains, and weakness. The cough can be severe and protracted, but generally the other symptoms are limited and the person recovers in two to seven days. Gastrointestinal tract symptoms such as nausea, vomiting, and diarrhea may also occur.

There are two types of influenza: type A and type B. Tamiflu® is a prescription medicine for type A influenza (but not for type B), and may help prevent symptoms after the person has been exposed and does not have time to get immunized. It can also be used to treat influenza if given early during the illness. Consult a physician or pharmacist for further information.

The mode of transmission for influenza is by airborne particles, especially after coughing and sneezing, that spread among crowded populations in close spaces. Transmission also occurs by direct contact with droplets that have fallen to surfaces. The incubation period is usually short, from one to five days, and the period of communicability is usually three to five days before the fever begins.

Homeopathic remedies have been used for many years to help influenza sufferers.

Aconite. Sometimes useful in the very early stages of influenza, especially as symptoms come on after exposure to cold, dry weather or to winds or drafts. There may be initial bouts of sneezing, and the person may feel chilly followed by a fever. The nose is often dry and stuffy, and the person is often thirsty. The person is agitated and fears getting very sick. *Aconite* must be used very quickly in the first three hours of the initial symptoms, after which it will not help.

Allium cepa. The nose is sore from burning discharge and becomes worse in a warm room. The eyes water profusely, but the fluid does not irritate the cheeks below. There is excessive sneezing, and the throat and larynx feel raw.

Arsenicum alb. A helpful remedy for the flu that was also used for many flu epidemics in the past. The eyes, nose, and throat burn. A thin, watery nasal discharge makes the upper lip sore. The person is restless and feels chilly. The sore throat that accompanies this type of flu is burning and is relieved by sips of warm water. The person, however, may also want to drink large amounts of cold water. Restlessness may be experienced, and the person paces the floor. This is accompanied by a feeling of extreme weakness. There is general aggravation from midnight until 2:00 or 3:00 A.M.

Baptisia. Useful for a rapid onset of influenza that is accompanied by great weakness and prostration. Confusion, delirium, and often disassociation are present, and the person sometimes feels as if he or she is not one person but two people. The person is restless and tosses about. There is muscle soreness, and putrid smells emanate from the mouth along with other bodily secretions (such as perspiration). The head feels large, numb, and heavy. The face appears mottled with a dark red appearance. The person has a very sick look, almost to the point of being septic with a high fever. This remedy is particularly helpful when influenza takes on a gastrointestinal form accompanied by putrid diarrhea and increased amounts of offensive-smelling stools.

Belladonna. Useful for sudden onset of fever that rises quickly. The face is red, hot, and flushed, and the eyes are dilated. The person may be delirious and hypersensitive and have a throbbing headache. Any kind of noise, touch, or light is disliked. Fever is accompanied by lack of thirst and, at times, the person perspires profusely only to become red, hot, and dry again. Useful in the very early stages after *Aconite* for influenza.

Bryonia. Helpful when the person does not want to move because any type of movement hurts the limbs and back. The body feels extremely weak, and the person wants to lie on the painful area. The person is irritable and does not want to be bothered. Conditions are better when the person remains still, but are extremely irritated otherwise. A bursting, splitting headache gets worse with any motion. The person has a thirst for excessive amounts of cold water, and all the mucous membranes are dry. A cough is present, and pains in the chest have a stitching or tearing feeling. The lips are dry and cracked. There may be excessive thirst. The joints may become sore, tender, and stiff. The person feels worse from any motion and better with rest. There may be constipation.

Dulcamara. Useful when influenza comes on after exposure to cold, damp weather in the late summer and early fall, especially after being outdoors for an extended amount of time or after sitting on damp ground. The throat is sore, and coughing hurts due to sore muscles in the chest wall. The eyes and nose drain excessive amounts of clear, watery fluid.

Eupatorium perf. Helpful for extreme aching in the bones. (*Eupatorium perf* is often referred to as Boneset because of its usefulness for this problem.) The eyeballs are sore. There is pain in the back of the head when lying down, accompanied by a sense of great weight. A hoarse cough is accompanied by soreness in the chest. The bed feels hard and uncomfortable, and the person is restless.

The back and legs feel as though the bones will break. These symptoms often come on in warm, mild weather. The soreness in the skin and aching in the bones tend to be relieved by perspiring, although the headache is not relieved. There is a characteristic chill between 7:00 and 9:00 A.M., preceded by thirst and aching in the bones.

Ferrum phos. Useful when the onset of influenza is gradual and the fever is not yet high. The skin is moist, and the face alternates between being pale and being flushed. The person is congested, and the skin looks inflamed. There may be nosebleeds, a feeling of fullness and aching in the ear, and a mild cough. There are very few mental symptoms associated with this remedy.

Gelsemium. Useful for the gradual onset of influenza with symptoms of chills, aching, extreme weakness, and fever. The person feels tired and aches in all the muscles. Heat is desired. A hard, painful cough is present. A general feeling of apathy and a curious lack of anxiety and fear are experienced with this remedy. The eyelids are heavy, sneezing is accompanied by burning discharges from the nose, and there is extreme weakness. Apathy and indifference to the condition are characteristic, and the person lies quietly with drooping eyelids trying to sleep. The person is not thirsty, and the face is flushed.

Hepar sulph. Useful when nasal discharge becomes thick, green, or yellow, signaling a bacterial infection that may complicate the flu. (Any person with yellow or green infected-looking discharges should be evaluated by a physician.) The person feels extremely cold, especially on the back of the neck, and tends to cover the neck. Pains (as stitches) run from the throat to the ear when swallowing. The person is irritable, nasty, sensitive to pain, and may perspire often. Symptoms may be brought on by cold, dry, and windy weather.

Mercurius sol. Usually helpful when influenza is accompanied by a bacterial infection. (Any person with yellow or green infected-looking discharges should be evaluated by a physician.) Pus accumulates in the throat and tonsils. A foul smell comes from the mouth, and perspiration is heavy and foul-smelling. The person feels worse at night, and there is often much nasal discharge and sneezing. The tongue is thickly coated and feels flabby. Teeth imprints can be seen on the sides of the tongue.

Nux vomica. Helpful when the person is irritable and sensitive to any kind of disturbance, noise, or odor. The person is chilly and feels worse from exposure to cold or open air. Conditions are better when the person is warm and lying down. The person is particularly affected at 3:00 A.M. and often cannot sleep until morning. Nighttime stuffiness may be accompanied by a sore throat, and pain stitches travel from the throat to the ear when swallowing. The person has a fever (the face is especially warm), but cannot move or uncover without feeling a chill. Sudden chills, shivers, and muscle aches may appear after exposure to east or northeast winds.

Phosphorus. Often useful in influenza epidemics, and especially for excessive coughing. There is a tickling, dry cough and tightness in the chest. Complete laryngitis or hoarseness and general weakness of the entire body are common.

Pulsatilla. Useful for influenza that often begins from getting the feet wet. The person experiences the feeling that cold water is being poured over the back, and chills run up and down the spine. Yellow, non-irritating nasal discharge is excessive. There may be a fluid discharge from the eyes. The person is weepy and desires company and consolation. The person is chilly, yet wants to be outside in the cool air. There is a lack of thirst, and the person feels worse in the evening.

Rhus tox. Useful when the person experiences restlessness and wants to keep moving. These symptoms often come on after exposure to cold, wet weather. Aching muscles and joints improve when warmth is applied and are worse with cold.

Sticta. Useful in the later stages of influenza, especially for a barking cough that gets worse at night and in the morning. Postnasal discharge causes irritation of the throat leading to a cough. There is dull, heavy pressure and a feeling of fullness at the root of the nose. The person feels like blowing the nose, which does not provide much relief, and little discharge is produced.

INSOMNIA (INCLUDES SLEEP DISTURBANCES)

Insomnia is a very common problem—up to one-third of Americans suffer from it. The two basic types of insomnia are difficulty falling asleep and frequent or early awakening.

Causes of insomnia are varied. Medications such as beta-blockers, oral contraceptives, and thyroid medicines can be the cause; caffeine in any form, such as chocolate, coffee, and tea, can also cause insomnia. Alcohol or any recreational drugs, such as marijuana, can also contribute to insomnia. Other causes of sleep loss are anxiety, stress, and dwelling on problems or events of the day. Pain in any form can also be a contributor. Depression is another cause, as are hyperglycemia, sleep apnea, and nocturnal cramping or movements of the legs. The fear of insomnia and preoccupation with loss of sleep will actually keep the person up longer.

One natural method to induce sleep is to avoid eating too close to bedtime, since this can lead to episodes of hyperglycemia, causing the person to awaken during sleep. Exercising in the morning, late afternoon, or early evening can be helpful in improving the sleep quality and general well-being of the person. Exercising right before bed should be avoided because it stimulates the nervous and cardiovascular systems. Avoiding anxiety-producing situations before bed, such as watching scary movies and reading books that may agitate a person, can help avoid potential problems. Avoiding naps late in the day or early evening is important, because they can cause a person to be awake too late into the night. It is important to develop regular sleep habits, such as going to bed at the same time and getting up with regularity. Stress management techniques, rest and relaxation techniques, and breathing exercises can also help the person relax so it is easier to fall asleep. Certain herbs, supplements, and vitamins are known to help insomnia.

Over-the-counter sedatives and prescription medications are commonly used to treat insomnia. Consult a physician or pharmacist for further information. Homeopathy has long been useful for people who have problems with insomnia. The homeopathic remedies listed here can be useful if the symptoms are matched carefully.

Aconite. Insomnia is often associated with the first stages of a fever or inflammation. The person is sleepless with restlessness and tossing about. If this insomnia occurs in children, the child wakes up feeling fearful, anxious, and restless. Fear of death may be present. When sleep occurs, the person is extremely restless. Talking in the sleep and muscular jerking interrupt sleep.

Aloe. With this type of insomnia, the person wakes at 5:00 A.M. with a sudden urge to have a bowel movement, usually diarrhea.

Antimonium crud. May be helpful in treating continual drowsiness in the elderly.

Apis. Helpful for the person who screams and is startled suddenly during sleep.

Argentum nit. The person is sleepless from an overactive imagination. The person is fearful of something serious happening, and worries about being overcome with an impulse toward self-injury, such as jumping out of a window. Fantasizing before falling asleep is a common characteristic.

Arnica. The person is sleepless and restless from being overtired or overexerted. The entire body feels sore. Great drowsiness and an inability to fall asleep until 2:00 or 3:00 A.M. is common. The person may even fall asleep while answering questions.

Arsenicum alb. Useful when the person wakes up short of breath with asthma or other respiratory problems and is very restless. The person must have the head raised by pillows and sleeps with the hands over the head. Lying on the left side causes problems. The person must often sleep sitting up, especially if respiratory problems are present. The person sleeps deeply after a chill from a fever. Sleeplessness until about 3:00 A.M. that is associated with great anxiety and burning in the veins is common. The person is sleepless from being overtired or from perspiring after shock.

Baptisia. The person fears sleep because nightmares and a sense of suffocation may occur. Sleeplessness and restlessness are present. The body feels broken or doubled over, and the person tosses about trying to put the pieces back together. The person seems delirious, with wandering thoughts and muttering. An unusual symptom is that the person falls asleep while answering a question.

Baryta carb. One of the most important remedies for sleeplessness in elderly people. A sensation of internal heat interrupts sleep.

Belladonna. One of the most important remedies for difficulty sleeping due to fever and headaches. Frightful images often appear just as the person tries to fall asleep, causing a dread of sleep. Throbbing in the head prevents sleep. This remedy is also very useful in treating the restless sleep of teething babies. The child sleeps with the eyes partially open, twitches, and startles easily. Sleep is extremely restless and is interrupted by muscular jerking and spasmodic motions. The person grinds the teeth and has a hot head and dilated pupils. Dreams cause the person to wake up from sleep. Sleeplessness with drowsiness is an unusual characteristic. The person startles when closing the eyes or during sleep. Another unusual characteristic is that the person yawns while coughing. The person may sleep with the hands under the head.

Borax. The affected person, especially if a child, cries out during sleep as if frightened. Sleeplessness occurs most often between 3:00 and 5:00 A.M. because of a feeling of heat, especially in the head. The person cannot sleep on the right side.

Bryonia. One of the most useful remedies when business problems and everyday worries keep a person awake at night. The person tends to think a lot about what was just read. Unusual symptoms include sleepiness when alone and yawning before dinner.

Calcarea carb. Especially useful for insomnia in women. Ideas crowd the mind, preventing sleep. The person startles at every noise and has an irrational fear of going crazy. The person experiences heart palpitations and fears heart disease when trying to go to sleep. Unpleasant ideas arouse the person from a light sleep. There is frequent night waking. The person tends to fall asleep before noon and is sleepy after supper. Sleeplessness occurs at 3:00 A.M. The person may find it difficult to wake up in the morning because of a restless sleep.

Calcarea phos. The person sleeps on the abdomen or knees, with the face forced into a pillow. Waking in the morning is difficult. The person is sleepy during dinner.

Carbo veg. The feet are cold, causing sleeplessness. Coldness in the limbs causes the person to wake from sleep.

Causticum. The person often yawns at night and when listening to conversations of other people. Waking up at 2:00 A.M. is common. Anxiety causes sleeplessness.

Chamomilla. Useful for treating sleeplessness due to severe pain in children, especially teething infants. The child is drowsy, and moans and weeps during sleep. *Chamomilla* is also helpful for treating insomnia of a nervous person who suffers from hypersensitivity to pain. The person sleeps with the limbs either drawn to the body or spread apart. Lying down is sometimes impossible.

China. Useful for treating sleeplessness associated with much bleeding or loss of fluids, such as from diarrhea. The affected person is worried and has an overactive mind. Dreams are anxious and frightful. The person wakes up with a confused consciousness; the fear of the dream remains. Snoring, especially in children, is another characteristic. Sleeplessness can also result from hunger, especially after bouts of diarrhea. Sleep is restless before a chill when a person has a fever.

Cina. This type of insomnia is characterized by night terrors in children, who cry out and wake up frightened. It is helpful for children with pinworms who cannot sleep due to itching of the rectum. Screaming and talking during sleep are common characteristics. The child grinds the teeth and tends to yawn a lot. The child may get on the hands and knees and sleep face down. The child is sleepless unless rocked or kept in constant motion.

Cocculus. One of the most important remedies for treating the insomnia of a person who watches over or nurses someone who is sick, in a coma, or dying. The person yawns a lot and is very drowsy because of lack of sleep, especially after lying down and in the morning. Lying on the left side is difficult.

Coffea. An important remedy for sleeplessness. The person is wide awake, and the senses are extremely active and acute (as though just after a cup of coffee). Insomnia is brought on by excitement or good news. Great mental activity and the flow of ideas with nervous excitability causes sleeplessness. Sleep also can be disturbed by itching of the anus. If the person does fall asleep, he or she often wakes up around 3:00 A.M.; then the person dozes on and off. This remedy is also useful for the sleeplessness of a person who nurses the sick. High potencies of this remedy are needed for insomnia. Note that high-potency remedies are not recommended for home prescribing. Consult a physician or skilled homeopathic consultant for potencies above 30c.

Cuprum met. The person wakes with cramps in the calves and soles of the feet. During sleep, the abdomen may rumble. A feeling of fright may rouse the person from sleep.

Gelsemium. One of the more important remedies for people who do a lot of mental work, such as a business person. The affected person passes many restless nights and wakes early in the morning to worry about business matters. This is similar to *Bryonia,* though it is more associated with being thirsty and there is more irritability if disturbed. The person tends to worry about upcoming events, such as giving a speech or flying in an airplane. The person cannot sleep fully and the insomnia gets worse with exhaustion. Smoking tobacco can also lead to insomnia. Itching may cause sleeplessness. Sleepiness is seen in students who have stayed up late to study and cannot stay awake any longer, although the student may wish to. When the person is sick with the flu or another upper respiratory infection, the body aches. The person is lethargic and sleeps during the day, but is up at night full of worries, cares, and thoughts of the coming day.

Graphites. The person is sleepy at noon after eating. The same idea is repeated in the mind constantly, causing sleeplessness. The person tends to be overweight, constipated, and have dry skin or eczema.

Ignatia. This type of sleeplessness occurs from grief, depression, and general cares and worries. The person yawns constantly. The limbs jerk and the person may sigh while falling asleep. When the person does fall asleep, the sleep is very light. Troubling dreams continue for a long time. Hunger causes sleeplessness; coughing causes sleepiness.

Kali carb. The person wakes up at 2:00 or 3:00 A.M. and cannot sleep again. The person tends to fall asleep after the least amount of mental activity. Sleepiness occurs during eating, especially at dinner. Sleepiness also occurs during the menstrual period. Twitching legs accompany sleeplessness.

Kreosote. Sleep is disturbed by tossing about. A sensation of paralysis in the legs is felt when waking up. Sleepiness occurs with a cough followed by yawning.

Lachesis. The person always feels worse physically and emotionally after sleep. This includes waking from naps or waking in the morning. There is sudden startling when falling asleep. The person is sleepy but cannot sleep. In the evening, the person is wide awake. After a night of sleeplessness, the morning sleep tends to be quite heavy. Excitement causes sleeplessness. The person usually sleeps on the right side, since sleeping on the left side is impossible.

Lycopodium. The person is drowsy during the day and tends to startle when sleeping. The person may fall asleep during sex. There is a tendency to wake up at 4:00 A.M. Mental stimulation causes sleeplessness. Hunger causes the person to wake up. The person yawns after dinner. Sometimes the person wants to yawn but cannot. Generally, the most comfortable sleeping positions are either on the right side or on the knees with the face forced into a pillow.

Magnesia carb. This type of insomnia is characterized by an unrefreshing sleep. The person is more tired after waking up than when going to bed. Falling asleep after dinner, especially when standing or talking, is an unusual symptom. Generally the person is sleepy while talking. Sleeplessness occurs after 2:00 or 3:00 A.M. Sleeplessness is accompanied by uneasiness, anxiety, and a sensation of heat. The person must uncover, which causes chilliness.

Mercurius sol. The person is sleepless from itching and excessive perspiration from before midnight until 3:00 A.M. Dreams and heart palpitations cause the person to wake up. (Note that if palpitations are new and have not been evaluated before, a physician should be consulted.) The person has difficulty sleeping on either side of the body.

Mezereum. Sleeplessness is caused from itching and being too cold.

Natrum mur. The person is sleepless from grief, especially because of past events rather than recent events. Great worry and brooding over past events keep the person awake at night. Heart palpitations from disappointment and shock cause sleeplessness. (Note that if palpitations are new and have not been evaluated before, a physician should be consulted.) The person tends to fall asleep while reading, especially when sitting down. Sleepiness occurs in the evening at 6:00 p.m., during a chill, and after dinner. The person frequently wakes from sleep feeling frightened and worried.

Nux vomica. An extremely important remedy for sleeplessness and sleep disorders, especially for those who drink too much alcohol, abuse coffee and cigarettes, and are overworked, especially at night.

People who need this remedy are often bothered by stomach or abdominal problems such as flatulence, indigestion, or belching. In general, the person feels sleepy in the early evening and cannot stay awake; however, this sleep is not sound or restful and the person wakes up after 3:00 A.M. At that time, the person feels somewhat refreshed, but soon falls back to sleep and wakes up at the usual time feeling worse than ever. The person tends to be drowsy after meals and better after a short nap. If aroused from a nap, the person may be irritable. Sleep can also be disturbed by frightening visions. The person tends to be sleepy after abdominal problems such as diarrhea. Sleeplessness results from too much mental strain, from the slightest noise, and after abusing wine. Sleepiness is overpowering after eating, especially after dinner. The person yawns a lot after rising in the morning.

Phosphorus. This type of insomnia is characterized by sleepiness that follows intense mental activity and overwork. These people tend to get scattered, spacey, and have difficulty focusing. The sleepiness occurs with anxiety, confusion, headaches, and vertigo. The person feels great drowsiness, especially after meals. Sleeplessness is especially common in older people. The person goes to sleep late and wakes up feeling weak. There is a tendency to take short naps during the day. The person feels sleepy during and after eating. Cold feet, hunger, and mental shocks cause sleeplessness. For women, sleepiness during the menstrual period is common.

Pulsatilla. The person is sleepless in the evening and tends to fall asleep very late at night. Sleep is restless and the person wakes up frequently. Medication, tea, and even iron supplements can cause sleeplessness. Sleep position is important; the person tends to sleep on the back with the hands over and under the head or with the limbs (especially the legs) stretched out.

Rhus tox. The person is extremely restless and sleepless before midnight. Changing positions constantly and moving from bed to bed in the house is common. Itching may also cause sleeplessness. Once the person does sleep, it is very heavy.

Sepia. Sleeplessness occurs after 3:00 A.M. The person yawns without feeling sleepy. Yawning also occurs during a chill. Sometimes the person sleeps on the knees with the face forced into a pillow.

Silica. Sleeplessness is associated with heat in the head, and occurs during the full moon. The body pulsates, particularly in the abdomen, causing insomnia. The person tends to be most sleepless after midnight, especially after 2:00 A.M. The person may sleepwalk.

Staphysagria. Sleeplessness occurs after a person has been embarrassed or has repressed angry feelings. The person stays up late dwelling on these feelings. Sleeplessness can also occur when the person is thinking about and dwelling on sexual issues.

Sulphur. The person is drowsy during the day but sleepless at night (particularly between 2:00 and 5:00 A.M.). The person takes cat naps, sleeping for short periods of time and waking frequently during the day. The person is particularly tired around 11:00 A.M. Sleeplessness often accompanies nervous excitement, itchy skin, and an overheated feeling. The feet are often hot and sweaty, and the person likes to stick them out of the bedcovers at night. When sleeping, the person tends to talk, jerk, and twitch. The person may wake up singing. At 5:00 A.M., the person wakes up with an urge to have a bowel movement. There is sleepiness after eating, during the menstrual period, after a stool, and after walking in the open air.

Thuja. Sleeplessness occurs after 3:00 A.M. Sleep is disturbed by unpleasant visions after closing the eyes.

Zincum met. Extremely restless legs at night prevent sleep. While asleep, the person cries out and the body jerks and moves nervously. Often the person screams out at night without waking. Sleepwalking is a characteristic of this type of insomnia. The person wakes in a frightened state.

JOINT PAIN (INCLUDES ARTHRITIS AND RHEUMATISM)

Joint problems have many different causes. Pain can originate from the joint, or the ligaments, tendons, or muscles that surround it. The most common causes of joint pains are osteoarthritis, osteoporosis, rheumatoid arthritis, injury, weakness of the supporting structures around the joints, viral illnesses, gout, and collagen vascular diseases such as ankylosing spondylitis or lupus.

Osteoarthritis, or degenerative joint disease, is probably the most common source of joint pain. It is usually seen in people over the age of fifty. It is more common in women than in men due to the loss of estrogen after menopause, which causes a disruption in calcium metabolism.

Weight-bearing joints and hand joints are the most affected by the degenerative changes seen in osteoarthritis. Calcium absorption problems are followed by bone spur formation in the joint's margins. This can lead to pain, deformity, and a limit to the joint's ability to move properly. As aging occurs, there is a decrease in the ability to restore normal collagen tissues associated with the joints.

Besides normal wear and tear on the joints that occurs through aging, other factors can lead to osteoarthritis; these include congenital problems in the joints, repeated trauma, weight on the joints, and other inflammatory diseases such as rheumatoid arthritis or gout.

Pain with osteoarthritis is associated with joint stiffness in the morning, which is worse with high levels of activity and relieved by rest. There are usually no signs of redness or inflammation. Limitation of the use of the joints involved, such as the hand, knee, or hip, can occur.

People sometimes recognize that refined sugar can cause joint pain, so it is important to eat high-fiber diets. Some people find that eliminating nitrate-rich foods, such as potatoes, tomatoes, eggplants, peppers, and tobacco, is beneficial. Swimming and other forms of isometric exercise are important. Heat therapy and physical therapy can also be helpful.

Osteoporosis is another source of joint pain. Osteoporosis is a weakening and thinning of the bone due to low calcium absorption from the bloodstream. This generally occurs in women, especially after menopause. Joint pain, back pain, and fractures of the hip and vertebrae are sometimes seen with severe osteoporosis.

Bone loss prevention is possible by natural methods. Because vegetarians tend to have fewer problems with osteoporosis, it would seem that a diet low in protein and phosphates is helpful in decreasing the amount of bone loss. High-protein diets, especially in people who eat a lot of meat, are associated with increased amounts of calcium excreted in the urine. Sugar intake also causes an increase in urinary excretion of calcium; therefore, it is important to avoid sugar. Exercise is extremely important in osteoporosis because it helps take calcium from the bloodstream to the cells. Walking is a good exercise because it is easy on the joints, yet mobilizes calcium into the bone.

Rheumatoid arthritis is a chronic inflammatory disease that affects the entire body, especially the synovial membranes. The most commonly affected joints are the hands, feet, wrists, ankles, and knees. It is more common in women and usually starts between the ages of twenty and forty-five. Juvenile rheumatoid arthritis, which is seen in children as young as two or three years of age, causes symptoms similar to adult rheumatoid arthritis.

Symptoms of rheumatoid arthritis are fatigue, weakness, joint stiffness, and low-grade fever. This is followed by appearance of red, hot, swollen, and painful joints.

There is evidence that rheumatoid arthritis is an auto-immune disease, where antibodies within a person's body actually attack and destroy the tissues around the joints. The cause of this auto-immune problem is a mystery but speculation includes genetic predisposition, viral illnesses, intense stress, and other lifestyle factors.

Natural approaches can help minimize the symptoms of rheumatoid arthritis and decrease pain. A diet low in animal fat is important to help diminish the problematic effects of rheumatoid arthritis. Vegetarian diets tend to have low levels of arachidonic acid, a fatty acid found only in animal products, which is responsible for the production of prostaglandins. These prostaglandin hormones cause inflammation in the body and contribute to the pain associated with arthritis. Fish from cold water (such as salmon, mackerel, sardines, and herring) are high in another type of fatty acid called EPA, which competes with arachidonic acid for prostaglandin production, causing a reduced inflammation in the body.

It is important to do joint exercises and other weight-bearing exercises to help decrease joint stiffness and contractions. Swimming is an excellent form of exercise because the cool water helps reduce pain when the joints are inflamed. Certain vitamins, oils, supplements, and herbs are known to help with joint pain.

Homeopathy has a rich and important history in the treatment of joint problems and pain. The homeopathic remedies listed here help joint pain associated with arthritis and other inflammatory conditions. Some of the remedies are associated more with rheumatoid arthritis, others with osteoporosis, and others with viral illness or trauma. It is important to note these differences when choosing a remedy.

Aconite. Helps the very early stages of joint pain, especially when the person's problems begin after exposure to cold, dry wind. Joint inflammation is worse at night when the joint is red, swollen, and sensitive to touch. Joint pain is often associated with great fearfulness and anxiety.

Apis. Useful for joint pain accompanied by stinging, soreness, and swelling. The skin around the joint is a rosy, light red color. Joint pain gets better when cold is applied and worse when heat is applied. The joints are stiff and painful when pressure is applied. There may be edema and swelling of the tissues around the joints. This remedy is particularly helpful for stinging pain associated with knee and ankle problems. *Apis* usually does not affect the joint itself, but helps the tissues around the joint, like the synovium, ligaments, and tendons.

Arnica. Useful for joint, muscular, and tendon pain caused by overstretching, overexertion, or an injury. The affected part feels sore and bruised. The person is afraid of being bumped in the sore muscle or joint. There may also be a sprained or dislocated feeling of the affected area. Joint or muscular pain becomes worse when exposed to cold and damp weather, especially when a joint or muscle group is injured or overstressed.

Belladonna. Useful for red, swollen joints often associated with fever. *Belladonna* was useful in the days before antibiotics for the first stages of scarlet fever. In modern times this picture is sometimes seen in acute arthritis associated with viruses. The person experiences tearing pain and stiff joints. The joints are swollen, red, and shiny, and joint pain is worse from touch, the slightest motion, and at night. Pain comes on suddenly and disappears suddenly. Joint pain is often associated with other symptoms of *Belladonna*; these include: mental agitation; a red, hot, and flushed face; dilated pupils; and a lack of thirst.

Bryonia. Helps joint pains that are worse from the slightest movement. Light touch and pressure also aggravate the symptoms, but firm pressure helps. The joints feel better when the person remains still. Warmth also relieves the pain. *Bryonia, Colchicum, Ledum,* and *Nux vomica* are the four main remedies useful for joints that are aggravated by motion, and *Bryonia* is the most important. The pain stays in the area and does not travel. Also, the person is thirsty for large amounts of cold water at infrequent intervals. *Bryonia* helps inflammation of the joint itself, as well as the surrounding muscle tissue. The joints are inflamed, swollen, shiny, and hot, and the muscles are sore and swollen. The pain is described as stitching or cutting.

Calcarea carb. Helpful for the chronic arthritis sufferer who has acute exacerbations of the problem. *Calcarea carb* is helpful for arthritis that worsens in cold, damp weather. The areas affected by the rheumatic pain feel wrenched or sprained. The person often has cold and damp feet and hands. The areas where this remedy is most helpful are the upper back, shoulders, and knees. This remedy is also useful for previously sprained ankles and other recurring joint injuries. *Calcarea carb* may also be helpful for an elderly person who develops minor swelling on the last joint of the fingers and who has osteoarthritis, especially when it gets worse in cold, damp weather or before a storm.

Calcarea phos. Useful for joint and muscle problems that appear with a change of weather and from drafts of cold air. The sacroiliac joint is stiff, sore, and feels broken.

Caulophyllum. Useful for erratic joint pains that change place every few minutes. The small joints are the most affected, especially the fingers, toes, and ankles. Joint and muscle pain is often associated with uterine or ovarian problems in women. The pain sometimes seems to alternate with asthma, so that when the asthma gets better, the joints get worse, and vice versa. The pain is severe and drawing. The joints feel stiff. The wrists ache, and the person feels cutting pains when clenching the fists. The joints often crack when the person walks.

Causticum. People who benefit from this remedy have joint stiffness. The tendons feel short and contracted. There are many similarities to *Rhus tox* in the treatment of joint problems, especially because both are relieved by warmth and both are useful for treatment of rheumatoid arthritis. There are also important differences: *Causticum* is useful for nighttime restlessness, while *Rhus tox* is useful for the person who is constantly restless day and night. Also, the pain is worse in cold, dry air (*Rhus tox* worsens from cold, damp air). There is a need to be in constant motion, but this does not relieve the symptoms or the pain (*Rhus tox* is associated with motion that does provide temporary relief). There may be burning and rawness in the joints, and the legs are often restless at night. The joints in surrounding tissues, including the tendons, feel as though they are extremely tight, shortened, and paralyzed.

Chamomilla. Helps the person who is extremely sensitive to joint and muscle pain. The pain actually drives the person out of bed, compelling him or her to walk around. The person is anguished and irritable. The pain is worse at night and when warmth is applied to the joint, and the pain gets better in warm, wet weather. There is particular soreness of the right deltoid muscle in the arm.

Cimicifuga. Useful for deep aching pain in the muscles, especially in the fleshy part of the muscle belly rather than farther out in the extremities. The pain seems to affect the larger muscles of the trunk. Pain in the muscles comes on suddenly with great severity and worsens at night and in wet, windy weather. There is restlessness that is aggravated by motion (unlike *Rhus tox,* where motion temporarily relieves the symptoms). Similar to *Caulophyllum,* rheumatic problems often accompany uterine problems in women. Unlike *Caulophyllum,* which affects the small joints, *Cimicifuga* affects the large muscles.

Colchicum. Useful for joint, tendon, and ligament pains that shift and move from joint to joint. The pain seems to start on one side of the body and moves quickly to the other side. The pain is worse in the evening and night, as well as in warm weather and in the springtime. Joints are swollen and dark red. *Colchicum* is often useful for gout, especially in the big toe and heel when the person cannot touch or move the joint. The person is irritable and aggravated by the slightest motion, and the pain seems unbearable (like *Bryonia*). This remedy may also be useful for the person who is weak. Generally, *Colchicum* is useful for the smaller joints (like

Caulophyllum, Ledum, and *Rhododendron*). Similar to *Pulsatilla, Kali bich,* and *Sulphur,* this remedy is useful for pain that seems to wander throughout the body.

Dulcamara. Useful for joint and muscular problems that come on with sudden changes of weather, especially when the weather turns cold and damp. *Dulcamara* is useful for the person who gets joint problems in the late summer or early autumn when the days are warm and the nights are cool. Muscle and joint pains sometimes alternate with diarrhea.

Kali bich. Useful for pains that move quickly from one place to another (similar to *Pulsatilla* and *Colchicum*). Pain can also occur in small areas of a muscle or joint. Useful for pain, swelling, stiffness, and cracking of all joints. Joint pain is also aggravated in hot weather. The pain is worse from cold applications and better from hot applications and gentle motion. Joint problems alternate with diarrhea, burning in the stomach, or lung problems (such as asthma or bronchitis). The person may have a problem with a cold or cough, and the discharges are thick, sticky, and yellowish-green.

Ledum. One of the most important remedies for arthritis and gout. *Ledum* is useful for pain that often begins in the smaller joints of the feet (such as the ball of the great toe or the small bones in the foot) and travels upward into other joints. The pain is worse in a warm bed and gets better when cold is applied (even ice water). The pain also gets worse from any kind of motion, at night, or in a warm bed. While the pain associated with this remedy gets better from cold, there is also a feeling of coldness on the surface of the joint. Nodes form, especially when the person has gout; *Ledum* helps alleviate the pain associated with these nodes. Particular areas of discomfort are: the ball of the big toe, which swells during gout; painful soles of the feet, on which the person is unable to step; an ankle, which sprains easily; and the right shoulder, which throbs and gets worse from motion.

Lycopodium. Useful for the person with chronic muscle and joint problems, especially for an elderly person who experiences an acute flare-up. The pain gets worse during rest and in damp weather and gets better with slow, gentle movement and the application of warmth. Joint problems often start on the right side and can sometimes travel to the left. Joint pain may be accompanied by excessive gas.

Magnesia carb. Useful for pain in the right shoulder. The pain gets worse when the person lies in bed and better when warmth is applied. The pain is described as a tearing in the shoulder accompanied by the feeling that the shoulder is dislocated. The person finds it difficult to raise the shoulder. In general, the whole body feels tired, especially the legs and feet.

Manganum aceticum. Useful for inflammation of the joints accompanied by digging or boring pains. The pain worsens at night. The body feels sore when it is touched. The person finds it difficult to walk because of a tendency to fall forward; because of this, the person tends to walk stooped forward. There may be red, shiny swelling of the joints. Muscle and joint pain tends to shift from joint to joint, often across the body. *Manganum* is particularly helpful for pain in the heels when the person cannot bear to put any weight on them.

Mercurius sol. Useful for joint and bone pain that worsens at night and is accompanied by excessive perspiration, which aggravates the condition. The person is sensitive to cold, and the extremities tremble, especially the hands. The legs feel cold and clammy at night. The joint pains often are part of a larger problem when the person is sick with an infection, such as sinusitis, and the discharges are green, yellow, and odorous.

Phytolacca. Useful for joint and bone pain below the elbows and knees. The pain moves quickly from one location to another and feels like electric shocks (similar to *Pulsatilla* and *Kali bich*). The muscles feel stiff and the discomfort is worse at night and becomes even worse in damp weather. This remedy is particularly helpful for problems with pain in the bones and around the bones in the connective tissue, or periosteum, rather than in the joints. The areas particularly affected are the heels, which are relieved by elevating the feet, and the right shoulder, which has shooting pains accompanied by stiffness and inability to raise the arm.

Pulsatilla. Useful for pain in the extremities and joints that moves rapidly from joint to joint. The mood of the person is the typical *Pulsatilla* picture of weepiness, oversensitivity, and wanting consolation and comfort. The person is chilly, yet feels better in open, cool air. The pain worsens when the person begins to move but is relieved from slowly moving around. The pain worsens in the evening and in bed. The lower extremities are particularly affected, especially the knee, ankle, and small bones of the feet. The legs feel worse when hanging. Elevating the legs relieves the pain, especially if the person has varicose veins.

Rhododendron. Helps joint and muscle pain that is aggravated by cold, damp, and windy weather. Pain is also aggravated before a thunderstorm and gets better after the storm breaks. Tearing pain is generally worse on the right side of the body. The pain is worse during rest and better with movement and warm clothing. Muscle and joint pain is generally worse in the small joints and ligaments.

Rhus tox. Probably the most important remedy for joint and muscle pain. The symptoms become worse from sitting, after rising from a sitting position, and when the person first begins to move; continuous motion relieves the discomfort. The person is restless and often paces because of the pain, especially at night. Warmth relieves the pain, and there is aggravation from cold, damp weather as well as from approaching storms (*Rhododendron* also helps the aggravation brought on by approaching storms). The person is stiff and sore and may experience tearing pains. One of the areas of the body most affected by *Rhus tox* is the deep muscles of the back, especially when the person complains of a crick in the back. This remedy is also used for pain associated with overexertion (such as wrenching the back or spraining an ankle or other joint area). Some specific joints affected are the temporomandibular joint (the joint in the jaw associated with TMJ Syndrome), the wrist, and the fingers. The fibrous tissues around the joints and the sheaths around the muscles are most helped by this remedy. The joints may actually appear red and swollen, although the problem is actually in the tissues around the joints (tendons, ligaments, and fascia).

Ruta. Useful for joint and muscle pain that stems from an inflamed and sore tendon. *Ruta* specifically helps with pain in the wrist (such as carpal tunnel syndrome), ankles (such as a sprained ankle), or the small muscles of the eyes (such as eye strain and soreness after reading or using the computer too much). A sore feeling is present in the small of the back, and the legs can give out when the person rises from a chair because the hips and thighs feel weak. This remedy is often helpful for ganglia forming on the back of sore wrists. The pain worsens in cold, wet weather.

Sanguinaria. Useful for pain in muscles near sore, stiff joints. These pains feel like they are moving, flying from one place to another, or stitching. *Sanguinaria* is particularly helpful for the nape of the neck, the right shoulder, and the left hip joint.

Sulphur. Useful for acute joint and muscle pain, as well as chronic, recurring pain. Mentally, the person is irritable, disorganized, and easily frustrated. The inflammation often starts in the feet and moves up. The pain is worse with rest, when the person is in a warm bed or bathing, at 11:00 A.M., and at night. The pain gets better in warm, dry air. At night the person has hot, sweaty, burning hands and soles of the feet. Itching may also occur in the joints. The person cannot walk straight or erect because of lower back pain and stiff ankles and knees. The person is often stoop-shouldered.

KIDNEY STONES

Kidney stones occur when normal minerals of the body that are usually passed out through the urine and kidneys crystallize and consolidate into stones. There are many causes of kidney stones, although a genetic predisposition seems to be important. The two main minerals in kidney stones are uric acid and calcium oxalate. Kidney stones are a relatively common condition; an important symptom is pain that radiates from the lower back around the side, toward the lower abdomen, and then down toward the groin and bladder. It may take weeks or months to pass a stone, and the pain can be intense and occur in spasms. The pain is considered one of the worst of any condition. A kidney stone can lead to a kidney infection, blood in the urine, and an enlarged kidney, especially if there is complete blockage, causing stretching of the ureters, kidneys, bladder, or urethra.

There are several methods of treatment. One is watchful waiting, as a kidney stone will often pass on its own. If a stone is lodged in the urinary tract system, a medical professional may administer medication such as morphine and intravenous fluids to relax the urinary collecting system and help the stone pass. A technique that uses ultrasound, called lithotripsy, can break up the stones. Occasionally surgery is needed if the stone is unable to be broken up or passed.

There are many natural ways to treat and prevent kidney stones; the most important is to increase fluid intake. Drinking at least six to eight glasses of water a day is very important. Eating a low-protein diet is important, and since protein increases the levels of uric acid and calcium excreted in the urine, vegetarians generally have fewer kidney stones than those who eat meat.

It is important when a person has kidney stones that are composed of calcium to avoid high levels of calcium. Dairy products, calcium supplements, foods with excess salt, and coffee should be avoided since they may increase the amount of calcium in the urine. Foods that are high in oxalate (including rhubarb, peanuts, spinach, chocolate, and black tea) should also be avoided. Foods containing uric acid (most meats) should be avoided. Eating foods that are high in magnesium (such as corn, buckwheat, barley, oats, soy, many types of beans such as limas, and potatoes) is helpful. Eating foods such as watermelon that are naturally diuretic can also be helpful. Certain vitamins and supplements are known to help kidney stones.

Berberis. Particularly helpful for kidney stones that are made from calcium oxalate (the more common type of kidney stone) as well as kidney stones made from uric acid. This remedy can be used during a kidney stone passage or the period between the passage of stones to help relax the urinary tract structures (kidney, ureter, bladder, and urethra) to allow the stone to pass more easily. *Berberis* may also help decrease the formation of sediment into stones. The left kidney is often more affected. There may be aching or burning kidney pain. Worse from deep pressure, the pain radiates around the back to the abdomen, then down to the hips and groin. The kidney region becomes stiff, which makes it difficult to sit and rise after sitting. There is a constant urge to urinate, accompanied by the sensation that urine remains after urinating. The urethra burns when the person is not urinating, and this symptom gets worse when the person stands. The symptoms get worse from motion, stooping, and lying down. *Berberis* can be used in a potency (such as 30c potency) and as a tincture. A person may drink a mixture of twenty drops in a quarter glass of water every ten minutes during the passage of the kidney stone. If *Berberis* is used after the kidney stone has passed, it can be used three or four times a day.

Calcarea carb. Useful for kidney stones, especially in the period between the passage of stones. *Calcarea carb* is particularly useful when stones are composed of calcium. It helps the person who is overweight, sluggish, chilly, and tends to form stones in other parts of the body (such as gallstones, cysts, or calcium deposits under the skin). This remedy is helpful for the person who tends to worry and is fearful.

Lycopodium. Useful for right-sided kidney stones accompanied by a severe backache. The backache is relieved by passing urine that contains a large amount of red, sandy sediment. *Lycopodium* can be used for the passage of kidney stones from the right kidney as well as in the period between kidney stone attacks.

Sarsaparilla. Useful for kidney stones passed from the right kidney. Pain from the right kidney extends around the right side and down to the groin. This type of stone causes the person to scream before and during urination. The person can urinate only when standing; the urine dribbles while sitting. *Sarsaparilla* is not as useful between kidney stone attacks, it is more helpful during an attack.

Sepia. Useful between attacks of passing kidney stones. A dragging sensation in both the bladder and kidney is accompanied by the constant desire to urinate. The sediment in the urine is red and has an offensive smell.

LABOR

Take special care. While homeopathic remedies are safe during pregnancy, labor, and breastfeeding, a pregnant woman should confer with her obstetrician or midwife to coordinate treatment.

When a woman goes into labor, it is important that a health care professional, such as a doctor or nurse midwife, be managing the care. Natural childbirth is a wonderful way to have a baby if the mother's health is good and there are no complications.

Homeopathic remedies should only be used by qualified people who have delivered many babies as an adjunct to normal medical intervention. The homeopathic remedies listed here can be used in conjunction with medical care to both prepare the uterus for labor and relax and stimulate the uterus during labor.

Aconite. Useful for frequent labor pain that is extremely intense and seems unbearable. The person is anxious and restless and is afraid of dying while in labor. There is a feeling of being unable to breathe or bear any kind of pain. Body tissue tends to be dry and tight, including the vulva, vagina, and cervical opening, which does not dilate.

Arnica. Useful during and after labor, especially for a bruised, sore feeling in the uterus, vagina, bladder, pelvis, or abdomen. *Arnica* helps heal and soothe a uterus that is fatigued from contracting and helps it to regain its strength to continue the labor process. This remedy helps heal tissue damaged during childbirth.

Belladonna. Labor pain that comes on suddenly and ends suddenly can be helped by *Belladonna.* There is a bearing-down feeling, as if the uterus will come out of the vagina. The cervical opening does not dilate well and is hot, tender, and rigid, but is also thin (this is different from *Gelsemium,* which also has a rigid cervical opening but is thick and rounded). While labor pain is very intense, it is also ineffectual because of the spasmodic condition of the cervical opening. There is a red, hot, flushed face, and the heart and carotid artery throb. The person experiences great agony and heat, and is sensitive to noise and jarring of the bed.

Caulophyllum. Useful for intensely sharp, cramping labor pain in the uterus, lower extremities, groin, and bladder. The pain tends to travel quickly from place to place, exhausting the person so much that she is barely able to talk. *Caulophyllum* is also used during the last weeks of pregnancy for false labor and is a specific remedy that can be used at any time for false labor. When labor pains are weak or irregular, *Caulophyllum* will help improve the quality of contractions; this remedy will increase energy and strength. This remedy also helps pain that comes in spasms and shoots in all directions;

the contractions are usually short. Useful for women who are nervous and experience pains that feel intolerable to them.

Chamomilla. Useful for labor pain that is felt in the back. The person is extremely irritable and angry, and strikes out verbally when bothered or criticized. The pain drives the person almost frantic because of the extreme sensitivity. The pain may also extend down the back into the legs.

Cimicifuga. Useful for pain that travels quickly across the abdomen from side to side, causing the person to double up; this pain seems so severe that the person almost faints. The cervix does not dilate properly. *Cimicifuga* is useful for joint pain or muscle pain around the joints during pre-labor and labor periods. This remedy can be used in 30c potency to prepare and tone the uterus before labor begins. It is often given once or twice daily for three weeks before labor begins.

Coffea. Useful when the person is extremely nervous and overexcited. The person may stay up late at night and experience insomnia during labor or possibly before. The pain is distressing, and the person cries and is afraid of dying. The main difference between this remedy and *Chamomilla* is that the person who needs *Coffea* is not as irritable or angry.

Gelsemium. This remedy can be used in two different labor circumstances. One circumstance is when labor has been in progress for many hours and the cervix is slow to dilate. The cervix feels hard and rigid, and the cervical opening tends to be thick and rounded (*Belladonna* also has a rigid cervical opening, but it is thin). Another circumstance is when the uterus is soft and flabby and the cervix is dilated, yet labor pain has stopped because the uterus is weak and unable to contract. Sometimes the membrane (bag of water) around the baby actually bulges out through the cervical opening, but the uterus is too weak to expel the baby. The person is drowsy, tired, dull, has heavy eyelids, and feels an aching sensation all over.

Ipecac. Labor pain accompanied by excessive nausea and vomiting can be helped by this remedy. The person experiences sharp pains around the navel that move down toward the uterus. There may also be pain that travels from the left side of the abdomen to the right.

Kali carb. Useful for early labor pain that begins in the back, especially in the sacral area, and runs down the thighs. The back is weak, and the legs feel as if they will give out. The person is anxious, tends to perspire, and feels weak. Anxiety may be felt in the pit of the stomach.

Nux vomica. Useful for labor pain accompanied by the constant desire to pass stool and urinate; despite this desire, little comes out. The labor pain is severe and comes in spasms, beginning in the back and moving down to the buttocks and thighs. This pain may cause the person to faint (which may slow down the labor). The person may be hypersensitive and intolerant to noise, disruptions, and odor, and is sometimes constipated. The person may also feel the need to vomit, yet may only be able to in small amounts.

Pulsatilla. When labor pain is weak, slow, and irregular, and sometimes causes fainting, *Pulsatilla* may provide relief. The person feels suffocated, especially when in a small, warm room, and wants the windows and doors open with cool air blowing despite feeling chilly. The person cries easily. There is a desire for consolation, comfort, fuss, and to have family nearby. There is a lack of thirst despite a dry mouth. This remedy is also useful when the baby is lying crosswise or is breech; *Pulsatilla* (30x or 30c) given three times a day during the last week of pregnancy may help turn the baby to the proper position. Another use for this remedy is when bleeding is too light and seems suppressed after the placenta is delivered. This remedy also can be used when the placenta comes out too slowly. In general, *Pulsatilla* helps all conditions in which the ability to expel is slow and ineffectual (this can be true of delayed menstrual periods, slow labor, difficulty expelling the placenta, and suppressed bleeding after the placenta comes out).

LABOR PREPARATION

Take special care. While homeopathic remedies are safe during pregnancy, labor, and breastfeeding, a pregnant woman should confer with her obstetrician or midwife to coordinate treatment.

When a woman goes into labor, it is important that a health care professional, such as a doctor or nurse midwife, be managing the care. Natural childbirth is a wonderful way to have a baby if the mother's health is good and there are no complications.

Homeopathic remedies should only be used by qualified people who have delivered many babies as an adjunct to normal medical intervention. The homeopathic remedies listed here can be used in conjunction with medical care to both prepare the uterus for labor and relax and stimulate the uterus during labor.

Aconite. Useful for a pregnant woman who is restless, fearful, and anxious. The woman may be afraid of dying during the upcoming labor, or she may fear that the baby will die.

Arnica. This remedy may be given in the very early stages of labor, especially if the abdomen, uterus, and vaginal area are sore. *Arnica* is also used after labor to help reduce swelling and bruising and hasten the healing of the tissues after childbirth.

Caulophyllum. This remedy is helpful in toning the uterus to help ensure a smooth delivery. *Caulophyllum* 30c is often given two to three times a day for two or three weeks before the end of the pregnancy to help uterine contractions become more efficient.

China. Useful for the woman who has had excessive blood loss in past labors and childbirth. *China* may be given in the very early stages of labor as a preventive to avoid heavy blood loss after childbirth, especially when the person has a history of weakness due to fluid loss.

Gelsemium. Useful when the person is apprehensive about labor. Anxiety and being emotionally paralyzed about the upcoming event may be experienced. The person who needs *Gelsemium* tends to be less restless than when *Aconite* is needed, and the limbs become heavy, the eyelids droop, and the body weakens. It is also a helpful remedy for those who have had painful labors in the past. This remedy helps decrease the intensity of the upcoming labor if given in the last two weeks of pregnancy. *Gelsemium* helps to smooth the dilation of the cervix and smooth out uterine rhythms during labor.

Ignatia. Helps the person who becomes hysterical, weepy, and extremely anxious about upcoming labor. A lump in the throat, sighing often, and a nervous cough may be experienced.

Pyrogenium. Sometimes used as soon as labor begins to help decrease the possibility of infection. *Pyrogenium* is sometimes used each morning for up to ten days for continued prevention or treatment of infection.

LACERATED WOUNDS
(INCLUDES JAGGED CUTS AND LACERATIONS)

Lacerated wounds are jagged, irregular, and often have torn skin. The underlying tissue may also be damaged. This type of injury occurs after a blow to the skin or a cut by a dull object. This kind of wound is often contaminated by dirt and foreign debris. As with all wounds, watch for infection. Contact a physician if signs of redness, oozing of pus, or fever are seen.

Aconite. Useful for a laceration accompanied by extreme fear and panic.

Arnica. A laceration with great bruising can be helped by *Arnica.* The person has a tendency toward shock. The signs of shock include: a rapid, weak pulse; cool, clammy skin; lightheadedness; irregular breathing; confusion; or loss of consciousness. If any of these signs of shock are present, a doctor or person trained in emergency medicine should be contacted.

Calendula. Useful as a tincture, ointment, or lotion to help prevent infection of the wound. *Calendula* is taken internally as a 30c potency every two or three hours; it may also be applied externally on the wound itself.

Hypericum. Useful for treating a laceration in the 30c potency or as a lotion, tincture, or ointment (these dispensing forms are commonly found at stores carrying homeopathic supplies). This remedy is helpful when there is extreme pain from a wound in a rich nerve supply area.

MENOPAUSE

Menopause is a natural condition that women experience, usually between the ages of forty and fifty-five. This is when the ovaries begin to decrease the amount of estrogen produced, causing the menstrual period to stop. Symptoms associated with menopause include hot flashes, headaches, insomnia, wakefulness, vaginal dryness, and changes in sexual desire. Other problems include dry skin, wrinkling of the skin, increased cholesterol levels (estrogen decreases the cholesterol), and decreased amounts of calcium in the bones leading to softening of the bones or osteoporosis.

Some women develop severe symptoms with menopause; other women have few symptoms and notice few changes in the body. Hot flashes are perhaps one of the most uncomfortable parts of menopause. They occur as estrogen lowers, and the body reacts with sweating, palpitations of the heart, nausea, and anxiety. (If palpitations are new and have not been evaluated before, a physician should be contacted.) Women sometimes wake up at night having to change their wet sleepwear or bedsheets. It is sometimes difficult to concentrate, not only because of the estrogen lowering, but also because of the hot flashes and lack of sleep.

Controlling blood sugar is important because it can lead to hyperglycemia and increased hot flashes. It is important to get plenty of exercise to help the heart, lower cholesterol, and increase the strength of the bones. Exercise also helps reduce anxiety, stress, and hot flashes. Certain herbs, supplements, oils, and vitamins are known to help menopause.

The homeopathic remedies listed here can be very helpful for both the immediate and chronic problems associated with menopause.

Aconite. The face is flushed red and the person is fearful and anxious. There are many fears (death, the future, crossing the street, crowds), and the person is restless and scared.

Belladonna. Useful for hot flashes occurring mainly in the head, where heat and redness begin and end abruptly; this is often accompanied by profuse facial perspiration. The person is generally agitated and sleepless at night.

Bellis. Helps a person who is fatigued, persistently tired, always wants to lie down, and has a backache. There is no real specific disease, flushing, circulatory problem, or bone and joint problem that causes this fatigue, the person is simply tired all the time.

Calcarea carb. Useful for excessive, heavy bleeding accompanied by abdominal cramps and leg cramps, especially during the early stages of menopause. *Calcarea carb* is also useful after menstrual periods have stopped and the person has settled into post-menopausal life. There is a tendency to gain weight and the breasts may enlarge. The person may feel chilly and have cold, sweaty feet. There is a tendency to crave sweets. Anxious and fearful, the person may worry about contagious diseases, heart failure, and heart attacks. There may be a fear of crowds, flying in planes, and being in closed spaces. Despite anxieties and physical problems, the person maintains an interest in sex. This remedy is also associated with osteoarthritis when the joints hurt, especially the knees, back, and hands. These pains are aggravated by cold, damp weather and better in warm weather.

Caulophyllum. Useful for nervous tension and uneasiness during menopause. The person worries about minor things and wants to work all the time. The person who needs *Caulophyllum* does not have the excessive fear and anxiety seen when *Aconite* is needed; *Caulophyllum* is more associated with general worry.

Cimicifuga. This remedy is helpful for depression and sadness during menopause; the person may have the feeling that a cloud is enveloping her. There is great depression and a feeling of impending doom or evil. The person is restless, unhappy, and irritable; this is often associated with a sinking feeling in the stomach accompanied by frequent headaches.

China. Excessive bleeding during the pre-menopausal period can be helped by *China.* The person is pale, has low blood pressure, and feels extremely weak both mentally and physically. Loss of blood causes ringing in the ears and decreased vision, and the person perspires from the slightest effort. *China* may be associated with abdominal distention covering the entire abdomen, and passing gas or belching does not provide relief.

Glonoine. This remedy is similar to *Belladonna* because there is flushing in the face that starts and stops abruptly and is accompanied by facial perspiration. *Glonoine,* however, tends to be associated more with heart palpitations and high blood pressure. (Note that if palpitations are new and have not been evaluated before, a physician should be consulted.) This remedy is often associated with headaches during menstrual periods. The person may experience vertigo and ringing in the ears, especially during hot flashes.

Graphites. Useful during the pre-menopausal period while the person still has menstrual periods. The periods are late and light and sometimes consist only of a discharge of pale blood. There is also excessive, white, liquidy vaginal discharge that is irritating; this seems to replace the menstrual period and may cause vaginal itching. The person who needs this remedy tends to be pale, even when flushing during the hot flashes of menopause. The hot flashes may be associated with nosebleeds. Those who need this remedy are generally overweight, sensitive to cold, and are sad and indecisive. The person feels better when warm, yet likes to be outside in the cool air (similar to *Pulsatilla*). There may be recurring skin problems, especially eczema and cracks in the skin, which ooze a thin, sticky discharge and are very itchy.

Kali carb. Useful during menopause after menstrual periods have completely stopped. The person is tired, weary, anxious, and easily discouraged. There may be the unusual feeling that the legs will give out and the kidneys will stop functioning. There is weakness in the small of the back, and possibly swelling above the eyelid. The person is sensitive to changes in the atmosphere or barometer, intolerant to cold weather, and feels worse in the early morning. There is joint pain, especially in the lower extremities, and there may be some swelling or edema in the legs. The pain in the joints and muscles surrounding the joints is sharp and cutting. The pain gets worse from cold, drafts, and rest, and is improved by movement (similar to *Rhus tox*).

Lachesis. An important remedy for menopause and for those who have not felt well since the menstrual periods ended. When *Lachesis* is the correct remedy, the person is worse from suppression or slow appearance of bodily discharges. In this case, it is the stopping or suppression of the menstrual period during menopause that makes the person feel worse. Hemorrhoids and headaches with heat on the top of the head often occur. There are sudden hot flashes during the day, but the person feels cold at night; also, the head may feel flushed and hot, and the feet cold. Headaches, which are often left-sided and migraine-like, may be accompanied by heart palpitations. (Note that if palpitations are new and have not been evaluated before, a physician should be consulted.) The small veins in the legs may bleed spontaneously from the slightest contact. The person is very intolerant to tight clothes around the waist and tight collars around the neck. The skin is extremely sensitive. This remedy is often useful for those who have problems when the menstrual period slows down and stops for several months. These people always feel better when the menstrual period begins to flow (even if it is light and scanty) because this relieves congestion and circulatory problems. In general, the person feels worse after awakening from sleep and better when outside in the fresh air as long as the temperature is mild. Mentally, the person is bad-tempered and tends to be jealous, irritable, possibly vindictive, and talkative. The person changes subjects quickly with no pauses between sentences.

Sanguinaria. Useful for hot flashes associated with migraine-like headaches that move from the back of the neck, up the head, and around the right eye. The veins and arteries in the head are dilated, especially around the temples. The person feels better when lying down and sleeping. Headaches may appear every seventh day. Red cheeks and burning palms and soles of the feet often accompany the hot flashes and headaches. Also possibly associated with menopause are enlarged, painful breasts, a cough with burning in the chest, and periodic earaches. This remedy is often used for profuse menstrual flow during the pre-menopausal time. There may be months without a period, but when it does come, it is extremely heavy. There may also be offensive, burning vaginal discharge. The skin tends to burn and itch all over, and this condition gets worse from heat.

Sepia. Useful when the person is irritable, bad tempered, sad, and weepy during menopause. The person often shies away from people and prefers to be alone, even shunning the family and children. There may be a heaviness in the pelvic region and a feeling that the bladder and uterus may fall out of the vagina. There is often pain in the lumbar and sacral areas of the back. Menstrual periods are irregular and light, although sometimes they may be profuse with dark blood; this irregularity around the time of menopause increases the person's irritability. There is often flushing in the face, without perspiration. Sexual intercourse may be painful because the vagina is dry, and sexual interest decreases because of the depression that occurs.

Sulphur. Those in menopause who suffer from vascular problems (such as high blood pressure, hot flashes, hemorrhoids, and varicose veins) may find relief from *Sulphur.* The person may also suffer from skin problems (such as acne rosacea or eczema). All of these symptoms tend to get worse in the heat, and the person wants to be in cool or cold places. These symptoms are also relieved once the menstrual period begins, only to return when the period slows down. Those who need this remedy may become lazy and do not maintain their appearance or cleanliness. They may become stoop-shouldered and develop back and joint problems.

Thuja. Often overlooked when considering menopausal problems, *Thuja* is useful after menstrual periods have completely stopped and symptoms of aging quickly develop. The person develops warts, moles grow quickly, and age spots begin to itch and become black or brown. Varicose veins develop on the legs as well as the nose. The person gains weight, especially in the trunk, hips, and shoulders, and may develop tumors or cysts on the ovaries, fibroids in the uterus, and hard, benign lumps in the breasts. The skin may become puffy, greasy, and oily, although certain areas may be dry. Emotionally, the person tends to be depressed, and develops fears and obsessions about cancer and other degenerative diseases. There is a tendency to develop high blood pressure. This remedy is best prescribed by a physician skilled in homeopathic training who is familiar with chronic conditions, especially when there is a medical history of excessive use of antibiotics, birth control pills, or steroids.

Veratrum viride. An important remedy for hot flashes accompanied by no other mental or physical symptoms. This remedy may help control hot flashes better than any other.

MORNING SICKNESS

Take special care. While homeopathic remedies are safe during pregnancy, labor, and breastfeeding, a pregnant woman should confer with her obstetrician or midwife to coordinate treatment.

Morning sickness is the nausea and vomiting that approximately 50 percent of all pregnant women experience during the first trimester. The nausea often occurs early in the morning after rising from bed, but can also occur at any time during the day. Generally, some nausea and vomiting is considered tolerable by most women, but sometimes the problem can be severe. Prolonged vomiting can lead to dehydration and have serious consequences for the progress of the pregnancy. It can also lead to hemorrhages in the eye, which is a very serious problem that should be handled by a physician immediately.

There are many different theories about the cause of morning sickness. One prominent theory is that it is the body's defense mechanism to keep the woman from eating foods that could be detrimental to the growing fetus. Another idea is that during the early months of pregnancy, the liver is unable to filter out toxins from the body, which leads to nausea.

Mild morning sickness can be treated naturally by eating small amounts of dry toast or crackers first thing in the morning. Drinking water that has been drained from cooked rice or barley also helps decrease the amount of nausea. It is important to avoid fatty foods and have a small amount of food in the stomach much of the day. If the woman is stressed or depressed about being pregnant, this can contribute to increased nausea and vomiting. In such cases, counseling may be important. Certain vitamins, herbs, and supplements are known to help morning sickness.

Arsenicum alb. Helps nausea during pregnancy and when vomiting occurs after eating spoiled food (such as meat), drinking ice cold water, or after eating ice cream. There is nausea with retching and extreme irritation of the stomach with a raw, burning feeling. Warm drinks temporarily relieve the burning in the stomach area.

There is restlessness and pacing, but the person is weak and tires easily.

Bryonia. Helps nausea and vomiting associated with an intestinal virus or from overeating, especially when pregnant. There is extreme abdominal pain and bitter tasting, nauseating belches. As long as the person remains still, the nausea and vomiting are relieved. The person is extremely thirsty.

Colchicum. Associated with nausea during pregnancy, especially when the person smells cooking food during the first months of pregnancy. The person tends to feel better when curled up in a fetal position.

Ipecac. An important remedy for nausea and vomiting during pregnancy, especially when they are excessive. Extreme nausea eventually leads to vomiting, which does not relieve the nausea. The person feels nauseous after eating rich foods, pastry, pork, and fruit (in general, foods that are difficult to digest). Diarrhea may accompany vomiting. There is a clear, pink tongue and often profuse salivation.

Iris. Helps vomiting during pregnancy that causes burning in the entire digestive tract. Vomit is watery, extremely sour, and excoriates and burns the throat. The entire body sometimes smells sour. There is a profuse flow of saliva (similar to *Mercurius sol* and *Ipecac*).

Kreosote. Helps vomiting during pregnancy when there is an excessive flow of saliva. Food eaten three to four hours before is vomited up. There is a feeling of coldness in the stomach, as if ice water is sitting there. After vomiting, the stomach is burning and excoriated.

Natrum phos. Helps nausea with sour vomiting during pregnancy. In general, there are sour-smelling discharges in various parts of the body (including saliva, vaginal discharge, and perspiration). The tongue is characteristically yellow or cream colored, especially in the back of the mouth.

Nux vomica. Helpful when nausea and vomiting during pregnancy come on after overindulging in food, alcohol, or coffee. There is excessive retching, and it is often difficult to bring up vomit. These symptoms are similar to other *Nux vomica* symptoms regarding gastrointestinal tract problems (for example, there is an urging to have a bowel movement, but the person is unable to). One hour after eating, there may be a sensation that a stone is in the stomach.

Pulsatilla. Useful when the person vomits food eaten long ago. The person is weepy, tearful, and wants consolation and comfort. There is chilliness, but the person likes the blowing of cool air. The nausea gets better from walking outside in a cool breeze and is aggravated by ice cream and fatty foods. Nausea and vomiting leave a bad taste in the mouth. Vomiting gets worse in the evening and after eating and drinking.

Sepia. Helpful for morning sickness that is relieved by eating. The person tends to crave pickles and acidic foods. There is an empty feeling in the stomach and abdomen. The person becomes nauseous from the smell or sight of food and while lying on the side. Foods tend to taste too salty. Nausea may get worse in the morning before eating. Nausea and a faint feeling usually occur in the late morning, especially around 11:00 A.M. The person may be intolerant of milk and meat, especially when sick. Sour vomit may be mixed with undigested food. After vomiting, the esophagus burns. *Sepia* may be helpful for morning sickness during pregnancy when there is no vomiting.

Symphoricarpus racemosus. Helpful for persistent nausea and vomiting during pregnancy, when all other remedies have failed. Motion aggravates the nausea, and the person is averse to all foods. Lying on the back provides relief. There is a fickle appetite and bitter eructations in the throat. This remedy should be used in the 200c potency and may be repeated three to five times a day when nausea and vomiting are extreme and nothing else helps. Note that high-potency remedies are not recommended for home prescribing. Consult a physician or skilled homeopathic consultant for potencies above 30c.

Tabacum. Helpful during pregnancy for incessant nausea that is aggravated from the smell of tobacco smoke. The least movement causes the person to vomit. *Tabacum* is useful when the person feels faint with a sinking feeling in the pit of the stomach, followed by vomiting. Vomiting is accompanied by excessive spitting, which gets worse when riding in a car, boat, or airplane. Stomach pain extends up to the left arm. There is a sense of relaxation of the stomach with nausea (similar to *Ipecac*). The person feels excessively wretched, despondent, and depressed because of the extreme nausea and vomiting. She is pale, icy cold with sweat, and has an irregular pulse.

MOTION SICKNESS

Motion sickness is caused by repetitive horizontal, vertical, or angular motion, and is generally characterized by nausea and vomiting, which causes no permanent damage. The most common form of sickness occurs from traveling on water, in the air, or on the ground by car, train, or bus. In susceptible people, any motion causes excessive stimulation of the inner ear. The labyrinth system of the inner ear connects to the vomiting center of the brain stem. Visual stimuli and emotional factors, such as fear and anxiety, can also bring on motion sickness.

Symptoms include nausea and vomiting, which may be preceded by hyperventilation, increased saliva, paleness, cold sweating, yawning, and headaches. Weakness generally follows nausea and vomiting, and the person is unable to concentrate. Prolonged exposure to motion often allows the individual to adapt and gradually return to a sense of well-being. Short exposure generally causes the most problems.

Prevention is the most effective way to treat motion sickness. Susceptible people should always position themselves where there is least motion. This includes the middle of a ship or over the wings in an airplane. Lying in a semi-prone position with the head raised is best. Reading should be avoided. A person should keep his or her viewpoint at an angle of 45 degrees above the horizontal line. Alcohol or overeating should be avoided during or before travel. The person should drink small amounts of fluids frequently and eat easily digested foods during extended periods of exposure. During air travel food and fluid should be avoided.

The homeopathic remedies listed here have been known to help prevent and treat motion sickness.

Bryonia. Symptoms of nausea and vomiting are worse with any type of motion or movement and better when completely still.

Excessive irritability is another common symptom. The person is thirsty for large amounts of cold water.

Cocculus. One of the most important remedies for motion sickness or travel illness either by sea or land. The person does not want fresh air and is sensitive to any noise. The mouth has a metallic taste. The abdomen is greatly distended, and the sight or smell of any food is repugnant. On a moving boat, the person wants to remain inside. The person will lie down on the bed, facing the wall, unmoving. A headache will often occur in the back of the head and neck. Symptoms are worse from kneeling, bending, or stooping. Extremes of heat and cold also have a negative effect. Symptoms are better from lying still.

Nux vomica. Nausea with a constant urge to vomit but an inability to do so is a symptom of this type of motion sickness. The person is irritable and angers easily.

Petroleum. Useful for treating symptoms associated with motion sickness, especially those brought on by the smell of gasoline. The person is very irritable. The person does not want to be in the fresh air, but does prefer dry, warm weather. Eating seems to help the symptoms, while raising the head makes them worse.

Tabacum. With this motion sickness, leaning the head out of the car window in order to breathe fresh air is common. The person wants to sit wrapped up in warm clothes. Looking at moving objects makes the person nauseous. There is often a tight feeling around the head. The face is pale and covered with a cold sweat. A person is often depressed and weepy, but also can become restless and excitable. Any kind of tobacco smoke makes these symptoms worse. Fresh air makes the person feel much better and actually prevents vomiting.

NARCOTIC ABUSE

Many forms of drug abuse can be helped with homeopathic remedies; however, seeking medical attention is extremely important, especially if a person has overdosed. To help break the habit of taking cocaine, morphine, heroin, or marijuana, a person can use homeopathic remedies to help decrease the craving, minimize the symptoms of withdrawal, and improve the immune system functioning.

Belladonna. Useful for hallucinations during which the person may have delusions, especially visual delusions. The person may see monsters or frightening faces. The person rages and may strike and bite. There is a hyperacuteness of all senses. There may be a flushed, red face, and the person may experience headaches that are worse from light, noise, jarring, and lying down, and better from pressure.

Chamomilla. Useful when narcotics cause a hypersensitivity to pain, and the pain is out of proportion to the seriousness of the problem. There is often an accompanying feeling of numbness. The person who abuses narcotics is irritable, easily angered, moody, and hateful. There may be digestive disorders such as diarrhea. This is a useful remedy when a person attempts to wean from or stop taking narcotics (such as cocaine or heroin).

Coffea. Oten helpful for extreme sensitivity following drug abuse. The person experiences unusual activity of the mind and body and is overly affected by sudden emotions and surprises. The person may become overly excited, even when there are pleasurable experiences. The mind is full of many ideas, and the person is quick to act.

Ipecac. Useful when narcotic abuse causes extreme nausea and vomiting.

Lachesis. Useful when narcotic abuse causes the person to talk a lot. The person begins one subject and quickly moves to another, often not making any sense. There may be restless and uneasy feelings, and the person wants to be somewhere else all the time. Unusual jealousy and suspicion may occur. The person may have experiences of a religious nature, often having visions of deities. The person often feels worse after sleeping and feels unusual tight feelings in various parts of the body. Warm applications often help to relax these constrictions.

Nux vomica. As with almost all situations where narcotics are used and there is hypersensitivity to drugs, *Nux vomica* is one of the most important remedies. It is associated with the person who seeks stimulants in general (such as coffee, alcohol, drugs, and tobacco). The person stays up late at night and is irritable and sensitive to noise, odor, and light. The person does not want to be touched, and may become sullen and fault finding. This is probably the most important remedy to start the case.

NAUSEA AND VOMITING

Take special care. While homeopathic remedies are safe during pregnancy, labor, and breastfeeding, a pregnant woman should confer with her obstetrician or midwife to coordinate treatment.

Nausea and vomiting have many causes that are either benign and limited or serious and reflect more serious disease. Less serious problems of nausea and vomiting occur when there are viral infections in the intestinal tract, lasting for twenty-four hours and often associated with diarrhea. This problem comes on suddenly, causing the person to feel quite ill. Other types of nausea and vomiting occur from eating spoiled foods, ear infections, coughing and asthma, or headaches, especially migraine headaches. With coughing and asthma, nausea and vomiting help eliminate the mucus that has dripped into the stomach from the respiratory tract. If vomiting occurs after a head injury or there are severe stomach or abdominal problems with illnesses, such as hepatitis, these conditions should always be evaluated by a physician.

Many of the remedies listed here may help with the nausea and vomiting of early pregnancy. (See Morning Sickness for specific information.)

Antimonium crud. Useful for a nursing infant that vomits breast milk in curds and refuses to nurse afterward; the infant is irritable and angry because of this. *Antimonium crud* is useful for vomiting in adults caused by overeating rich, fatty foods. Belches taste like what was eaten. Bloating also occurs after eating. The person has a thickly coated, white tongue. Foods that cause nausea and vomiting are bread, pastry, acidic foods, and sour wine. This remedy may be associated with nausea during pregnancy.

Antimonium tart. Useful for nausea caused by great anxiety and fear. The nausea is followed by pressure in the chest and heart, a headache with yawning, watery eye drainage, and finally vomiting. The person often is thirsty for cold water, but drinks little. Nausea, retching, and vomiting get worse after eating, and are accompanied by extreme faintness and weakness. Vomiting occurs in almost any position, except when lying on the right side.

Arsenicum alb. Helpful for vomiting that occurs after eating spoiled food (such as meat), drinking ice cold water, or after eating ice cream. Nausea and retching are accompanied by an extremely irritated stomach with a raw, burning feeling; warm drinks temporarily relieve this burning. The person is usually restless and paces, yet is weak and easily fatigued.

Bryonia. Useful for nausea and vomiting associated with stomach flu or overeating. The person experiences extreme abdominal pain and bitter tasting belches which have a nauseating taste. As long as the person lies perfectly still, the nausea and vomiting are relieved; as soon as the person moves, the nausea returns. The person is very thirsty for large amounts of cold liquids, yet drinks at infrequent intervals.

Calcarea carb. Useful for infants who vomit immediately after nursing. Adults may either crave or dislike milk, but in general drinking milk causes nausea. There may also be a craving for eggs. Fatty foods cause nausea, especially when the person is already ill.

Chamomilla. A good remedy for babies who are irritable and agitated. *Chamomilla* may be associated with ear infections or teething accompanied by excessive vomiting and retching. Vomit tastes bitter, and belches have an odor similar to rotten eggs. Adults may become nauseous after drinking coffee. *Chamomilla* is helpful for nausea and vomiting after taking drugs, especially narcotics or cocaine.

China. Helpful for excessive nausea and vomiting that result in exhaustion and weakness. The person vomits undigested food; however, vomiting does not relieve extreme abdominal distention caused by flatulence. The person experiences nausea, vomiting, and generally ill feelings after drinking tea.

Cina. Useful when the person experiences nausea and vomiting immediately after eating or drinking. Diarrhea may also be present.

Children who need this remedy may also have pinworms or other types of worm infestation. Vomiting usually occurs with a clean tongue.

Cocculus. Useful for motion sickness accompanied by nausea, vomiting, dizziness, and a sick headache when riding in a car, boat, or airplane. The person becomes nauseous from smelling food or tobacco smoke or from being cold. The person feels better when warm.

Colchicum. Helpful for nausea that occurs when the person sees, smells, or thinks about food; this is particularly a problem when smelling cooking food. If the smell of food is strong, the person becomes nauseous and feels faint. *Colchicum* is also associated with nausea during pregnancy, especially when the person smells cooking food during the first months of pregnancy. The person tends to feel better when curled up in a fetal position.

Colocynth. Useful for nausea and vomiting, accompanied by abdominal pain in the center of the abdomen, that is relieved by bending double and by applying pressure. Abdominal pain is a strong symptom associated with nausea and vomiting.

Cuprum met. Helpful for stomach cramps accompanied by nausea and vomiting; these symptoms are improved by drinking cold water. The person experiences cramping in many parts of the body (such as the legs, calves, and the abdomen) and may also vomit while coughing.

Ipecac. An important remedy for excessive nausea and vomiting. Extreme nausea eventually leads to vomiting, which does not relieve the nausea. The person becomes nauseated after eating rich foods, pastry, pork, and fruit (in general, foods that are difficult to digest). Nausea may be accompanied by diarrhea. The tongue usually remains clear and pink. The person experiences nausea with profuse salivation.

Iris. Helpful for vomiting spells that occur in cycles (such as every month, six weeks, or every four to six months); these spells last for two to three days. Migraine headaches on the right side that are preceded by visual blurring often accompany the nausea and vomiting. Vomiting, which causes burning in the entire digestive tract, consists of a watery, sour fluid that excoriates and burns the throat. The entire body sometimes smells sour, and there is a profuse flow of saliva (similar to *Mercurius sol* and *Ipecac*).

Kali carb. Useful for nausea that is relieved when the person lies down. Anxiety is felt in the pit of the stomach. *Kali carb* is useful for nausea during pregnancy in which there is no vomiting; the nausea gets worse when the person walks.

Nux vomica. Useful for nausea and vomiting that come on after overindulging in food, alcohol, or coffee. There is excessive retching, and it is often difficult to vomit. These symptoms are similar to other *Nux vomica* symptoms regarding gastrointestinal tract problems (such as the person feels the need to pass a stool, but cannot). One hour after eating there is a sensation that a stone is in the stomach.

Phosphorus. Helpful for the person who becomes nauseous from smelling strong odors (such as flowers or chemicals). The person tends to vomit after drinking cold water when the water becomes warm in the stomach.

Pulsatilla. Useful when the person vomits food eaten more than four hours before. The nausea and vomiting leave a bad taste in the mouth and get worse in the evening and after eating and drinking. The person is weepy, tearful, desires consolation and comfort, and is chilly, yet likes to feel cool air blowing. The nausea gets better when the person walks outside in a cool breeze and becomes particularly bad after eating ice cream and fatty foods.

Sanguinaria. Helpful for nausea and vomiting accompanied by headaches. There is increased salivation and a sinking feeling in the abdomen. The person has migraine-like headaches on the right side; nausea and vomiting occur when the headache pain begins in the back of the neck, spreads upward, and settles over the right eye. Headache pain, nausea, and vomiting are relieved when the person lies down and while sleeping.

Sepia. Useful for morning sickness during pregnancy that is relieved by eating. *Sepia* may be helpful for morning sickness where there is little vomiting. When vomiting does occur, the esophagus burns. The person may crave pickles and acidic foods. There is an empty feeling in the stomach and abdomen, and the person becomes nauseous from seeing or smelling food. Lying on the side also causes nausea. The person is nauseous in the morning before eating. There may also be nausea and a faint feeling in the later morning, especially around 11:00 A.M. The person is intolerant of both milk and meat, especially when ill. Foods may taste too salty. Sour vomit is mixed with undigested food.

Staphysagria. An excellent remedy for nausea and vomiting that occur after abdominal operations.

Tabacum. Useful for persistent nausea and vomiting that gets worse from the smell of tobacco smoke (similar to *Phosphorus*) or when the person sits or looks up. There is vomiting with the least motion. *Tabacum* is helpful for seasickness when the person feels faint and has a sinking feeling in the pit of the stomach, followed by vomiting; the person feels better in fresh, cool air. The person feels wretched, despondent, and depressed because of the extreme nausea and vomiting. The person is pale and icy cold with sweating, and has an irregular pulse. There is extreme weakness and a deathly pale face. If nausea and vomiting occur in children, they want the abdomen uncovered, which seems to provide relief. There is increased saliva with nausea, especially during pregnancy. This remedy is also helpful for vomiting during pregnancy with excessive spitting. Stomach pain may extend up to the left arm, and there is a sense of relaxation of the stomach with nausea (similar to *Ipecac*).

Veratrum alb. Useful for excessive nausea and vomiting aggravated by drinking fluids and by the least motion. Great anxiety and anguish are felt in the pit of the stomach. The person is thirsty for cold water but vomits as soon as it is swallowed. *Veratrum alb* is also useful for extreme diarrhea accompanied by vomiting. Diarrhea with extreme vomiting along with chilliness may be helped by *Veratrum alb.*

NERVE INJURIES

The first thing a person should do after an injury is make sure there is no damage to deeper tissues such as blood vessels, nerves, tendons, bones, or organs. If not certain as to the extent of the injury, it is best to consult a physician or go to an emergency room. Bleeding should be controlled as quickly as possible by applying direct pressure to the site with a clean, moist cloth. For control of pain and swelling, a cold, moist application can be used, although ice should not be applied directly against the skin. When transporting a person who is injured, it is important not to aggravate the injury. Consulting a Red Cross first aid manual or taking a first aid course can be helpful.

Injuries to a nerve usually result from trauma, such as an accident or repetitive work-related activity. An example is carpal tunnel syndrome. The sciatic nerve is another nerve that is often injured, especially when a person falls or twists the back. Another nerve injury is to the coccyx, such as when a person falls on the tailbone. This area is rich in nerves and is close to the surface of the body, so its injury can cause excruciating pain. If there is any loss of function, numbness, tingling, or excruciating pain, a health care professional should be contacted.

Calendula. Useful as a tincture or ointment for torn or lacerated nerve tissue.

Hypericum. An important remedy for injuries to nerves. Nerve damage can occur in many different areas (such as the spinal cord, tailbone, and neck). An injury such as whiplash has shooting pain from the neck, down the arms, and into the fingers. This remedy can also be used for injuries to the fingertips. Pain tends to be severe, and symptoms may include muscle spasms and soreness.

PERIODS: EARLY OR FREQUENT

Causes of an early or frequent menstrual flow are usually the same as those of a heavy flow. Sometimes women have early or frequent flow with no physiological cause, and some women have early or frequent flow at each menstrual cycle due to excess estrogen stimulation. Sometimes early or frequent bleeding can represent more serious problems, such as ovarian cysts, fibroid tumors in the uterus, effects of birth control methods (especially birth control pills or IUDs), cervical polyps, endometriosis, or cancer. Recurrent problems with early or frequent periods need to be treated by a homeopathic physician who is skilled at treating chronic constitutional illnesses.

Certain vitamins and supplements are known to help early or frequent periods.

Belladonna. Helps early and profuse menstrual periods. There is a large amount of bright, red blood that feels hot as it passes out of the vagina. *Belladonna* is often associated with a throbbing headache. There may also be a bearing-down sensation that feels like the uterus or bladder will protrude out through the vagina.

Bryonia. Useful for menstrual periods that are too early and often too profuse. Before the period starts, headaches are accompanied by congestion in the head and a feeling that the head will split. There also may be nosebleeds and constipation. Abdominal pain gets worse with the slightest movement and is relieved when the person lies still. The person feels irritable when spoken to or bothered, and is better when alone.

Calcarea carb. Useful for early, profuse, and long-lasting menstrual periods. Physical exertion can aggravate and increase the intensity of the menstrual flow. Before the period, nervousness and anxiety are often experienced. The person may be extremely fearful of losing emotional control and also fears being seen in an anxious state. There is chilliness and a craving for sweets. The feet tend to be cold and damp, and the person perspires often and has a sour odor. *Calcarea carb* is often useful for women who are heavy.

Carbo veg. Useful for menstrual periods that come on too early, are too frequent, and may be either too profuse or light. The odor of the menstrual blood is quite strong and often smells like decaying flesh. The skin is often cold and clammy. The person is restless, anxious, and sometimes feels faint. *Carbo veg* is almost always associated with weak digestion in which eating the smallest amount of food causes indigestion. There is an excessive abdominal distention, especially in the upper abdomen; belching temporarily relieves this discomfort.

Causticum. Useful for a menstrual period that is too early and too profuse. The flow tends to occur only during the day and stops at night or when the person lies down. The flow is mixed with large clots that smell offensive and cause vaginal itching and rawness. When the period finally does stop, small amounts of blood continue to be passed occasionally for many days.

Chamomilla. Helps menstrual periods that are too early and too profuse with dark, clotted blood. The menstrual flow is abundant and it starts and stops often. The person tends to be irritable and easily provoked. The pain that occurs during cramps seems unbearable and causes the person to cry out. The person may be extremely sensitive to the pain.

Cocculus. Useful when menstrual periods are too early and profuse and are accompanied by extreme abdominal cramping. Doubling up, firm pressure, and heat relieve abdominal pain. The menstrual period is aggravated by anger and grief. Increased flatulence and distention may occur, and abdominal pain sometimes feels as though sharp stones were rubbing against each other in the abdomen. When the person stands, the menstrual blood tends to gush out in a stream.

Ignatia. Early menstrual periods that last too long but are not profuse are often helped by this remedy. Grief, the loss of a loved one, or a great disappointment are often associated with this remedy. The person may feel that there is a lump in the throat, and may sigh and cry when alone. The menstrual blood is dark, thick, and may smell offensive.

Kreosote. Useful for menstrual periods that arrive too early, are very heavy, and last too long. The flow starts and stops frequently. The person tends to feel better when menstrual blood is flowing and feels worse after the period ends. Lying down tends to aggravate the flow, causing it to become heavier. After the flow, an odorous discharge itches, burns, and irritates the vaginal tissue.

Natrum mur. Useful when menstrual periods are too early and profuse or too late, too short, and scanty. If the period is early, it is consistently seven days early. *Natrum mur* is associated with sadness and depression before the period starts and with the tendency to brood about disappointments and loss of love relationships. The person may also weep when music is heard because it causes sentimental feelings. The person often craves salt during this period of time.

Nux vomica. Useful for menstrual periods that are too early and last too long, although the amount of blood loss is not very much. Periods are irregular and never occur at the right time, but are generally early. The person tends to be irritable, angry, and hypersensitive to all sorts of stimuli. Constipation occurs; the person has an urge to have a bowel movement, but is unable to. Indigestion is also a prominent symptom when this remedy is indicated.

Phosphorus. Helps menstrual periods that are too early, too profuse, and last too long. The menstrual blood tends to be thin and does not clot very easily. The person may want to lie down, but feels worse when lying on the left side. There is a sensitivity to all sorts of external stimuli, such as thunderstorms, rainstorms, and weather changes. *Phosphorus* is often useful for tall, lean women and those who are creative, artistic, and tend to communicate feelings easily.

Sabina. Useful for menstrual periods that occur too early, are profuse, and last too long. The menstrual blood is bright red with thick, dark, offensive-smelling clots.

Sepia. Useful for menstrual periods that occur too early, are light, and flow only in the morning. Irritability and depression are experienced, and aggravation occurs when anyone tries to console the person. There is a great amount of weakness, which is worse indoors and better in open air.

PERIODS: HEAVY
(INCLUDES MENORRHAGIA AND METRORRHAGIA)

There are many causes for heavy menstrual bleeding (menorrhagia) and bleeding between menstrual periods (metrorrhagia). Sometimes women have a heavy flow with no physiological cause, and some women have heavy flows at each menstrual cycle due to excess estrogen stimulation. Sometimes heavy bleeding can represent more serious problems, such as ovarian cysts, fibroid tumors in the uterus, effects of birth control methods (especially birth control pills or IUDs), cervical polyps, endometriosis, or cancer. Recurrent problems with heavy periods need to be treated by a homeopathic physician who is skilled at treating chronic constitutional illnesses. Certain vitamins and supplements are known to help heavy periods.

Aconite. Useful for profuse and long-lasting menstrual periods. *Aconite* is often associated with fear of death, restlessness, and general anxiety. Often the menstrual blood begins to flow heavily after the person has been frightened. Heavy periods may also occur after exposure to cold, dry wind. Nosebleeds are associated with heavy periods.

Arnica. Helpful for heavy menstrual periods that come on after an injury (such as being hit in the area near the uterus) or after sexual intercourse.

Belladonna. Helps early and profuse menstrual periods. There is a large amount of bright, red blood that feels hot as it passes out of the vagina. *Belladonna* is often associated with a throbbing headache. There may also be a bearing-down sensation that feels like the uterus or bladder will protrude out through the vagina.

Calcarea carb. Useful for profuse and long-lasting menstrual periods, often due to weakness in the muscular activity of the uterus, especially in an older woman who tends to be overweight. The least excitement causes the menstrual period to return. The person is chilly and has cold, damp feet. The person is quite anxious and often has fears of losing mental stability during the period and that others will observe this. The person craves sweets, especially before the period begins. *Calcarea carb* is useful for heavy periods experienced during breastfeeding and for a heavy period brought on by physical exertion or exercise.

Calcarea phos. Useful for a heavy menstrual period brought on by physical exertion or exercise.

Causticum. Useful for a menstrual period that is too early and too profuse. The flow tends to occur only during the day and stops at night or when the person lies down. The flow is mixed with large clots that smell offensive and cause vaginal itching and rawness. When the period finally does stop, small amounts of blood continue to be passed occasionally for many days.

Chamomilla. Useful for menstrual periods that are too early and often very profuse. The person is very irritable. The blood tends to be dark and clotted and may smell offensive. Menstrual flow is often inconsistent and starts and stops, but is extremely heavy when it does begin. The cramps are excessive, causing the person to cry out.

China. Useful for a menstrual period that is early and too profuse, with a discharge that is dark and clotted. A great loss of blood causes anemia, causing ringing in the ears, fainting, and even decreased vision. The person feels very weak and trembles.

Cocculus. Useful for menstrual periods that are too early, profuse, and accompanied by cramping pains. When the person rises, the menstrual blood tends to gush out. *Cocculus* is also associated with a distended abdomen, which is worse at night and with movement. The menstrual period is also aggravated by feelings of grief and anger. The person experiences profuse menstrual periods that are worse when standing and are aggravated from walking.

Hamamelis. Helps heavy menstrual periods associated with a slow, gradual loss of blood. The blood tends to be dark and venous, rather than the bright red of arterial blood. Anemia results because of the long duration of flow. The vaginal area and abdomen tend to be sore, and the menstrual flow slows down or stops at night.

Ignatia. Useful for a long-lasting menstrual flow that comes on too early. The symptoms tend to occur after feelings of great loss or sadness. Much blood is lost, not because of heavy bleeding, but because the flow lasts for such a long time.

Ipecac. Helps profuse menstrual flow that is early and lasts too long. There is generally an association with excessive nausea and vomiting, resulting in great weakness and a desire to lie down. The period often occurs every two weeks and is quite heavy. The menstrual blood is bright red and tends to clot easily. The person is generally adverse to food, and the tongue is clean and pink, despite the nausea and vomiting. Profuse bleeding is accompanied by a feeling of faintness.

Kreosote. Useful for early, profuse menstrual periods that last a long time. The blood flow is intermittent; it is heavier when lying down and at night, and gets lighter or even stops when sitting or walking. The blood tends to smell offensive and irritate the vagina as it passes through. After the period ends, the woman actually feels worse mentally and emotionally. *Kreosote* is helpful for the person who has heavy periods that get worse when lying down.

Lachesis. Only helpful for profuse menstrual bleeding that occurs during menopause. *Lachesis* is useful for the woman whose menstrual period has stopped for some time, then starts again and is very heavy. When the period starts again, the person feels better emotionally and is less depressed, yet experiences general irritability after the period begins again during this menopausal time. Tight clothing is disliked around the abdomen or uterine area, and the person often feels worse when awakening in the morning. Sometimes profuse and heavy periods alternate with absent periods; the profuse periods tend to be of short duration.

Lycopodium. Useful for a menstrual period that is too profuse, too lengthy, and tends to flow excessively in the afternoon, especially around 4:00 P.M. *Lycopodium* is often associated with great abdominal distention and gas pains. The person often experiences great sadness before the menstrual period.

Magnesia carb. Useful for heavy menstrual periods, especially during the night and in the morning. The menstrual blood flow tends to get worse when lying down and stops when the person walks. *Magnesia carb* is also useful for the reappearance of the menstrual period in postmenopausal women. Useful for heavy periods that get worse at night.

Nux vomica. Useful for menstrual periods that often last too long, although the amount of blood loss is not excessive. It seems as though the period will start, but often does not. (This is typical of conditions that benefit from *Nux vomica,* which has the symptom of discharges that are characterized by ineffectual urging.) The periods are irregular and never seem to come at the right time. There is great irritability. *Nux vomica* is often useful for women who are up late at night studying or working or for those who drink too much alcohol, smoke too many cigarettes, or drink too much coffee. Often, heavy periods are associated with episodes of anger and excessive irritability.

Phosphorus. Useful for menstrual periods that are too early and too profuse. The person tends to bruise easily and also suffers from hemorrhoids that get worse during the menstrual period. *Phosphorus* is useful for tall women with narrow hips who have heavy periods and are sensitive to all sorts of events (such as thunderstorms, the emotions of others, or sad movies). Useful for heavy menstrual periods that occur during breastfeeding. Heavy periods may be associated with increased sexual desire. Heavy periods seem to be aggravated by thunderstorms.

Sabina. Helps when menstrual periods are too early and profuse. The menstrual blood is bright red with dark clots; its flow tends to increase with movement and motion and may decrease from walking. *Sabina* is useful during menopause when thick blood clots are passed, especially in women with uterine fibroids.

Sepia. This remedy is often associated with irregular menstrual periods and with heavy periods that occur during menopause. *Sepia* is often associated with pain and weakness in the small of the back. There is also a feeling during heavy flow that the uterus may actually fall out of the vagina; this feeling is alleviated by crossing the legs or lying down. The person often experiences profound sadness, depression, and weepiness around the time of the menstrual period. The menstrual flow tends to be heaviest in the morning.

Silica. Useful for menstrual periods that are often irregular and sometimes light, yet may be heavy at times (especially during breastfeeding). *Silica* is often associated with cold feet and general coldness throughout the body. The person feels weak and tired, especially while nursing. Useful for a profuse menstrual period that is short in duration.

PERIODS: LATE OR ABSENT (INCLUDES AMENORRHEA)

Late or absent periods have multiple causes that can either be serious or benign. Some serious causes are hypothyroidism, hyperthyroidism, congenital problems of the ovaries or adrenal glands, and problems with the endocrine system, such as tumors or cysts on the ovaries or adrenal glands.

A condition that is not serious but troublesome is delayed menarche, the first period of young girls. In some girls, it is delayed until after the age of sixteen because of genetic tendencies or hormonal deficiencies. Other reasons for delayed or halted periods include: crash dieting; obesity; anorexia nervosa and bulimia; stress; increased exercise such as strenuous training for running, gymnastics, and swimming; diabetes; or heart disease. Birth control pills, barbiturates, steroids, and some blood pressure medicines can also cause periods to be delayed or halted.

A physician should always evaluate when periods are missed to make sure there are no serious problems. If this is a recurrent problem, but serious illness or pregnancy are ruled out, natural methods can be helpful. Eating properly, cutting back on exercise, and stress reduction techniques can help restart the menstrual cycle and keep it regular. A chronically delayed period represents a constitutional problem and should be treated by a skilled homeopath. Occasional late or missed periods can be treated with homeopathic remedies on an acute basis.

Aconite. Useful when the menstrual flow stops because the person is scared or frightened.

Apis. Useful for late menstrual periods that may be accompanied by stinging pain in the right ovary. The vaginal tissue tends to be swollen and feels better with cold water. When the period does not come, headaches often occur. This is often seen in teenagers or young women who tend to be whiny, tearful, restless, and tend to change boyfriends on a whim or change jobs frequently. During the time before the period comes, the person who needs *Apis* tends to be awkward and clumsy.

Bryonia. Useful for nosebleeds that occur instead of the menstrual period. The person is irritable and does not like to be bothered, especially when the period is late. The person tends to be constipated and experience abdominal pain and cramps that are worse from movement and feel better when resting. There is thirst for cold liquids.

Dulcamara. Helpful when menstrual periods are late and very short. The menstrual blood is watery and thin, and a rash or pimples often appear before the period begins.

Gelsemium. Useful for a delayed or suppressed menstrual period. A sense of heaviness in the uterine area is accompanied by drowsiness, apathy, and extreme tiredness. Sometimes there is pain across the back in the sacral area, as if the period is about to start. The person often loses her voice during the menstrual period.

Graphites. Helps when menstrual periods are too late, too light, and too short in duration. *Graphites* is often useful for heavy women who tend to be anemic, cold, constipated, and have eczema or other skin problems. Useful when ongoing constipation and delayed menstruation occur simultaneously.

Kali carb. Often indicated in young girls who have delayed or difficult menstrual periods, with long intervals between periods. There tends to be weakness in the back, and the legs often feel like they are giving out.

Natrum mur. Useful for menstrual periods that are late and often too short and light. When the period does come, the blood tends to be dark and flows day and night. Before the menstrual period, the person experiences sadness, depression, anxiety, and even palpitations and a fluttering sensation in the heart.

Pulsatilla. One of the most important remedies for absent or delayed menstrual periods. The menstrual blood flow tends to be scanty and often starts and stops. The flow increases during the day or when walking, and lessens at night. Various events tend to suppress the period (such as disappointment in a love relationship or, oddly, getting the feet wet). The person feels chilly most of the time, even when in a warm room; the person does, however, like to have cool air blowing and will often go outside or open a window. Sometimes a nosebleed occurs in place of the menstrual period. *Pulsatilla* is useful when the first menstrual period (menarche) does not arrive in girls who are in the middle adolescent period (ages thirteen to fifteen).

Sepia. Useful when menstrual periods tend to be late, too light, and flow only in the morning. The periods also can be regular, but are very light and last only one day. The person is weak, irritable, and weepy. When the period does come, pains often shoot up the vagina into the uterus. There may also be the sensation of a ball or round object in the uterus or vagina. The person tends to feel weak in the small of the back and there may be a coldness between the shoulders. She generally feels better with exercise and activity, and when pressure and warmth are applied to the uterine area.

Sulphur. Helps when menstrual periods are either late or suppressed and are often too short and light. *Sulphur* tends to be associated with burning feet and heat on the top of the head. The person tends to feel worse around 11:00 A.M. and prefers not to bathe or have any water come in contact with the body. There is a tendency to be disorganized and messy.

PERIODS: LIGHT OR SCANTY

Some women have lighter periods than others; this is a normal physiological difference. However, especially when there has been a change in the flow, lighter periods can represent illnesses or a problem with the female reproductive tract. Homeopathy can be helpful if the problem is occasional and without serious symptoms.

Light or scanty periods have multiple causes that can either be serious or benign. Some serious causes are hypothyroidism, hyperthyroidism, congenital problems of the ovaries or adrenal glands, and problems with the endocrine system, such as tumors or cysts on the ovaries or adrenal glands. Other causes for light or scanty periods include: crash dieting; obesity; anorexia nervosa and bulimia; stress; increased exercise such as strenuous training for running, gymnastics, and swimming; diabetes; or heart disease. Birth control pills, barbiturates, steroids, and some blood pressure medicines can also cause periods to be light or scanty.

A physician should always evaluate light or scanty periods to make sure there are no serious problems. If this is a recurrent problem, but serious illness or pregnancy are ruled out, natural methods can be helpful. Eating properly, cutting back on exercise, and stress reduction techniques can help regulate the menstrual cycle. A chronically light period represents a constitutional problem and should be treated by a skilled homeopath. Occasional light or scanty periods can be treated with homeopathic remedies on an acute basis.

Carbo veg. Helps light menstrual periods that often come too early. The menstrual blood is quite odorous. *Carbo veg* is often associated with cold and clammy skin, anxiety, a desire to be fanned (the person does not seem to be getting enough oxygen), and excess gas formation (especially in the upper abdomen), which is temporarily relieved by belching.

Graphites. Light menstrual periods that are often late and very short in duration are helped by this remedy. *Graphites* is generally associated with worn out, tired women who are constipated. These women are constantly cold, often overweight, and have rough, dry skin and eczema.

Lachesis. Useful for menstrual periods that are scanty, light, and often irregular. The menstrual blood tends to be very dark. The person feels better mentally and emotionally when the flow starts. The only time the period is heavy with this remedy is after menopause begins and the person bleeds a heavy, dark flow. *Lachesis* is often associated with hot flashes and a need to talk. Symptoms are better when the menstrual blood flows and worse when it stops.

Magnesia carb. Useful for menstrual periods that are light, especially during the day after rising. Menstrual flow tends to increase at night when the person is lying down. *Magnesia carb* is also associated with a light flow during menopause when occasional bleeding is experienced.

Natrum mur. Useful for menstrual periods that are scanty, light, too short, and often late. The menstrual blood is dark and tends to flow both day and night. The person perspires, is irritable and depressed, and often craves salt before the period begins. The person feels vulnerable and wants to take care of others. *Natrum mur* is often useful in the helping professions (such as teachers, librarians, and health care professionals), who overwork and have delayed, light, and irregular menstrual periods.

Pulsatilla. Helps light menstrual periods that are either late or are completely absent and suppressed. There is great weepiness, chilliness, and a desire to be consoled and cared for. The menstrual blood flow tends to increase during the day when walking and lessens at night. The person tends to avoid stuffy rooms and wants to be outside in cool air.

Sulphur. Useful for menstrual periods that are too light, too short, and often late. The period tends to get worse in the early morning. Menstrual bleeding often causes the vaginal area to become red and inflamed, and there is heat all over the body, especially in the feet and the top of the head. The person who needs this remedy is often disorganized and generally does not like to bathe or shower. The skin tends to be itchy and red.

PERIODS: PAINFUL
(INCLUDES DYSMENORRHEA AND MENSTRUAL CRAMPS)

Many women suffer from painful menstruation (dysmenorrhea) and menstrual cramps. The intensity of the pain may change, and it is often difficult to find its origin. An intense muscular contraction of the uterus may be from nerve irritation due to trauma. Irritation of the uterus from fibroid tumors, as well as emotional stress, can sometimes initiate or aggravate painful menstrual cramps.

More serious causes of menstrual pain include: infection of the uterus, pregnancy in a fallopian tube, cysts in the uterus or ovary, fibroid tumors, endometriosis, and cancer. Pelvic pain should be evaluated carefully by a physician. If the cause of the pain is not a chronic condition, homeopathic remedies can be helpful. If the problem recurs each month, a skilled homeopath can be helpful in treating the person with deep-acting remedies to change the intensity and help heal the irritated uterine tissues and nerves.

Apis. Useful for intense menstrual cramps that have a labor-like, bearing-down sensation. *Apis* is usually associated with stinging ovarian pains that are worse on the right side. The abdomen tends to swell before the menstrual period, and the body feels full of water. Swollen labia are relieved when cold water is applied.

Belladonna. Useful for cramps preceding the menstrual period. The cramps are accompanied by a sensation of heaviness in the uterus, as if the pelvic organs might protrude from the vulva (similar to *Sepia*); this sensation is relieved by sitting upright (unlike *Sepia,* which is better while sitting down with the legs crossed). Uterine pain tends to start and stop suddenly. The vagina is hot and dry, and the menstrual blood is odorous and clotted. Cramps are described as cutting and travel through the pelvis horizontally.

Bromium. Can help when early and heavy menstrual periods are extremely painful. The left ovary often hurts and feels swollen, and there may be a left-sided headache during the menstrual period, especially in those who are thin, blonde, and sensitive to heat. The person who needs this remedy tends to feel better when near the ocean. There is a tendency to be depressed before the menstrual period starts.

Calcarea carb. Useful for menstrual cramps accompanying heavy periods. The calves or legs tend to cramp during the pain. *Calcarea carb* is also useful for menstrual cramps that come on when the person is overexcited. It is generally indicated in those who are overweight, chilly, and subject to anxiety, especially regarding health.

Calcarea phos. Useful for menstrual cramps, especially for young girls whose periods are just beginning. The period tends to arrive too early and last too long, and it may often become worse after urination or bowel movements. *Calcarea phos* is useful for slender teenage girls who have low energy levels and feelings of weakness.

Caulophyllum. Useful for painful menstrual cramps when pain travels to other parts of the body (such as the groin or legs). There may be needle-like pains in the cervix. The menstrual periods are generally very light. These people tend to be weak, sensitive to cold, and often have problems with joints, especially the smaller joints of the fingers and toes.

Chamomilla. Useful for menstrual cramps that seem unbearable to the person, causing her to cry and scream (the pain is out of proportion to the actual condition). *Chamomilla* is also used for painful periods that come on after anger. The person is sensitive, irritable, thirsty, hot, and numb in various parts of the body. There is a tendency to have diarrhea during the period. The person is impatient, intolerant of being spoken to, and oversensitive in any kind of interaction.

Cimicifuga. Useful for menstrual cramps that travel across the pelvic region from side to side. There may also be pain in the ovarian region that shoots upward and also down the front of the thigh. The cramps tend to get worse during the menstrual period; in fact, the more profuse the menstrual flow, the greater the abdominal pain. While the pain is bothersome and unusual, it is not as severe or intense as what is felt during the *Chamomilla* type of pain.

Cocculus. Useful for menstrual cramps that are spasmodic and often associated with hemorrhoids. During the menstrual period, the person is weak and almost unable to stand. *Cocculus* is often useful for those who experience menstrual cramps while on a trip, especially in a car, boat, or airplane where there is nausea, vomiting, and general motion sickness. This remedy may also be helpful for menstrual cramps that occur while the person is caring for someone who is sick or dying. Abdominal pain sometimes feels as though sharp stones are rubbing against each other, and the abdomen is distended because of an accumulation of gas. The cramps tend to get worse at night, awakening the person and causing irritability. *Cocculus* is also associated with nausea, especially when the period arrives too early.

Colocynth. Uterine cramps that cause the person to double up can be helped by this remedy. The person feels better when warmth and pressure are applied to the stomach. The pain extends from the navel to the vagina and starts and stops suddenly. There is usually irritability with this remedy and any criticism is taken as an insult; the person becomes angry, and this intensifies the menstrual cramps.

Cuprum met. Useful for violent and extreme menstrual cramping. There is cramping in the uterus, thighs, calves, and even the chest muscles. Uterine cramping is better from stooping and when pressure is applied to the abdomen. The menstrual flow tends to be profuse at night and light during the day.

Ipecac. Can provide relief from menstrual cramps accompanied by severe nausea and vomiting.

Lachesis. Useful when uterine cramps occur before the menstrual period starts. *Lachesis* is useful for those whose cramps improve when the menstrual flow begins. It is also useful for those in menopause who have cramps in their uterus because the menstrual period has stopped. This remedy can help the menstrual flow begin sooner and thus decrease cramping. Cramping tends to get worse when the person awakens from sleep. Tight clothing around the lower abdomen bothers the person. When the menstrual flow begins, it tends to be dark and slow; there may also be left-sided ovarian cramps that get better when the flow starts. The person tends to be irritable, talkative, and jealous before the onset of the period and, as soon as the period begins, the emotional tension is relieved.

Magnesia phos. Useful for cramping menstrual pain that starts several hours before the period and continues throughout the period. There is relief from doubling up and from applying firm pressure and warmth. *Magnesia phos* is often used in the 6x potency by dissolving twenty tablets in one cup of warm water and sipping the mixture slowly throughout the day.

Natrum mur. Useful for menstrual cramping that causes a bearing-down sensation in the uterus and gets worse in the morning. The menstrual periods generally are late and often too light. The breasts become sore before the periods. There is often a premenstrual headache that persists after the period begins. Heart palpitations can occur before the period. (If palpitations are new and have hot been evaluated, a physician should be consulted.) A backache is relieved when the person lies flat on the back or presses something firmly against the back while in a seated position. Feelings of sadness, depression, and irritability are experienced, and the person wants to be alone and does not like to be consoled.

Podophyllum. This remedy helps when there is pain in the right ovary that radiates to the right thigh; this is associated with abdominal cramping and diarrhea. The ovarian pain is worse when stretching the right leg.

Pulsatilla. Useful for menstrual cramps associated with late periods or periods that stop and start frequently. The pain causes the person to double up and possibly cry, and the person feels better when consoled and when bent over. The person is chilly, but does not like to be in hot, stuffy rooms, preferring the windows to be open or to walk outside in the cool air. The mouth is dry, but the person tends to be thirstless. One peculiar symptom is that when the feet get wet (such as in a rainstorm), the severity of the abdominal cramps tends to increase.

Sabina. Useful for menstrual cramps that travel from the lumbosacral area of the back to the pubic bone. This pain tends to be stabbing and moves up into the vagina. Menstrual periods are generally heavy, with a discharge of red blood with dark clots. Menstrual flow is aggravated by the slightest movement.

Sepia. Useful for menstrual cramps that are described as bearing down in the abdomen and lower back. The pelvic organs and uterus feel extremely heavy, as if they might fall out of the vagina; this feeling is relieved by sitting with the legs crossed and aggravated by standing or walking. Cramping in the uterus causes the uterus to feel as if it is being squeezed by a hand. There may be the sensation that a ball or lump is in the uterine area. Cramping pain may shoot up the vagina into the uterus. *Sepia* is often associated with menstrual periods that are late and light.

Veratrum alb. Useful for painful, heavy periods that are often accompanied by diarrhea and vomiting. There is heavy cramping and a sensation of icy coldness in the body, with cold sweat on the forehead, exhaustion, and cramps in the calves as well as thighs. The person may actually faint from the pain or from the least exertion. A peculiar symptom is that sexual desire may increase before the period is due.

PMS (ALSO CALLED PREMENSTRUAL SYNDROME)

Premenstrual syndrome (PMS) is a common problem that usually occurs seven to ten days prior to menstruation. Causes of PMS are increased estrogen and decreased progesterone levels before the menstrual period. Prolactin levels and hormones, such as aldosterone, are also elevated in women who have PMS problems.

Typical symptoms include decreased energy, fatigue, irritability, anxiety, depression, mood swings, and altered sex drive. Physical symptoms include bloating, diarrhea or constipation, change in appetite, craving for chocolate or sugar, enlarged breasts, backache, swelling of the hands and feet, headaches, and acne. Sometimes the symptoms can be very severe, causing women to feel they cannot control either their emotions or physical body. In most cases, however, the symptoms are mild and manageable.

Some natural approaches can be helpful for PMS problems. It is important to avoid caffeine since it can affect the mood with cyclical changes and mood swings. Sugar in high concentrations can cause hyperglycemic reaction, which affects the mood and energy levels and leads to headaches and irritability. Eating a moderate amount of carbohydrates and low-fat protein are also recommended. Alcohol and salt retain fluids and should be avoided. Certain herbs and vitamins are known to help PMS.

Apis. Useful for excessive premenstrual swelling, which can occur in the abdomen, hands, legs, and eyelids. There may be pain in the ovaries, especially a stinging pain in the right ovary. The person is awkward and drops things easily. She is often tearful, feels excessive jealousy and rage, and tends to whine. At other times the person may be listless and unable to concentrate and think clearly.

Calcarea carb. Helpful for premenstrual headaches, abdominal cramping, chilliness, and a milky vaginal discharge. The breasts are usually tender and swollen before the onset of the period. *Calcarea carb* may be associated with women who are heavy and chill easily. The person tends to be anxious and worries about health problems (such as the heart and contagious diseases).

Dulcamara. Useful for premenstrual rashes, eczema, and itching, especially during cold, wet weather. There may also be intensified sexual excitement before the menstrual period.

Lachesis. The mental symptoms associated with this remedy are talkativeness, increased jealousy, and unreasonableness. Headaches get worse after awakening from sleep. The face may be bloated and have a bluish-purple color. Tight clothes are not tolerated well, especially around the waist and neck. The person may experience palpitations accompanied by a sense of faintness. As soon as the period begins, the person feels much better.

Lycopodium. Associated with a person who is hard-working, likes to be in control, and is veryorganized. However, an underlying insecurity and decreased sense of self-worth become exaggerated before the menstrual period; this can lead to episodes of rage and verbal striking out at family members or colleagues if the person is stressed or insulted. The person is irritable and cries before the period begins. *Lycopodium* is associated with women who suffer from indigestion, abdominal distention due to gas buildup, and constipation. These symptoms may get worse before the period begins. The person seems to become worse emotionally and physically in the mid- to late afternoon, especially between 4:00 and 8:00 P.M.

Natrum mur. The person who needs *Natrum mur* broods and thinks about past insults; these feelings intensify before the period begins. The person becomes withdrawn, self-absorbed, irritable, and does not want comfort or consolation. Noise or any kind of mental activity are bothersome. The symptoms generally get worse around 10:00 A.M. *Natrum mur* is associated with migraine-like headaches, nausea, vomiting, and vision difficulties. There is great abdominal distention and a craving for salt. The person may experience palpitations and fluttering in the heart. (If palpitations are new and have not been evaluated, a physician should be consulted.)

Phosphorus. Helpful for the person who feels fearful and anxious at night, especially when alone. Fears and anxieties are all exaggerated during the premenstrual time. The person is hypersensitive to external influences (such as sad stories, other people's comments, or even electrical storms and thunderstorms). There is a tendency to startle easily and be weepy because of hypersensitivity. *Phosphorus* is often indicated in tall, thin, narrow chested women who tend to bleed easily. When the periods do come, they last a long time, but are not profuse. The person tends to have a lot of indigestion and vomits easily. Cold drinks relieve the indigestion, but the person vomits as soon as the water gets warm in the stomach. Painless diarrhea that causes great debility and weakness afterward is common. All symptoms tend to get worse when the person lies on the left side. The person tends to feel warm and feels better in cool, open air.

Pulsatilla. Helps during the premenstrual time when sadness, weepiness, and depression are experienced.The person tends to cry a lot and seek company and sympathy. Moods are changeable. The person may have diarrhea and indigestion. The person is chilly, yet likes to be outside in the cool air or to have the windows open with a cool breeze blowing in. There is usually a lack of thirst, despite a dry mouth.

Sepia. Helps premenstrual problems when the person is irritable and ornery, while at the same time is sad, depressed, and weeps easily when discussing problems (similar to *Pulsatilla*). The person does not want consolation when feeling bad or unhappy (similar to *Natrum mur*). The person tends to be indifferent and withdrawn, especially with those she loves the most, including her own children. The sensation that the uterus and bladder are heavy and may fall out of the pelvis may be experienced. Possible headaches on the left side are accompanied by nausea and vomiting. The sight and smell of food causes nausea, and this is accompanied by an empty feeling in the stomach that eating does not relieve. The person feels better with exercise and movement in general.

Sulphur. Can be helpful during the premenstrual time when the person is irritable and possibly lazy, not wanting to take care of herself, her family, or her business. The person does not want to bathe or maintain a neat appearance. Headaches occur, especially with heat on the top of the head. The body tends to itch and feel hot, and the skin burns. The person feels weak and faint around 11:00 A.M. and must eat something, especially before the period begins.

Zincum met. Helps the person who is adverse to working and talking before the menstrual period begins. The person is lethargic, yet at the same time is restless and hypersensitive to noise in particular. The person is depressed, anxious, and weepy. The body feels cold, and there is aching and burning along the spine. The nape of the neck feels tired when writing or from any exertion. A guiding symptom to this remedy is that the feet are extremely restless and in constant motion; the person cannot keep them still, even at night before bed. Fitful sleep is experienced in that the body jerks and the person wakes up frightened.

POISON IVY AND POISON OAK

Poison ivy and poison oak are related plants that cause similar allergic reactions when a person comes in contact with them. Reaction to the irritants can range from no symptoms at all, if the person is not sensitive to the substances, to severe systemic problems, with great breakouts of itching rashes and difficult breathing. The rash is usually red and itchy, and forms blisters.

Poison ivy is often not spread after the first hour or two of contact with the plant, since the chemical actually binds itself to the skin. What most people experience within the first hour is the spreading of the irritant to other exposed parts of the body, either through touching the plant or rubbing the skin with clothes or hands that have been contaminated. The body then breaks out at different times, depending on the local area's specific sensitivity.

When first exposed to poison ivy or poison oak, it is important to clean the skin thoroughly. This may diminish or even stop future breakouts. When prescribing homeopathic remedies, it is important to observe the modalities, such as whether the eruptions are better from cold applications or warm applications, whether the person is restless or not, and what the skin actually feels like.

Because the two plants cause similar reactions, the listings here speak of poison ivy only. Both plants are included, unless specified otherwise. Also, the term poison ivy is used here to denote the skin rash caused by contact with either plant.

Anacardium. The affected area itches intensely and might swell (such as with hives). The person with poison ivy is overly anxious, fearful, demanding, and easily offended. The person may become confused about the poison ivy and how severe it really is. Pain and itching are worse when hot water is applied. Gently rubbing the area makes the person feel better.

Croton tig. This remedy is particularly helpful when poison ivy occurs on the face or genitals. The skin feels tight, and the affected area itches intensely, followed by painful burning. Scratching is painful. Sometimes the person has watery diarrhea that is forcibly shot out after much urging. Symptoms are worse from heat, touch, and washing.

Graphites. This type of poison ivy sometimes appears in the bends of the elbows or knees, behind the ears, on the neck, or in the groin area. It is characterized by sticky discharges that ooze out of the eruptions.

Grindelia robusta. Useful as an external wash for poison ivy. Mix ten drops in a quart of water. Soak sterile gauze in the mixture, and apply it to the irritated area.

Ledum. This type of poison ivy is worse from warm applications and the heat of a bed. It is better from cold applications.

Rhus tox. This remedy is actually made from poison ivy.

Characteristic symptoms are restlessness and agitation with a continual change of position, especially at night. The person cannot remain in the bed. Symptoms are worse from cold applications and better from warmth. Gentle rubbing may help the itching.

PROSTATE DISORDERS

The prostate is a walnut-sized gland that surrounds the urethra in men. Most men after the age of forty-five develop an enlargement of the prostate gland, called benign prostatic hyperplasia. Symptoms include difficulty starting the urine flow, a slower stream of urine, and dribbling after urination with a feeling that some urine remains. As men age, the enlargement of the prostate increases. They wake up at night with the urge to urinate, but pass only small amounts. Generally this problem is more a nuisance than a great concern, although if the enlargement is too severe, it may cause an obstruction leading to the inability to urinate, a kidney infection, or bleeding. Another problem common in men is prostatitis, which can be caused by bacteria, viruses, or irritation from sports or injury. This can lead to symptoms similar to benign prostatic hyperplasia.

Prostate disease is diagnosed by several different methods. A blood test to determine the concentration of prostate-specific antigen (PSA) can help diagnose prostate disease. It can also help determine if cancer is a possibility, since the level of PSA becomes dramatically higher in people who have cancer. Elevated levels of PSA can also indicate prostatitis or benign prostatic hyperplasia. A digital rectal examination may determine if the prostate is enlarged and an ultrasound of the prostate gland can also determine if there are enlargement problems. To rule out cancer, which can have symptoms similar to hyperplasia, a biopsy of the prostate gland is sometimes performed.

It is important to drink plenty of fluids and avoid alcohol, since one of the hormones that causes the prostate to enlarge is increased by the consumption of alcoholic beverages. There seems to be lower incidence of enlarged prostates in men who have low cholesterol, indicating that eating foods low in fat, especially saturated fat, is helpful. Hot sitz baths can be helpful for glands that are acutely swollen, especially when there is prostatitis. Certain herbs and supplements are known to help prostate problems.

Aconite. Useful for the very first stages of prostate inflammation and infection. Symptoms can occur after exposure to cold, dry air and wind, and possibly after an experience that causes fear.

Apis. An enlarged, inflamed prostate can be treated with *Apis,* especially when the person feels stinging pain during urination. When the person urinates, the last drop burns as it comes out. There may be swelling in the legs or hands.

Baryta carb. An enlarged prostate (especially in older people) can be treated with *Baryta carb.* The urethra burns during urination. A peculiar symptom is that each time the person urinates, the hemorrhoids come down. Sexual desire decreases. Often, symptoms of memory loss and a decrease in self-confidence are seen (especially in older people).

Belladonna. Useful for treating inflammation of the prostate gland that may occur with fever. There may be hot, red skin, a flushed face, glaring eyes, and an excited mental state. Urinary retention is a common symptom. A peculiar symptom is that the bladder feels as though a worm is inside it. Pain in the prostate gets worse from any kind of jarring motion.

Chimaphila. Useful for acute prostatitis with retention of urine and a feeling that there is a ball in the perineum. The person is unable to urinate without standing with the feet wide apart and body bent forward. The person must strain before urine flows.

Lycopodium. Useful for an acute exacerbation of chronic prostatitis. The person emits prostatic fluid after urination (without an erection). Urine is slow to come. Impotence is sometimes a symptom with this problem. Flatulence and aggravation between 4:00 and 8:00 P.M. are typical. Back pain occurs before urinating. Urine may contain a reddish sediment. The frequency of urination increases during the night.

Pulsatilla. Helpful for treating an enlarged prostate accompanied by acute prostatitis. The person feels pain in the prostate gland after urination, which gets worse from lying on the back. The urine stream seems interrupted and urine may pass only in drops. The person is often emotionally sensitive and cries easily. There may be chilliness, yet the person wants to be out in the open air. The person is generally thirstless.

Sabal serrulata. Useful for an enlarged prostate. There may be either an acute, swollen prostate or a chronically enlarged prostate associated with benign prostate hyperplasia. This latter condition, which is associated with older men, makes urination difficult. *Sabal serrulata* can help decrease the size of the prostate gland.

Silica. A prostate infection with pus formation can be treated with this remedy. The prostatic fluid often contains infected material that comes out when the person strains for a stool.

Staphysagria. Useful for prostate enlargement and inflammation. A peculiar symptom is the sensation that a drop of urine is continually rolling down the urethra. The urethra burns when the person is not urinating. Obsessive sexual thoughts and a tendency to dwell on sexual matters are common with this problem.

Thuja. Used for chronic cases of prostate infections. The urine stream is poor and often forked or split. The person has a frequent, urgent desire to urinate. The area between the rectum and bladder burns.

PUNCTURE WOUNDS

Puncture wounds are caused by sharp, penetrating objects such as needles, thorns, or nails. Bacteria or other infectious materials may be forced under the skin, causing pain and infection. A tetanus shot may be necessary, especially if the puncture is caused by a dirty or rusty object or an object contaminated by animal feces. Bites and stings are other forms of puncture wounds (see Bites and Stings for specific information).

Aconite. Useful if the person with a puncture wound is fearful or panicky. A physician should be contacted regarding a tetanus shot for puncture wounds, especially if caused by a dirty or rusty object or an object contaminated by animal feces.

Arnica. Helpful when a wound is excessively sore or bruised or if the person is in shock. The signs of shock include: a rapid, weak pulse; cool, clammy skin; lightheadedness; irregular breathing;

confusion; or loss of consciousness. A doctor or person trained in emergency medicine should be contacted.

Calendula. Can be used as a tincture, ointment, or lotion on the site of the puncture. Immediately after the puncture, the wound should be cleaned with *Calendula* tincture to reduce the risk of infection.

Hypericum. Useful for a puncture located in a nerve-rich area, when pain travels up from the limb or the site of the injury, or when the wound is on the chest or abdomen. The pain travels toward the center of the body. When red streaking moves from the injury upward (such as in puncture wounds from thorns or nails), this remedy is often used. This could be a serious condition because infection may be spreading to the blood or lymph glands. A physician should be contacted. A tetanus shot for the puncture wounds may also be required, especially if caused by a dirty or rusty object or an object contaminated by animal feces. Before the tetanus vaccine was invented, *Hypericum* was alternated with *Ledum* in a potency of 30c to prevent tetanus.

Ledum. A classic homeopathic remedy for puncture wounds and generally the first remedy used after any puncture unless there is great fear (use *Aconite*), soreness, or shock (use *Arnica*). Note that a physician should be contacted regarding a tetanus shot for puncture wounds, especially if caused by a dirty or rusty object or an object contaminated by animal feces. The injured part feels cold to the touch, although it feels hot to the person who is injured. The wound is better from cold bathing, ice water, cold dressings, cold air, and uncovering. The pain gets worse from warmth and touch. *Ledum* can be alternated with *Arnica* every two hours if much bruising occurs, or with *Hypericum* if there is great pain or injury to the nerve tissue. Puncture wounds that are treated by *Ledum* include: injections (such as vaccinations) or lumbar punctures (spinal taps); nail, splinter, or pin wounds; and animal or insect bites.

RADIATION SIDE EFFECTS

Radiation can cause many types of injuries to the body. The most severe damage is to the genetic part of the cell's nucleus, because of the structural alterations of DNA in the chromosomes. Because of the loss of chromosomes, cell death occurs. Most exposure to radiation in humans has occurred over the last seventy-five years. Early cases were in the 1920s and 1930s, when some 2,000 luminous dial workers, mostly young women in the United States, inadvertently ingested large amounts of radium on their tongues and lips; this lead to development of cancer in their sinuses. In Germany during the mid-1940s, children with tuberculosis of the bones and adults with rheumatoid arthritis were injected with radium; several years later, they developed bone cancer. Increased mortality from leukemia and multiple myeloma has been documented in radiologists during the early years of the use of X-ray equipment. Increased rates of thyroid cancer and leukemia have been reported in adults treated with X-rays in the 1940s and 1950s for thymus enlargement or eczema of the scalp. There has been an increase in lung cancer among uranium miners. The most serious form of radiation sickness occurred following weapons testing in the Marshall Islands and after the atomic bomb was dropped in Japan near the end of World War II.

There are many forms of radiation sickness, including loss of appetite, nausea and vomiting, diarrhea, excessive abdominal cramps, and dehydration. Effects after excessive exposure can be lethargy, weakness, seizures, convulsions, and death.

Radiation treatment is used for many types of cancer, including breast, uterine, and prostate. While it sometimes can help slow the cancer growth and improve long-range survival, radiation can also cause problems with nausea, vomiting, weakness, and pain. Radiation exposure can be a very serious problem; a physician or emergency room should always be contacted immediately regarding radiation side effects.

It is interesting to note that radiation and its effect on the body is similar to the homeopathic idea of disease causation. Radiation can cause cancer, yet it also can help cure cancer in smaller doses. This is similar to the homeopathic idea of the law of similars. The homeopathic remedies listed here can help diminish the side effects from radiation exposure or after radiation treatment for various illnesses.

Cadmium sulphuratum. Vomiting and diarrhea occur after radiation treatments. The vomit may be black or full of mucus and blood. The person is extremely exhausted. Note that if there is red or dark blood or black material in the vomit, a physician should be contacted.

Ipecac. Often used for people who are undergoing radiation treatment for cancer. Severe, persistent vomiting and nausea after radiation are typical symptoms. The tongue is clean.

Nux vomica. Useful for diarrhea with an intense urge for a stool. The person may be unable to pass any stool despite a sensation that there is more to pass. Anxiety, irritability, and sensitivity to touch, smell, and odors are common.

Phosphorus. The person is extremely weak and tired. The physical energy prior to radiation is gone. The person is unable to do daily chores because of the extreme weakness.

SCARS

Scarring can occur from any injury to the skin, including accidental injury, surgery, or acne. Scars can sometimes become thick, fibrous keloids, especially in dark-skinned individuals. Several homeopathic remedies help decrease inflammation of scars, and some are even known to dissolve scars and adhesions within the body.

Calendula. To keep future scar formation soft and help decrease the possibility of infection, *Calendula* ointment is useful. The ointment can be used liberally two or three times a day, and will help the body absorb excess scar tissue, which is often seen when there is a sticky discharge early in scar development, or when a scar occasionally breaks down and oozes a sticky material. *Calendula* is particularly helpful when hard scars are caused by burns. The scar is painful and gets worse when exposed to open air; *Calendula* can help keep the scar soft.

Causticum. Particularly useful when a scar reopens (especially a scar from an old injury). Helpful when the skin and tendons of an old burn that did not heal well contract. *Causticum* may help heal the scar and relax the contracted areas that were injured.

Lachesis. Useful when scars bleed, become painful, and are quite red.

Nitric acid. Useful when a wound becomes painful (especially with a sticking pain). The pain is often worse when the weather changes.

Silica. One of the most important remedies for scar tissue formation, because it helps soften scar tissue. The scar may be shiny with sharp edges, and it may become sore even months after it has formed. This remedy can be used in the 6x potency for a long period of time (up to one or two months).

Thiosinaminum. Can help dissolve scar tissue deep inside the body (such as adhesions from previous surgeries). Scarring of the eardrum after a rupture and numerous infections are also helped with this remedy. *Thiosinaminum* 30c is often alternated with *Silica* 6x throughout the day at three- to four-hour intervals, so that each remedy is taken twice during the day.

SCIATICA

Sciatica is a condition in which the nerves that run from the back to the legs are stretched or irritated. The sciatic nerve is a large nerve in the body and a composite of many nerve roots that come out the spine in the lower lumbar and upper sacral regions. Back trauma, disease of the spinal vertebrae, herniated disks, muscle spasms, and arthritis can all lead to irritation and inflammation of the sciatic nerve.

One symptom of sciatica is pain in the lower back that radiates into the buttocks and thighs, especially the back and outside of the leg. There can be burning and tingling in the area and a sensation of numbness in the feet. When the numbness gets severe or there is a diminished reflex in the knee, the pressure on the sciatic nerve has become severe and a physician should be contacted.

Milder forms of sciatica tend to be recurrent and chronic. Treatment includes bedrest, traction to open up the vertebrae, ice when an injury has recently caused a problem, or heat when there are spasms in the lower back. Massage, physical therapy, chiropractic care, and acupuncture can help decrease inflammation, decrease spasms of the muscles around the nerve, and help with circulation in the area. Certain vitamins and supplements are known to help sciatica.

Aconite. Only useful in the beginning stages of sciatica. Useful for sciatica that comes on after exposure to cold, dry air. The person is restless and afraid, and may experience tingling or numbness along the nerve. The pain is excruciating and becomes worse at night.

Arnica. Useful for pain that comes on after overexertion, injury, straining, or lifting. The pain travels from the buttocks to the leg. The person changes position often and feels as though everything lain upon is too hard. There is soreness and a sensation of feeling bruised.

Arsenicum alb. Useful for burning pains that run down the sciatic nerve and become worse at night (especially after midnight). The pain is unbearable, and the burning is aggravated by cold, but feels momentarily better when warmth is applied. Vigorous activity increases the pain, and gentle motion provides relief.

Belladonna. Useful for a sciatic nerve that is inflamed and has pain that comes on suddenly. The nerve is irritated. The pain is especially severe at night and worse from touch, the least jarring, and drafts of air. The person is agitated and has to change positions often. The pain gets worse with motion, noise, or contact (even contact with clothing). The pain is relieved by letting the limb hang down, warm applications, and by sitting up straight.

Bryonia. Useful for shooting, stitching pains in the back, which move down the leg. These pains are aggravated by motion and exposure to cold and are relieved by lying perfectly still and applying hard pressure.

Causticum. Useful when the person experiences burning, rawness, and soreness of the sciatic nerve, especially on the left side, accompanied by numbness and the feeling that the leg is paralyzed. The leg feels contracted, and the tendon feels shortened. The pain gets better when warmth is applied, and becomes worse from lying in bed and walking in the open air. The person experiences a constant desire to move the feet, although this does not provide relief.

Chamomilla. Useful for left-sided sciatica accompanied by excruciating pain that seems exaggerated for the actual problem. The pain is associated with a numb feeling that gets worse at night and from motion.

Colchicum. Useful for right-sided sciatica when pain shoots down the leg, to the knee. The person must keep still because the pain gets worse with motion. The pain comes on suddenly, and is constant and very severe. Sciatica may be associated with gout, inner stiffness, and heat in the joints.

Colocynth. One of the most important remedies for sciatica. Pain travels along the sciatic nerve, extending down to the knee or heel. The pain gets worse from any kind of motion and from cold. Sharp, cramping pain comes in waves and is followed by numbness that can even lead to partial loss of sensation in the lower part of the foot. The person may feel as if the thigh is bound with iron bands or clamped in a vice. The muscles are tense and contracted. The pain is particularly worse on the right side, and the person has difficulty walking and can find no comfortable position for the leg.

Hypericum. Useful for sciatica caused by injury to the nerve. The pain is excruciating and gets worse in cold, damp weather.

Iris. Useful for sciatica in which there is a feeling that the left hip joint was wrenched. The pain extends down to the back of the knee.

Kali bich. Useful for left-sided sciatica that gets better from motion. The person experiences light pains that travel rapidly from one area to another. These wandering pains seem to run along the leg bone and get worse when exposed to cold. Along with this kind of sciatica, there can be soreness of the heels when walking. This type of sciatica gets worse from a change of weather, standing up, and pressure. The pain comes and goes suddenly and wanders up and down the leg. Walking alleviates the pain.

Kali iod. Useful for sciatica in which the pain becomes worse at night and when lying on the painful leg. The sciatica becomes better in the open air.

Lachesis. Useful when the sciatica is worse on the right side and the person feels better lying down. This is an unusual symptom for this remedy since *Lachesis* is usually a remedy associated with left-sided problems. The person is nervous and very talkative. The pains are worse after waking in the morning.

Ledum. Useful for sciatica in which the pain seems to originate in the foot and spread upward, rather than the typical downward spread. The leg feels cooler than the rest of the body, and the pain gets worse when the leg gets warm, especially when the person is in bed and under the covers. The heels and soles of the foot are tender, and the person, as a whole, feels better when chilly.

Magnesia phos. Useful for right-sided sciatica with painful lightning-like shocks that travel along the nerve. This pain can actually cause the person to cry. The pain is worse from touch, pressure, and exposure to cold air, and gets better when external heat is applied.

Nux vomica. Frequently used for sciatica because of its gentle action on the spinal cord. Pain is violent and lightning-like, shooting down into the foot and causing the leg to be cold, to stiffen, and contract. The leg feels numb and paralyzed, and the calves and soles of the foot are cramped. The person may actually drag the foot when walking. The pain gets better from lying on the side of the sciatica and from application of hot compresses or water.

Phytolacca. Useful for sciatica in which the pain feels like electric shocks along the nerves. The pain shoots and shifts to different areas, appearing and disappearing rapidly. The pain can occur on the outside of the thigh. The person experiences a desire to move, but any attempt to move aggravates the pain.

Pulsatilla. Useful for mild forms of sciatica in which the person experiences aching in the hips and a sense of heaviness and fatigue in the leg and lower back. The person is weepy and wants company. This remedy may be associated with women who have problems with varicose veins, hemorrhoids, or painful menstrual periods. This sciatica often occurs on the left side and is worse on beginning movement, in the evening, in a warm room, and also from letting the leg hang down when sitting in a chair. The sciatica gets better in the open air and with gentle motion such as walking around, rubbing the affected area, and applying pressure.

Rhus tox. Helpful for sciatica that worsens during rest and is aggravated when the person begins to move. Continual motion alleviates the pain, but as soon as movement stops, the sciatica returns. Pain comes on after wrenching the back or from overexertion. Note that *Arnica* should be the first choice for this type of pain; *Rhus tox* is useful when the pain becomes more chronic. Pain is also aggravated from exposure to cold, wet weather; the person experiences relief from warmth and rubbing. The person is usually restless and is often in constant motion. The muscles become tense, causing tearing and burning pains. Sciatica helped by *Rhus tox* is sometimes accompanied by other joint and muscular problems.

Thuja. Useful for left-sided sciatica. When the person walks, the limbs feel as if they are made of wood or glass that could break easily. *Thuja* is useful for sciatica that gets worse when the person bends forward.

SHINGLES (ALSO CALLED HERPES ZOSTER)

Shingles is a localized eruption that represents a recurrence or reactivation of the chickenpox infection and is caused by the herpes zoster virus. Blisters with a red base break out along a sensory nerve in certain parts of the body, often in the face, side, or back. Shingles most often occurs in older adults, but can also occur in healthy children and children who have immune system problems such as kidney disease, cancer, or HIV infection and are taking steroids.

Shingles is very painful. The person complains of pain in a specific area before the breakout occurs. Researchers hope that mass immunization with the chickenpox vaccine will make shingles a less serious problem.

Apis. Useful for shingles with large, stinging blisters. Cold compresses relieve the pain. The person is generally not thirsty.

Arsenicum alb. Useful for treating eruptions from shingles that burn like hot coals and are relieved by heat and warm compresses. Blisters may join together. Pain usually occurs at night (especially between midnight and 3:00 A.M.). Great restlessness and anxiety occur because the person feels like the condition is serious and incurable. Extreme weakness accompanies this restlessness. The person is generally thirsty for small amounts of water at a time.

Belladonna. Useful in the very early stages of shingles. The area where the shingles break out is red and burning. The person is extremely sensitive to contact, and the pains are worse from warm applications.

Hypericum. Useful when shingles have dried and begun to heal. Pain radiates along the nerves, causing excruciating pain. This pain is aggravated by any kind of jarring or motion. Useful for any type of injury to the nerve that causes pain, swelling, irritation, or inflammation.

Iris. Useful for shingles accompanied by gastric problems (such as nausea and vomiting) and a headache preceded by blurred vision. The pains usually begin over one eye (especially the right eye). Thick, ropy saliva may drop from the mouth during conversation. Generally, this type of shingles is on the right side and affects the eye area.

Lachesis. Useful for shingles accompanied by dark blue or purplish eruptions. This remedy is particularly helpful for shingles located on the chest wall and back. Pains are often left-sided and are worse from any kind of pressure and after waking up. Eruptions tend to bleed.

Magnesia phos. Useful for spasmodic, cramp-like, post-herpes pain that starts and ends suddenly. Intense pain often makes the person cry out. Heat and bending forward generally relieve the pain. This remedy is particularly helpful for post-herpetic facial or eye neuralgia (especially when located on the right side). A low potency of this remedy (such as 6x) can be useful when dissolved in one cup of warm water and sipped during the painful episodes.

Mezereum. Shingles with small, extremely itchy blisters that dry quickly and form thick scabs can be relieved with *Mezereum.* When pressure is applied, the white or brownish crusts may release yellow or white pus from small ulcers under the crusts. The person is extremely chilly and the itching is intense. The person is worse from scratching, from heat, and at night. *Mezereum* is particularly useful when the shingles are located around the ribs, the intercostal muscles, and the face. Oddly, although the symptoms are worse at night and from the warmth of a bed, the warmth of a heating duct or heater relieves the symptoms. This remedy is also very useful for pain that occurs after the blisters have healed.

Petroleum. Useful for the burning pains of shingles. Characteristics include great itching and a raw feeling.

Rhus tox. Shingles characterized by very small eruptions (about the size of a pin head) can be treated effectively with *Rhus tox.* The base of the eruptions is red, very itchy, burning, and contains a clear liquid. The itchiness is not relieved by scratching, but is relieved temporarily by constantly changing position, hot showers, and hot compresses. *Rhus tox* is often useful for shingles located on the right side of the body. The symptoms are worse at night, in damp weather, and in cold months (such as late fall and winter). Useful in the early stages of shingles and particularly helpful for shingles of the chest and back.

Sulphur. Helps facilitate the eruption of shingles. The more the body erupts, the less likely the virus is to travel along the nerve, reducing the chance of post-herpes neuralgic pain. Itching and burning are worse from heat and bathing, and relieved by scratching. Useful for large, itchy, burning eruptions that are relieved from cool temperatures and cool compresses and worsened by warmth.

SINUS INFECTION (ALSO CALLED SINUSITIS)

A sinus infection, also called sinusitis, is the inflammation of the sinus cavities that make up about one-third of the skull capacity. When the tiny holes that drain the sinuses get blocked because of infections or allergies, the mucus remains in the sinus cavities and becomes infected with bacteria. This causes pain, congestion in the head, and a thick green or yellow discharge; a fever may accompany this condition. Allergies can cause pain in the sinus area with a clear discharge. If a fever and green or yellow discharge continue after a few days, a physician should be contacted.

If sinusitis is chronic, with no fever and tolerable pain, then simple, natural methods can help heal the sinuses. It is important to drink plenty of fluids, such as hot teas and soups, and at least six to eight glasses of water a day. The environment that the person is living in should be humidified with a cool mist vaporizer. Often, steaming the face with hot water or taking a hot shower can help drain the sinuses. Using warm compresses over the sinus area can help relieve the pain and initiate drainage. Massaging the forehead and face can help increase circulation and diminish the discomfort. Certain vitamins and herbs are known to help sinusitis.

Arsenicum alb. A thin, watery nasal discharge burns and irritates the upper lip. Sinuses burn. The nose feels stuffed up, and sneezing does not relieve the stuffiness. The person craves warm drinks, which temporarily relieve the burning sensations in the nose and sinuses. The mental state is very important in that the person is anxious, fearful, restless, and feels chilly. The problems tend to be worse between midnight and 2:00 or 3:00 A.M. Nasal discharge is more profuse in the open air and less profuse indoors. The person generally feels better by placing hot applications on the face and elevating the head.

Calcarea carb. This type of sinus infection comes on when there is a change of weather. Glands around the neck get enlarged, and the head tends to sweat. A headache extends from the front part of the head to the nose. A yellowish, thick pus drains from the sinuses and nose and has an offensive odor (similar to manure or rotten eggs). The nostrils are sore and ulcerated, especially at the wings of the nostrils. The sinuses and nasal membranes are dry during the day and tend to drain at night. The nose drains while in the cold air, but stuffs up in warm air. The person feels thirsty, chilly, and anxious.

Hepar sulph. The type of sinusitis relieved by *Hepar sulph* is associated with a green or yellow discharge that drains from the sinuses into the nose. This discharge is blown out frequently. The person is very sensitive to cold winds and will cover the neck and face for protection from the wind. An aching pain at the base of the nose and above the eyes is common. Swollen, tender lymph glands along the neck are often present. The pains are worse upon waking and from motion, stooping, and moving the eyes. Symptoms are relieved by warmth.

Hydrastis. Can be used for sinusitis associated with a thick, sticky, yellowish discharge that drains from the sinuses into the nose. There is a pressing, dull pain in the forehead on the side of the infection. Pain in the scalp and the neck muscles is sometimes present. Symptoms are often accompanied by a feeling of weakness and sometimes weight loss.

Kali bich. One of the most important remedies for sinusitis. This type of sinusitis is associated with a thick, greenish-yellow, very sticky, ropy, nasal mucus. The mucus may also be bloody. Crusts of mucus may form inside the nose and are difficult to dislodge. The nose may be completely obstructed, and very little air can get in and out. Post-nasal dripping is profuse. Great pain in both the frontal and maxillary sinuses causes soreness in the cheekbones and forehead. The person is worse in cold, damp air between 2:00 and 3:00 A.M. Symptoms are better from heat and continual motion.

Kali iod. Profuse, hot, watery, light-green nasal discharge irritates the skin below the nose. The pain is often located in the frontal sinus, causing pain on the side of the infected sinus.

Lachesis. Sinus pain occurs when the nose is stuffed up and is relieved when the nose begins to run. The pain is most often felt in the face (maxillary sinuses) and is usually located on the left side. Sometimes the pain moves to the right side after starting on the left side. Symptoms are worse when waking from sleep or a nap.

Mercurius sol. This type of sinusitis generally affects the frontal sinuses on the right side. Bloody, greenish-yellow, pus-like discharge drains from the sinuses into the nose, causing the breath to smell foul. The nostrils can become raw and ulcerated from this discharge. The person is thirsty. Salivation and perspiration increase, but do not bring relief. Symptoms are worse at night, when overheated, lying on the right side, and from cold and damp weather. Symptoms are better in moderate temperatures.

Natrum mur. This type of sinus infection is an inflammation without bacteria, rather than a true infection. It may be associated with the beginning of a head cold or with a severe allergy. The frontal sinuses are most affected. A blinding headache is worse from sunrise to sunset. Nasal discharges are clear and copious, lasting from one to three days. Discharges are followed by a stoppage of the nose, which makes breathing difficult. The person loses the senses of smell and taste, and is thirsty and chilly. The person feels pressure and heaviness in the frontal sinuses. Symptoms are often worse in heat and between 9:00 and 11:00 A.M. Symptoms are better in cool weather.

Nux vomica. This type of sinus infection occurs in a person who is angry, impatient, irritable, and easily chilled. *Nux vomica* can be used to treat sinus infections associated with a stuffed-up feeling, especially at night and when outdoors. Nasal discharges are more runny during the day. Nasal blockage alternates between nostrils. The person has a frontal headache and wants to press something hard against it. The infected person's resistance is often weakened from drinking too much alcohol or coffee or from taking drugs. This weakness leads to recurring sinus infections, especially when exposed to cold air and drafts.

Pulsatilla. Can be used to treat sinusitis that has a yellow, non-irritating mucus that is worse in the morning. The person is weepy, wants consolation, and is very sensitive. Although thirstless and chilly, the person wants to be out in the cool air. Frontal sinuses are most affected, often on the right side. The nostril on the same side as the sinus pain is blocked. Symptoms are changeable. Pain moves between the face, teeth, and frontal and maxillary sinuses quickly and alternately. Pain is worse in the evening.

Pyrogenium. A foul-smelling discharge drains from the sinuses into the nose. The person has a high fever and is extremely weak.

Sepia. This type of sinusitis is often associated with chronic post-nasal drip that must be coughed up into the mouth. Thick, sticky, green discharges plug up the nose. The person is very sensitive and irritable and wants to be alone. Symptoms generally occur in the left sinus.

Silica. Helps to promote drainage of pus from the sinuses and is sometimes used to complete drainage started by another sinus infection remedy. Discharges tend to be yellow or green, bloody, and form hard, dry crusts in the nose that bleed when loosened. This remedy is most useful for maxillary sinusitis. The face is red, and the throbbing pain is worse in cold and damp conditions.

Sulphur. The person who needs *Sulphur* for sinus infection is irritable and disorganized. He or she can be adverse to taking showers and has a strong body odor. The nose is stuffy indoors and runny outdoors. The nose tends to obstruct on alternate sides. The person is thirsty, and is worse with heat and better from cool air.

Thuja. Useful in the treatment of acute and chronic sinusitis. This type of sinusitis is more often associated with the left sinus than the right. An important characteristic is a thick, green mucus with blood and pus. On blowing the nose, the person often feels pain in the teeth.

SORE THROAT (INCLUDES STREP THROAT)

A sore throat is one of the most common problems in both children and adults. It is often caused by a viral infection and accompanied by other viral symptoms, such as coughing, sneezing, and runny eyes. At other times, the sore throat can be caused by a strep infection caused by streptococcal bacteria. The symptoms of strep throat are sometimes difficult to identify. A person can feel very sick with a high fever and have a sore throat that is worse than usual, but it is also possible for a person to have strep with mild symptoms that are similar to another virus. Strep throat should be treated with antibiotics since it can be a serious illness. Untreated strep throat can lead to rheumatic fever, heart disease, or a kidney infection.

Sore throats can also be caused by sinus infections that drip mucus down the back of the throat, causing it to feel irritated. A stuffy nose that leads to breathing through the mouth is also a cause; these sore throats tend to be worse in the morning upon waking and better during the day. Another cause of sore throats is too much acid being secreted by the stomach, which causes acid regurgitation into the throat and esophagus. Allergies can be a cause of sore throats, especially when there is itching in the nose, roof of the mouth, or back of the throat.

It is important to treat infections of the sinuses, allergies, or stuffy nose. Keeping the mouth clean and treating any kind of dental or gum disease can be helpful. Changing toothbrushes every few months is important, since they harbor bacteria and viruses. Gargling with either salt water or a mixture of half water and half hydrogen peroxide can help fight the infection; it is important not to swallow these mixtures. Drinking hot water with lemon is often soothing to the throat. If dryness is the cause of a stuffy nose, a humidifier can be run at night to increase moisture in the nose. Certain vitamins and herbs are known to help a sore throat.

Aconite. Given in the first stages of a sore throat when it comes on suddenly, especially after exposure to cold, dry wind. The mucous membranes are hot and burning, and the fever can be very high. The person is thirsty, anxious, restless, and fearful.

Allium cepa. Useful for a sore throat accompanied by hay fever-type symptoms that include watery, irritating nasal discharge that reddens the upper lip and the bottom of the nose, a non-irritating watery discharge from the eyes, excessive sneezing, and a raw throat.

Apis. Useful for stinging pain in the throat accompanied by swelling. The uvula hangs down and looks like a little bag of water. The throat is puffy and fiery red. There is great constriction and tightness in the throat. There is an absence of thirst, and the pain is worse from warm drinks and better from cold drinks.

Argentum nit. Useful when the person experiences the sensation when swallowing that a splinter or stick is in the throat. The throat is dark red, sore, and feels rough. *Argentum nit* can also be used for sore throats in those who use the voice a lot, such as singers and lecturers. The pain is raw, and the throat secretes a clear, thick, and sticky mucus. The pain may be worse on yawning.

Arsenicum alb. Useful for burning throat pain that is relieved by hot drinks. Despite being thirsty, the person only drinks small amounts of liquid at a time. There is great restlessness, agitation, and pacing, and the symptoms are worse at night, especially between midnight and 2:00 A.M.

Arum triphyllum. Useful for a raw feeling at the base of the mouth and the soft palate. The throat feels constricted, swollen, burning, and raw. The person clears the throat often. The glands under the mandible swell. The corners of the mouth are sore and cracked, and the person picks at the lips until they bleed. The saliva is very irritating. The sore throat may occur sometimes after exposure to a northwest wind.

Baptisia. Useful for an inflamed sore throat accompanied by very bad breath and possibly a high fever. Mouth ulcers are often present, and solids cause the person to gag when swallowing. The mouth is dry and the person is constantly thirsty for cold drinks. There is a bitter taste in the mouth. High fever is accompanied by extreme weakness. The most important symptoms in this remedy are putrid odor coming from the mouth and a feeling of great sickness and weakness.

Baryta carb. Used for acute tonsillitis and helps the child who has tonsil problems whenever a cold is present. Generally, this child has chronic enlargement of the glands around the neck, and the problem occurs mostly on the right side. It is interesting to note that many children who need this remedy are a bit delayed in both physical and mental development, although this is not always the case (children who develop normally may also need this remedy).

Belladonna. An important remedy for sore throats. There is a dry throat, and the soft palate and throat are highly inflamed and bright red. The tonsils are red, swollen, enlarged, and worse on the right side. There is a constant need to swallow accompanied by a constricted feeling in the throat. The throat feels worse when swallowing liquid, and there is an aversion to drinking anything. The person is red, hot, and flushed, and the pupils are dilated. The tongue is either bright red or has the appearance of a strawberry. The person is restless, agitated, and, if the fever is high enough, delirious.

Bryonia. Useful for a dry, constricted throat. The lips are dry, and the tongue is coated white. Excessive thirst for large amounts of cold water is accompanied by a desire to remain motionless and be left alone. The person is easily irritated.

Calcarea carb. Useful for a sore throat that is worse when swallowing. The pain makes its way down the esophagus to the stomach. Throat pain is worse in the morning, and in damp weather as well as during weather changes. Sore throats that come on during the menstrual period may be helped by this remedy. *Calcarea carb* is often used for chronic swelling of the tonsils and lymph glands in the neck. There is a constricted feeling in the throat. This remedy is more often used for chronic sore throat problems (rather than acute throat problems).

Calcarea sulph. Useful in the later stages of a sore throat for ulcerations or tonsillitis accompanied by yellow, infected discharge. *Calcarea sulph* may help tonsil abscesses, especially when the abscess drains, since this remedy helps promote the continued drainage.

Cantharis. Useful for burning in the mouth and the throat, with a feeling like they are on fire. There are blisters in the mouth and on the tongue, and the person finds it difficult to swallow liquid. *Cantharis,* when there is burning during urination, may help urinary tract infections that occur at the same time.

Ferrum phos. Useful for a sore throat associated with a fever. The throat is sore, red, dry, and inflamed. There is a lot of pain and burning. There are no strong mental symptoms, so this remedy is often used when there is only a sore throat. Singers and people who speak a lot and get sore throats often need this remedy.

Gelsemium. Useful for a sore throat that often develops slowly over a long period of time, especially on warm summer days. The most important symptoms are sluggishness, weakness, swollen tonsils, and a throat that feels rough and burning. Swallowing sometimes causes pain that travels from the throat to the ears. Chills run up and down the back, and the legs are weak and aching. The eyelids are heavy, and the person gets dizzy when trying to get out of bed.

Hepar sulph. Useful for a sore throat that comes on after an established cold. When swallowing, the person feels like a splinter, stick, or fish bone is caught in the throat. Pain shoots from the throat to the ear. Throat pain is worse from cold drinks and better from warm drinks. The person is irritable, angry, and sensitive to drafts, often covering the neck to keep it warm and away from drafts. *Hepar sulph* may help tonsillitis when there is yellow or green pus coming from the tonsils. The person is usually irritable and easily angered.

Hydrastis. Useful for raw, burning pain in the throat. The person expectorates yellow, thick, and sticky mucus from the back of the throat. A child will often be suddenly aroused from sleep by thick, post-nasal drainage. There is a bitter taste in the mouth, and the person may hear a high-pitched noise due to fluid in the eustachian tube. *Hydrastis* often helps sinusitis, as well as sore throat.

Ignatia. Useful when the person feels as if a lump is stuck in the throat; this feeling gets worse when swallowing, which is often painful. *Ignatia* may help globus hystericus, a tightness or lump in the throat that may be a problem for a person who is under stress or extremely anxious. This remedy can sometimes help with small yellow or white ulcers on the tonsils.

Kali bich. Useful for a sore throat accompanied by swollen tonsils and ulcers on the tonsils. There is an accumulation of sticky, thick, greenish-yellow mucus in the throat that is difficult to cough up. Sinus drainage often accompanies or causes the throat pain. The nose is blocked with mucus, and there is pain in the eustachian tube. The throat is burning, dry, and raw, and there is a feeling that something is sticking in the throat. The pain is often worse on waking (like *Lachesis*).

Kali carb. Helps the person who is always clearing the throat, coughing up mucus, and has a feeling that a fish bone or needle is stuck in the throat. Symptoms of sore throats may be aggravated at 3:00 A.M.

Kali iod. Helpful for people who have sore throats that are worse from speaking and swallowing. There may be an associated nasal discharge, sinus drainage, and a headache in the front of the head. Fever is usually absent.

Kali mur. Useful for swollen glands and tonsils. The throat can have ulcers with a white or grayish appearance. The tongue is also coated white or gray. *Kali mur* is used when no clear picture is found from other remedies, since there are few mental symptoms indicating this remedy. *Kali mur* may help thrush or yeast infections of the mouth and throat. The glands around the throat are swollen.

Lachesis. Useful for a sore throat that often begins on the left side and either stays there or moves to the right side. The throat and neck feel so constricted that the person does not want the throat touched or to wear a turtleneck or other tight collar. The pain is worse with any pressure and from hot drinks, and it feels better from cold drinks. Pain travels to the ear, especially when swallowing. The throat is a purplish-blue color and does not look as swollen as it feels. There is a sensation of a lump in the throat that moves up and down when swallowing. The throat symptoms are better either when there is discharge from the nose or when the person is able to expectorate mucus. The person feels worse after waking up. The person may be overly talkative and somewhat hyperactive.

Lycopodium. Useful for a sore throat on the right side, which either remains on that side or moves to the left. The pain is aggravated by cold drinks and relieved by hot drinks. The throat is very dry, and there may be increased gastrointestinal symptoms (such as flatulence). The pain is often worse from 4:00 to 8:00 P.M. The person is quite chilly.

Mercurius sol. Useful for a sore throat accompanied by offensive breath and swollen, sore glands around the neck. The pain is raw and burning, there is increased saliva from the mouth, and the person tends to perspire excessively. The sore throat comes on later during a cold and can be accompanied by swollen tonsils that discharge green or yellow pus. The pain is generally on the right side, and the person is usually very thirsty.

Natrum mur. Useful when a person with a sore throat has a feeling that a hair or plug is stuck in the throat or that the uvula is too long. The tongue may have small bubbles of saliva on the sides, and cold sores may be on the lips.

Nitric acid. Useful for sharp pains that occur while swallowing (as though there are splinters in the throat); this is due to ulcers that form in and around the throat. There may be a sensation of bread crumbs in the throat. The saliva can be bloody, and the person wants to constantly expectorate the mucus. The pain travels to the ears when the person swallows. Any blood in the saliva should be evaluated by a physician.

Nux vomica. Useful for sore throats that occur in the morning after drinking, smoking, or using the voice too much. The throat is described as having a rough, scraped feeling. The person experiences a tickling sensation in the throat after waking up, and stitching pains are felt in the ear. The person is generally irritable and very sensitive to noise, touch, and bright lights.

Phosphorus. Helps sore throats that tend to be burning but are relieved by cold drinks. The throat pain is aggravated by sneezing. Pain and soreness tend to be on the left side.

Phytolacca. Useful for a sore throat accompanied by aching, soreness, and restlessness. The glands feel hot and inflamed around the throat, which is dark red or bluish-red and feels rough, narrow, and hot. The person feels shooting pains in the ears when swallowing. The pain is often worse on the right side. There is pain at the base of the tongue, soft palate, and tonsils. The throat pain is worse when swallowing hot liquid. A grayish-white or thick, sticky discharge in the back of the throat is difficult to dislodge when coughing. Both the uvula and tonsils are swollen and burning. The person is indifferent to others. The sore throat generally feels better with cold drinks, rest, and warm, dry weather. Cold and damp weather, nighttime, changes in weather, and exposure to electrical storms make the throat feel worse.

Pulsatilla. This remedy helps a sore throat that is accompanied by the typical *Pulsatilla* emotional picture of weepiness and liking consolation and comfort. The person tends to be chilly yet likes the open, cool air. He or she has little thirst. The throat is dry, raw, and has a purplish-blue appearance because the veins in the back of the throat are engorged. (There are often symptoms of enlarged and swollen veins when *Pulsatilla* is the right remedy.)

Rhus tox. Useful when the throat and glands around the neck feel stiff. There may be hoarseness from overusing the voice. The person is restless and the body aches; he or she may move around or stretch to try to get comfortable. The sore throat is worse when swallowing and in damp weather and better from warm drinks (like *Arsenicum alb, Lycopodium, Hepar sulph,* and *Sulphur*).

Sabadilla. Useful for a sore throat that usually begins on the left side and may move to the right (like *Lachesis*). The person finds it difficult to expectorate the phlegm. Warm liquids can relieve the pain (unlike *Lachesis,* which is worse from warm drinks and better from cold drinks). The pain is worse when swallowing saliva. The throat is dry, and the person has the sensation of a lump, bread crumbs, a string, or a hair in the throat accompanied by the constant need to swallow. The pain gets worse from cold air, and the person is generally sensitive to cold. The person is nervous, shy, and easily startled. Allergy symptoms and nasal discharge accompanied by sneezing and a runny nose may also be experienced.

Sulphur. Useful for a burning, red, and dry throat. The person feels a pressure in the throat as from a lump, splinter, or hair. There is a sensation that a ball is rising up from the esophagus and closing off the throat. *Sulphur* is often associated with a person who is hot, flushes easily, and has a red face and lips. The person tends to be disorganized, irritable, and lazy.

Wyethia. Useful when the person must clear the throat constantly, trying to expectorate the mucus. The throat feels swollen, dry, and burning. The person has difficulty swallowing, and there is a constant desire to swallow saliva. The uvula feels elongated. *Wyethia* may also be helpful for a sore throat in singers and public speakers. An important accompanying symptom is itching in the back part of the nose and soft palate. Hoarseness may also accompany the sore throat.

SPRAINS AND STRAINS

Sprains and strains result from stretching the tendons, ligaments, and muscles. They can be painful and lead to difficulty walking or using the extremities. Ankle sprains should always be evaluated for a possible fracture. Wrists are another area that is commonly sprained. Athletes often experience strains, especially of the thighs, calves, fingers, arms, or shoulders.

Apis. Often used for a joint sprain or strain. The joints are hot and swollen. The stinging pain gets better with cold applications and worse from touch, pressure, and warm applications.

Arnica. This is usually the first remedy given to help initiate healing of a sprain or strain. If there is a feeling of intense bruising or soreness, and especially if the person is in shock, *Arnica* is the best remedy. (The signs of shock include: a rapid, weak pulse; cool, clammy skin; lightheadedness; irregular breathing; confusion; or loss of consciousness. If any of these signs of shock are present, a doctor or person trained in emergency medicine should be contacted.) *Arnica* ointment can be used on any soft tissue or muscle that is bruised or sore, but should never be used when the skin is broken.

Bryonia. Useful for sprains or strains, especially when the strain is to the joint or soft tissue. There is extreme pain and swelling (often swelling with fluid) in the affected area. *Bryonia* is particularly useful when the affected area is painful with the least motion and better from complete rest.

Rhus tox. Useful when a strained area of the body (especially the joint) becomes hot, swollen, and red. The pain is often tearing. This pain gets worse from cold applications and better from warm applications. Movement is painful at first, but gets better as motion continues. (In contrast, a strain relieved with *Bryonia* is worse from both early and later motion.) Gentle rubbing often lessens the pain. The person is restless and constantly wants to change position, which temporarily relieves the pain. *Rhus tox* is particularly useful for problems with the ankles and knees, and it is often helpful after overlifting or overstretching.

Ruta. Particularly helpful for tendon and ligament strains. It is often used if the bone is close to the surface of the body (such as the wrist, shin, or ankle). This remedy is also useful for overstretching and overlifting (especially the wrist and ankle). The aching pain is worse from movement of the injured part. When the muscle is stretched, the injured tendon is painful. The person is restless (but not as restless as one with a sprain or strain relieved by *Rhus tox*). If the person has a constant tendency toward a sprain, *Ruta* can be used as a preventive aid as well as a treatment.

Symphytum. Useful when the strain or sprain is closer to the bone (periosteum) and is slow to heal. The bone feels broken but does not appear broken when X-rayed. *Symphytum* is also useful for a broken bone or when a tendon is partially or completely detached from the bone. A physician should always be contacted if a broken bone is suspected.

STYES

A stye is an infection of the follicle at the base of the eyelash. It can also occur in the oil gland where tiny particles clog the gland or follicle on the eyelid. A stye consists of a small boil or pustule, usually caused by the bacteria staphylococcus; it can often be associated with blepharitis. Characteristics include a discharge, watery eyes, sensitivity to light, and a feeling of a foreign object on the eyelid. The symptoms usually begin with pain, redness, and tenderness of the eyelid, followed by a small, round, tender area of swelling. Swelling, however, may occur on the entire eyelid. To help bring down the swelling and to help unclog the gland or follicle, a warm washcloth can be used. This should be pressed gently against the stye to help it come to a head and burst, which will eventually relieve the pain. It is important not to rub, squeeze, or irritate the stye. Warm compresses can be repeated four or five times a day. If the stye does not heal in a week, a physician should be consulted.

Apis. Useful for styes that form with sudden, stinging pains. The eyelids are red and swollen and feel better with cold water. *Apis* helps to prevent the recurrence of styes.

Calcarea sulph. Useful after *Silica* when the stye comes to a head and starts to drain. *Calcarea sulph* helps the drainage continue, especially yellow and infected-looking drainage.

Ferrum phos. Helpful in the initial signs of a stye when there is redness of the eyelid margin but no actual swelling.

Graphites. Useful for styes associated with eczema. The eyelids are dry, red, scaly, and sometimes ooze a sticky substance. The eyes are sensitive to light.

Hepar sulph. Helps very sensitive styes that get better when warm washcloths are applied.

Hypericum. Useful as a tincture to help soothe the eyes, especially if there is great pain. The person has a tendency toward styes in the left eyelid.

Kali mur. Useful after the eyelid begins to swell. It is often used after *Ferrum phos.*

Lycopodium. Useful for styes that form in the inner corner of the eye. It is also useful when the eyelid becomes red and ulcerates.

Pulsatilla. Useful for inflamed eyelids that stick together. Creamy white or yellow discharge is present. *Pulsatilla* helps when styes form on the upper eyelid. This remedy is usually associated with the *Pulsatilla* temperament of weeping, changeable moods, and chilliness.

Silica. Helps the stye form a head, and is often used continuously until the stye drains or disappears. The eyes are sensitive to light, which causes sharp pains that run through the eyes. *Silica* is usually used in the 6x potency.

Staphysagria. Useful for recurring styes, and may be repeated weekly or monthly. The styes often form hard lumps (chalazion) that do not disappear. The eyelids itch, and the eyes appear sunken with blue rings around them.

Sulphur. Helps recurring styes in which the eyelids are red, sore, burning, and get worse from washing.

TEETHING (ALSO CALLED DENTITION)

Babies often suffer from pain when their teeth are coming in. This pain is often worse at night and causes great distress. When teething, babies want to bite on things and they often have profuse salivation coming from the mouth. Because the gums are swollen and inflamed, babies are more susceptible to infections at this time. Teething is often associated with ear and throat infections.

Homeopathic remedies can be very helpful to mothers, fathers, and babies during the wakeful nights and days when teething pain is most severe.

Aconite. The child whines constantly. Pain seems to come on suddenly, especially after coming indoors from the cold, dry air. The child may constantly gnaw at the fingers or fist. A fever is sometimes present.

Belladonna. The gums are swollen and inflamed over the area of the erupted tooth. The baby moans and groans. While asleep, he or she jerks suddenly as if frightened. The face is red, the eyes are dilated, and the baby is generally agitated.

Calcarea carb. This remedy is used for children with delayed eruption of teeth. The head sweats during sleep, and the feet are cold and damp; these are characteristic symptoms. Sour vomiting with large curds is sometimes seen.

Calcarea phos. Teething pains are worse from having either cold or warm food or drink in the mouth. The child often whines and is fearful. The child constantly wants to nurse. Green, loose, slimy, and somewhat hot and watery diarrhea is very common.

Chamomilla. The most frequently used remedy for teething.

Irritability is excessive. The child may demand toys or other objects, but throws them as soon as they are given. The child is thirsty and wants to be carried. Diarrhea looks like eggs and spinach. Sometimes one cheek is hot and red while the other is pale and cold.

Cina. Teething will cause restless sleep in the child, and often, he or she cannot fall asleep unless rocked. The child tends to pick and bore into the nose. This type of teething may be associated with watery diarrhea.

Coffea. This type of teething is associated with great anguish and insomnia. Toothaches in little children are very painful. These pains are better when holding cold water or ice in the mouth. Warm liquids make the pain worse.

Kreosote. This painful type of teething is associated with red, soft gums. The child is very restless and constantly wants to be in motion; he or she often screams all night. *Kreosote* is a particularly good remedy for teething problems in children whose teeth decay quickly and tend to look yellow.

Phytolacca. When the teeth hurt, the child wants to clench the teeth or gums together or bite on something hard.

Podophyllum. The child sleeps restlessly with the eyes half closed. A profuse, watery, painless stool is associated with these teething problems, especially in the summer.

Staphysagria. Useful for teething in older children, especially for rapid growth and eruption of the teeth. The teeth seem to decay as soon as they are cut. The child is very sensitive to every harsh look or word from the parents. Irritability is also a common symptom. The child may demand toys or other desired objects, but will throw them away when given.

TESTICULAR CONDITIONS

There are several causes of enlarged, painful testicles. Two of the most common are inflammation of the epididymis (epididymitis) and inflammation of the testes (orchitis), due to an infection that may also cause either prostatitis or urethritis. Viruses can also cause inflammation of the testicle, including mumps. The testicle can also swell due to hydrocele, a problem associated with fluid accumulating around the testicle. This is usually the result of an injury or a congenital problem that occurs early in life.

Any testicular swelling should be evaluated by a physician, since this may be an early sign of cancer. An evaluation can also determine if a venereal disease, such as gonorrhea, may have caused the inflammation. Antibiotics may be necessary. A physician should be contacted whenever there is swelling and pain.

Aconite. Useful in the very early stages of acute orchitis. The symptoms usually occur with the beginning of a cold (especially after exposure to cold, dry air or drafts). The person is restless and fearful. The pain is located either in the testicle or epididymis.

Belladonna. Useful for a sudden onset of testicular pain. The testicles are hard, drawn up, and inflamed. Also common are: fever; a hot, dry, flushed face; and glazed, dilated pupils. The person may be emotionally hypersensitive.

Clematis erecta. Helpful when the right testicle feels hard (like a stone) and is painful. The testicle tends to be drawn up, and the spermatic cord is sensitive. Becoming chilly or lying in bed may aggravate the testicular inflammation.

Hamamelis. The keynote symptom for using *Hamamelis* is extreme soreness of the testicles. This remedy can also be used for swelling, bruising, and discoloration (such as a black-and-blue area) after a blow or kick to the testicles. The person feels great pain in the spermatic cord, which extends down into the testicles.

Pulsatilla. Useful for pain and inflammation of the testicle and epididymis, especially on the left side. The person is highly sensitive and emotional, and cries easily. The testicle is retracted, enlarged, and sensitive. Dragging pain along the spermatic cord shoots down into the thighs.

Rhododendron. Useful for inflammation of the testicle, predominantly on the right side. The person feels as if the testicle has been crushed.

Spongia. Useful for epididymitis and squeezing pain in the testicles. The spermatic cord is swollen and painful, and shooting pain moves along it. This remedy often follows *Pulsatilla* and *Hamamelis* well. The testicles, scrotum, and spermatic cord feel hot. *Spongia* can be used for chronic orchitis (especially with acute exacerbations).

TOOTH AND GUM ABSCESSES

Abscesses or boils can develop either on the gums or at the root of the teeth. Pain, redness, and swelling of the gum next to a tooth are common. It is often difficult to know whether the problem is due to an abscess in the root of the tooth, a sinus infection, or allergies. Dental evaluation is extremely important in these situations.

Belladonna. Useful in the very early stages of the abscess. The person is agitated and flushed. The gums and teeth throb painfully. The mouth is dry and the area over the abscess is red and hot.

Hepar sulph. Often useful after *Belladonna* when the abscess has already formed. The person is often irritable, easily upset, and sensitive to drafts. Abscesses of both the gums and the roots of the teeth are associated with inflamed gums that are very painful to the slightest touch.

Mercurius sol. Abscesses and boils are seen, especially in decayed teeth. The breath is foul smelling. When the person enters a room, the odor can be easily smelled, even at a distance. Increased salivation and swelling of the lymph glands are aggravated at night and from the warmth of a bed.

Pyrogenium. Useful in cases where the abscessed teeth cause high fevers, weakness, and restlessness. Delirium accompanies a fever. The person cannot tell if dreaming takes place while awake or asleep. All discharges from the body, including the breath and sweat, are offensive. The abscesses burn with great intensity. This remedy may also be used for boils on the gums and abscesses at the root of the teeth. *Pyrogenium* seems to ripen the abscesses. The teeth are extremely sensitive to cold water, and the gums are extremely sensitive to cold air.

TOOTHACHE

A toothache can be extremely painful. There are many causes of toothache; however, the most important is dental decay, which is aggravated by cold food or drinks. Another cause can be an abscess or boil that forms at the root of the tooth; in this case, the pain is usually worse from warmth or hot foods and drinks. A toothache can also result from a problem in the sinuses, which causes pain near the root of the tooth. Still another cause can be gum disease, such as pyorrhea. Whatever the cause, it is important to see a dentist for the acute problem and have regular checkups to help prevent recurring problems.

Aconite. A toothache comes on very suddenly. The person is in great pain and appears frantic and fearful. The toothache is worse from cold drinks and exposure to cold, dry winds.

Antimonium crud. This type of toothache is characterized by decay, causing gnawing pains that are worse at night. The toothache seems to penetrate the head. The gums separate from the teeth and bleed easily. The tongue has a white coating (an important guiding symptom).

Arnica. Should be given after dental procedures such as teeth cleaning, crowns, or fillings. It will help after injuries to the teeth or mouth, and after extracting teeth to help decrease the bleeding and pain. This remedy is also used for swelling from wearing false teeth. The most important physical symptom is soreness.

Arsenicum alb. Helpful when the person is restless, agitated, and paces the floor. Toothaches are worse at night, especially between midnight and 2:00 A.M. The toothache is relieved by warm water despite a possible burning in the gums and teeth. This toothache is characterized by sharp, aching pains in the teeth and gums. Pains often extend to the cheeks, ears, or temples. Teeth may have the sensation of being loose and elongated.

Belladonna. A person with this type of toothache is irritable and excitable and may have a fever, a red and hot face, and dilated pupils. The throbbing and burning pains are aggravated at night, when chewing, and while outside in the open air.

Bryonia. Helps the toothache that occurs in healthy teeth. The affected tooth feels loose and too long, but is actually fine. Pain is often worse from taking warm liquids into the mouth and with any kind of motion (like chewing). Pain is improved by lying on the painful side. The person is very thirsty and has a white tongue. A person who chews tobacco may have the sensation of a jerking pain, and *Bryonia* may help the sensation stop.

Calcarea carb. Useful for children who have teeth that are slow to erupt or who have rapid tooth decay. The toothache is worse in cold, damp weather. In women, the toothache is worse during the menstrual period and pregnancy. Note that while homeopathic remedies are safe during pregnancy, labor, and breastfeeding, a pregnant woman should confer with her obstetrician or midwife to coordinate treatment.

Chamomilla. One of the most important remedies for a toothache and for teething babies who have unbearable pain that radiates to the ears. The person is hypersensitive to pain and has an aggravation at night. These symptoms are worse from any kind of warmth, especially after eating warm food or drinking coffee. *Chamomilla* is useful for infants and children who are irritable, want to be carried, and are very thirsty.

Coffea. Especially suitable for oversensitive and nervous people. Often a rapid flow of ideas in the mind prevents sleep. These toothaches cause great anguish because of the extreme pain. Pain is relieved by holding cold water in the mouth, but it returns when the water becomes warm. Pain is worse from anything warm.

Hepar sulph. The person helped by this remedy is very irritable and angry. Useful after treatments with *Belladonna* when the tooth pain is associated with infection. Pus and blood are discharged from the gums and teeth. The teeth are very sensitive to cold air or the slightest touch. (Note that these symptoms could be signs of pyorrhea and should be evaluated by a dentist.) *Hepar sulph* is also useful for treating tenderness where the tooth meets the gum, especially over an erupting tooth such as a wisdom tooth.

Ignatia. Helps toothaches associated with people who have undergone grief or shock, which aggravates the pain in the teeth. This type of toothache occurs after drinking coffee or smoking.

Lachesis. The person is talkative, irritable, and feels depressed on waking. The toothache is worse in the morning, upon waking, after hot drinks, and after dinner. The pain of this type of toothache seems to run from the jaw to the ear.

Magnesia phos. Useful for treating a toothache with intense shooting pains that are relieved with pressure and warm liquids. The pain is worse with movement of the head and with cold liquids. Dissolve twenty tablets of the 6x potency of *Magnesia phos* in one cup of warm water and sip slowly.

Mercurius sol. This toothache is associated with excessive salivation. The lymph glands often swell. *Mercurius sol* is especially important for treating the pain from decaying teeth. Associated symptoms include a beginning abscess or pyorrhea with swollen and ulcerated gums. (Note that pyorrhea should be evaluated by a dentist.) Pain is felt in the jaw and high in the root of the teeth. The pain is often associated with sinusitis. The breath and perspiration are foul smelling. The pains are worse at night and from the warmth of a bed. Pains are aggravated from either hot or cold foods, and better from lukewarm drinks or warm food.

Pulsatilla. The person is often weepy, sad, and thirstless. The pain is relieved from walking outside, with pressure on the aching tooth, and in the open air (especially when drawing cool air into the mouth). The pain is better by holding cold liquids in the mouth and worse from warm drinks. This toothache is worse in the evening, at night, and from the warmth of a bed.

Pyrogenium. This type of toothache is associated with an abscess, very bad breath, a high fever, and restlessness.

Rhododendron. Pain from this toothache is worse before a thunderstorm, in damp weather, and in bed. These tearing pains are better from eating and with warmth.

Rhus tox. The person is restless and often paces the floor. Tooth pain follows a sudden chill. The teeth feel as if they are being pressed into their sockets. The pains are worse at night and in the open air.

Spigelia. This tooth pain may actually be associated with an inflammation of the nerve that goes to the face, teeth, and jaw (trigeminal neuritis). It is worse on the left side. The person is unable to sleep at night; the severity of the pain actually drives the person out of bed. Pains generally set in after the person eats, smokes a cigarette, or relaxes before bed.

Staphysagria. This remedy is often useful for people who smoke too many cigarettes or have pyorrhea. This type of toothache is associated with unhealthy, retracted, diseased gums and a tendency toward decay of the teeth. Often teeth crumble and turn black as soon as they erupt, especially in children. The person feels gnawing pains in the roots of the teeth. The symptoms are worse after eating, chewing, or drinking anything cold and in the open air and late at night. The pain is often relieved by hard pressure. Note that a person experiencing these symptoms should be under the care of a dentist.

Thuja. Useful when the roots of the teeth decay while the crown remains healthy. Gnawing pain in the decayed teeth is made worse by cold things or chewing. Note that a person experiencing these symptoms should be under the care of a dentist.

URINARY TRACT INFECTIONS
(INCLUDES BLADDER INFECTIONS AND CYSTITIS)

Urinary tract infections include bladder infections and infections of the kidney and urethra. This section refers generally to bladder infections, because kidney infections should be evaluated by a physician.

A bladder infection, also known as cystitis, causes pain when urinating. There is often burning that occurs in either the urethra or bladder. There may be a frequent need to urinate, especially at night, and dribbling of urine may be common after urination. The urine may smell odorous, and there may be abdominal pain over the bladder area. Bladder infections can be serious if the bacteria that cause the problem migrate into the kidney area, causing a kidney infection. This is a serious condition and whenever back pain, fever, and weakness occur with urinary problems, a physician should immediately be contacted.

Bladder infections are most common in women because of the shortened urethra and because of the proximity of the rectal and urethral openings. In women, therefore, it is more common for the bacteria in stool to contaminate the urethra. It has been estimated that approximately 50 percent of women have experienced a urinary tract infection at some point in their lives.

Urinary tract infections in males are much less common and often indicate an enlarged or infected prostate or an anatomical or structural problem. They generally need to be treated by a physician rather than by using natural means or antibiotics.

The urine is usually sterile and does not contain bacteria. Bacteria can reach the urinary tract by rising up from the urethra into the bladder, or, less commonly, can reach the bladder through the bloodstream. Important risk factors that can cause bladder infections include irritation to the urethra (from an accident or vigorous sexual intercourse), structural abnormalities of the urinary tract (which blocks the outflow of the urine), or pregnancy.

Diagnosis of bladder infections is usually done by evaluating symptoms and by culturing the urine to see if bacteria is growing. The most common type of bacteria that affects the urinary tract is E. coli, a natural inhabitant of the large colon.

It is important to treat urinary tract infections quickly. Alternative and natural approaches include teaching women and especially young girls good hygiene. This includes wiping from the front to the back after a bowel movement, wearing cotton underwear, and avoiding unnecessary douching, bubble baths, tight clothes, and nylons. It is important to instruct women who are susceptible to bladder infections to wash themselves after intercourse. It is also important to urinate frequently; holding in urine may make the person susceptible to bladder infections. Drinking plenty of water (four to six glasses a day) helps prevent urinary tract infections. During a urinary tract infection, drinking six to eight glasses a day helps flush the urine and bacteria out of the urinary tract.

Certain vitamins, supplements, and herbs are known to help urinary tract infections. If these methods do not quickly relieve the symptoms, antibiotics are then often used.

Note that a physician should be contacted if blood is seen in the urine.

Aconite. Useful for urinary tract pain that comes on suddenly. The person experiences anxiety and is quite fearful when beginning to urinate. *Aconite* is of particular help for the child who develops urinary tract symptoms after exposure to cold wind. Urination is painful and difficult, comes out in drops, and feels scalding hot. The bladder burns and has spasms, and the urethra burns as urine passes through. Because of these problems, the person tends to retain urine, causing restlessness and possibly screaming and holding of the genitals.

Apis. Helps people who have stinging pain during urination, especially the last few drops that burn and sting. The person feels the need to urinate frequently, yet only a few drops come out at a time. There may be swelling in certain parts of the body (such as the ankles or hands), a lack of thirst, and a feeling of suffocation when lying down.

Berberis. Useful when the person experiences the sensation that urine remains after urinating. The person urinates frequently, and the urethra burns when not urinating. There is pain in the thighs and hips during urination. Often kidney stones form or there are crystals in the urine, which may irritate the urinary tract and cause cystitis. There may also be severe tearing pain in the kidneys that extends down the back as well as into the ureter, bladder, and urethra. The pain is worse while stooping, lying, or sitting, and is relieved by standing.

Cantharis. One of the most important bladder infection remedies and useful when the person experiences extreme pain when feeling the urge to urinate. The urine is often bloody and comes out in drops that burn before, during, and after urination. The person feels as if the urine is scalding hot, that it burns as though it is made of molten lead.

Causticum. Useful when a person involuntarily urinates when coughing or sneezing. The urine is expelled very slowly and at times cannot be passed at all. There is often involuntary passing of urine, especially from excitement or during the initial stages of sleep at night. *Causticum* is useful for retention of urine after surgical operations, and is associated with bladder paralysis and loss of sensation while passing urine. The entire muscular system of the bladder is weak; this is indicated by the fact that the person has to wait a long time before urination starts, and during urination the urine is expelled very slowly. Because of these symptoms, the person experiences involuntary loss of urine at night. Useful for a child who wets the bed, especially during the first few hours of sleep.

Chimaphila. Useful when the person is unable to urinate unless standing with the feet wide apart and the body bent forward. There is burning and a sense of scalding during urination, and straining afterwards. The person must strain a great deal before urination. The urine tends to be cloudy, offensive smelling, and contains bloody, stringy mucus. Note that a physician should be contacted if blood is seen in the urine. There is an unusual fluttering sensation in the kidney region. *Chimaphila* may also be associated with acute prostatitis and the feeling that there is a ball in the perineum.

Equisetum. Useful for dull pain and a feeling of fullness in the bladder that are not relieved by urinating. The person feels a frequent urge to urinate, and there may be severe pain at the completion of urination. The urine flows only by drops, not in a stream. There is a sharp burning and cutting pain in the urethra during urination. This remedy is also used for an incontinent child who has dreams and nightmares about urinating. This remedy is also useful for a urinary tract infection in a child who experiences pain that is worse after urination. *Equisetum* is helpful for a woman who has problems with urinary incontinence. There is pain deep in the right kidney region, extending to the lower abdomen, accompanied by the urgent desire to urinate. This pain is worse from movement, pressure, touch, and sitting down, and it gets better in the afternoon and when lying down. This remedy may be helpful during pregnancy and after delivery when there is urine retention and pain during urination. Note that while homeopathic remedies are safe during pregnancy, labor, and breastfeeding, a pregnant woman should confer with her obstetrician or midwife to coordinate treatment.

Ferrum phos. Useful for the first stage of urinary tract infections when there is fever and very few guiding symptoms. *Ferrum phos* is useful when there is blood in the urine, especially in the early stages of an infection. Note that a physician should be contacted if blood is seen in the urine. The urine tends to spurt when the person coughs. Burning during urination is worse at very early morning, from 4:00 to 6:00 A.M., and from touch or from jarring motion, and on the right side. All pain gets better when cold is applied to the abdomen over the bladder area.

Gelsemium. Useful for incontinence, especially with paralysis and bladder weakness (similar to *Causticum*). Profuse, clear, and watery urine is accompanied by chilliness and shaking. A curious symptom with this remedy is that blinding headaches are improved when the person urinates profusely. The person feels better in general when urinating. The body is heavy and the limbs ache.

Kreosote. Useful for intense burning during urination and for when the urine is extremely acrid and burns the skin as it passes out of the genitals. *Kreosote* is often associated with extreme itching of the vulva and vagina, especially during urination. The person must hurry when the desire comes to urinate; this is especially true during the beginning of sleep. Useful for a child who wets the bed (especially in the first part of the night) and who has dreams of urinating.

Lycopodium. Useful for pain in the back before urination; this pain stops after the urine starts to flow. The urine is slow in coming and the person must strain to begin urination. There is increased urination during the night. The urine is dark red and actually may leave a red discoloration in a diaper or on the bedsheets. *Lycopodium* is a good remedy for a child with a urinary tract infection who tends to cry before urinating. This remedy may also help kidney stones, especially those on the right side.

Mercurius sol. Useful for burning in the urethra at the beginning of urination that is often associated with a vaginal infection in women (vaginitis) or a urethral infection in men (urethritis). Greenish discharge may come from the urethra. The person feels burning pain in the urethra opening, and there may be pus and blood in the urine. Note that a physician should be contacted if blood is seen in the urine. The person often has a foul smell, increased perspiration, and nighttime aggravation.

Natrum mur. Useful when the person experiences pain only after urinating (similar to *Sarsaparilla*). The person experiences increased involuntary urination when walking or coughing. A peculiar symptom is that the person must wait a long time for the urine to pass when in a public restroom or if others are present in the next room.

Natrum sulph. Useful for the person who experiences a frequent, urgent need to urinate that only produces small amounts of urine. When the urine is not passed, the person may feel pain in the small of the back. The urine is dark and often loaded with bile, especially when a liver problem (such as hepatitis) is present. The urine can also be full of glucose (a form of sugar) in a person who is diabetic.

Nux vomica. Helps the person who feels a frequent need to urinate, but little comes out each time. During urination, there is itching in the urethra and pain in the bladder. Pain in the kidneys can extend to the genitals, especially during urination. *Nux vomica* is particularly useful for an irritable, nervous, and hyperactive person and for one who overindulges in tobacco, cigarettes, or alcohol. This remedy is also helpful for the person who does complex mental work, spends too much time at the office, is overly sensitive to noise, odor, and light, and is easily chilled and avoids the open air.

Pulsatilla. Useful for an increased desire to urinate that gets worse when lying down. The person is weepy, wants consolation, and tends to be sad. The person is chilly, yet likes the open air, and is generally not thirsty. The tip of the urethra burns during and after urination. There is involuntary urination at night that is worse when coughing or passing gas. The problems worsen when the person is exposed to cold, damp air and when lying on the back. *Pulsatilla* is particularly helpful during pregnancy when there is increased urination due to pressure from the weight or position of the baby. Note that while homeopathic remedies are safe during pregnancy, labor, and breastfeeding, a pregnant woman should confer with her obstetrician or midwife to coordinate treatment.

Sarsaparilla. Useful for severe pain in the urethra at the completion of urination. The urine dribbles out while the person is sitting. A child will scream before and while passing urine. The bladder has spasms and the urine passes in a thin, feeble stream. Pain from the right kidney extends downward. Bloody or sandy sediment in the urine may stain a diaper red.

Sepia. This remedy is associated with burning during urination and a bearing-down sensation above the pubic bone. Another unusual symptom is offensive-smelling urine. Adults taking *Sepia* tend to be depressed and want to be left by themselves, away from their loved ones. *Sepia* is also useful for a child who wets the bed at night, especially during the early part of sleep. There may be red, clay-colored sediment in the urine that is often passed in great quantities so that the child will scream while urinating. There is a general heaviness and dragging sensation in the bladder. This remedy is also useful after childbirth when the female organs seem to be heavy.

Staphysagria. May be useful for a woman after her first sexual intercourse experience. There is an ineffectual desire to urinate and pressure on the bladder, which feels as though it did not empty completely. An unusual symptom is that a drop of urine is rolling continually along the urethra. The person experiences great urging to urinate, and pain after urination. This remedy is also associated with prostate problems in men who experience frequent urination and burning in the urethra when not urinating (similar to *Thuja*). The person may be angry and irritable but may not be able to express emotions well.

Thuja. Often used for chronic urinary tract problems. An unusual symptom is that the urine flows out in a split stream. The urethra can be swollen and inflamed. This remedy is often used in urethritis in men. There is a sensation of urine trickling out after urinating. Severe cutting pains are felt in the urethra after urination (similar to *Sarsaparilla*).

Urtica. Useful for urinary tract pain, especially after passing uric acid stones. The urine is acrid, and causes the genitals to itch and burn.

VACCINATION SIDE EFFECTS

Vaccinations have been used since the 1700s when the cowpox vaccine was developed to immunize people against smallpox. A terrible disease for thousands of years, smallpox has been eliminated by the routine use of vaccinations. Routine immunizations now exist for the following illnesses: diphtheria, tetanus, pertussis (whooping cough), measles, mumps, rubella, polio, hemophilus influenza, hepatitis B, chickenpox, hepatitis A, pneumococcal diseases, rotavirus, meningococcal meningitis, influenza, and genital warts. Other immunizations are used in certain circumstances, such as during outbreaks of specific illnesses or when traveling to foreign countries. These include vaccines for yellow fever, typhoid, and cholera. These immunizations have proven to be very effective in preventing these diseases.

Homeopathic remedies can be used to counter some of the side effects of immunizations, including soreness, redness, infection at the site of injections, gastrointestinal problems, or neurological problems. Some homeopaths believe that taking a 200c potency of the specific immunization that was given is helpful. One dose is given before immunization and a second dose is given after. Other homeopaths will give a routine dose of *Ledum* 200c immediately after vaccination followed by *Thuja* 200c six hours later, to prevent side effects from developing. Still other homeopaths believe nothing should be done unless symptoms actually develop. Note that high-potency remedies are not recommended for home prescribing. Consult a physician or skilled homeopathic consultant for potencies greater than 30c.

Homeopathic remedies are, in a sense, similar to immunizations in that small amounts are used to stimulate the body's immune system. There is, however, no evidence that homeopathic immunizations are effective in raising antibody levels against disease; therefore, it is not recommended that these be used in replacement of the conventional types of immunizations. Homeopathic remedies can always be used if a person contracts one of these diseases due to the vaccine failing to create immunity or if immunization was refused for religious or medical reasons.

Antimonium tart. Useful for the effects of vaccinations, especially when there is asthma. *Antimonium tart* may help if there is excessive mucus during coughing, but the person is unable to expectorate it.

Hypericum. Can be used after *Ledum* for extreme pain in the vaccination area that seems to travel along the nerve. *Hypericum* was used in the past to prevent tetanus.

Ledum. Usually given right after a vaccination for the effects of the vaccination puncture wound. *Ledum* is always the first remedy given whenever there is an injection of any kind, especially when the injected medicine or drugs can cause side effects. This remedy seems to be preventive and is usually administered in the 200c potency immediately after vaccination.

Silica. Associated with many problems experienced after a vaccination. Abscesses can appear in the armpit near the site of the injection. *Silica* is also helpful for the side effects of vaccination, including asthma, backaches, diarrhea, seizures, fever, nausea, or vomiting. This remedy is especially helpful for hard swelling in the area of injection, especially if the site is red and inflamed.

Thuja. This remedy was used in the 1800s as a direct antidote to the side effects of the smallpox vaccination. At the time, the vaccine was quite crude and caused extreme reactions, and *Thuja* was used to help diminish some of the extreme skin reactions. *Thuja* is still used for ailments from allergy shots. This remedy is helpful for warts that develop along the vaccination site. *Thuja* is useful for asthma or coughing experienced after any kind of vaccination. Diarrhea may also be present, as well as headaches. Sleeplessness can also occur. *Thuja* is particularly useful for side effects of the influenza shot, and may help with emotional oversensitivity or mental changes resulting from use of some vaccines affecting the nervous system (such as pertussis). *Thuja* is often recommended in the 200c potency twelve to twenty-four hours after immunization to help prevent future side effects.

VAGINAL INFECTION (ALSO CALLED VAGINITIS)

The three different types of vaginal infection are irritating, hormonal, and infectious. Irritating vaginitis can come from chemicals, allergies, foreign objects, or trauma. Chemical vaginitis, a form of irritating vaginitis, is often due to the use of medications or other hygiene products that irritate the vaginal tissues. Another form, allergic vaginitis, is caused by an allergy to tampons, condoms, or other foreign objects. Irritating vaginitis can also be caused by injury or sexual activities that may cause inflammation of the delicate tissues of the vagina.

Hormonal vaginal problems are due to atrophic vaginitis or increased, irritating vaginal discharges. Atrophic vaginitis is a problem for women during menopause when there is a decreased amount of estrogen stimulation, causing the vaginal tissues to become thin and irritated. This can lead to itching, burning, and a thin, watery discharge. Normal vaginal discharges may have a secretion that can be irritating; it fluctuates because of hormonal stimulation during the menstrual cycle.

Infectious vaginitis includes bacterial vaginosis, yeast infection, trichomoniasis, chlamydia, gonorrhea, herpes, or warts (caused by the human papillomavirus). These vaginal infections can be promoted by sexual transmission, antibiotics such as penicillin, diabetes, birth control pills, pregnancy, steroids, wearing noncotton underwear, or immune deficiency problems causing an increase in the tendency to get an infection. Between 80 and 90 percent of all vaginal infections are caused by bacterial vaginosis, yeast infection, or trichomoniasis.

Bacterial vaginosis, caused by Gardnerella vaginalis, is characterized by a milky, bubbly discharge with a very distinct fishy odor. It causes itching and irritation and is worse after sexual contact. If the infection is detected early, a combination douche of hydrogen peroxide and water in a one-to-one ratio (one-half quart of each) used through the menstrual period can be helpful. Taking lactobacillus acidophilus tablets orally is also helpful (two tablets thirty minutes before eating, twice daily).

Yeast infections, caused by Candida albicans, are often associated with dry, irritated vaginal tissue and cottage cheese-like discharges. The vagina is itching, burning, and irritated. To treat this condition, a douche made with one quart of water and two tablespoons of apple cider vinegar can be used through the menstrual period. Lactobacillus acidophilus should also be taken thirty minutes before eating. Women should avoid eating foods that are heavily yeasted or fermented and should avoid refined white flour.

Trichomoniasis is often associated with a foul, thin, yellow-green discharge that causes great amounts of corrosiveness in the vagina and cervix. The cervix often looks like a strawberry with red dots on it. Sometimes a hypersaline solution, with a quart of water and a tablespoon of salt, is used for trichomoniasis to help burst the protozoa.

Chlamydia is another type of vaginitis. It often causes cervical infections or cervicitis. The cervix is red and crumbly, with a creamy yellow discharge. Because chlamydia is sometimes asymptomatic and is transmitted usually through sexual intercourse, it is sometimes not diagnosed unless a physician is specifically looking for it. Generally, antibiotics are given for treatment.

Gonorrhea is a disease that was treated homeopathically before antibiotics, but is presently almost always treated with the appropriate antibiotic therapy. Homeopathic remedies have been used in the past for people who never felt well after being treated for gonorrhea. Homeopaths continue to use remedies for physical or emotional changes after being treated with antibiotics for gonorrhea and other sexually transmitted diseases.

The homeopathic remedies listed here can be very helpful in treating acute or recurring vaginitis, and they are usually used in combination with natural methods. Certain herbs and vitamins are known to help vaginitis. Even if antibiotics are used, homeopathic remedies can help decrease the susceptibility to yeast infections.

Take special care. Note that a person with vaginal herpes should be under the care of a physician.

Arsenicum alb. Useful for vaginal discharge that burns and irritates the vaginal tissue, causing it to become raw and foul smelling. The discharge is not profuse, can be either thick or thin, and is generally yellow. Burning pain in the vagina caused by the discharge is relieved by warm compresses. Two types of people typically experience this kind of discharge: elderly women who have chronic diseases and extreme weakness, and women who are anxious, restless, and meticulous about their habits and critical of themselves and others. Similar to their bodily discharges, which are raw, irritating, and corrosive, the people who need this remedy emotionally may act and speak in an irritating, caustic way. *Arsenicum alb* may be useful for vaginal herpes, especially when the pain is burning and gets worse at night, causing the person to be agitated, restless, fearful, and weak.

Borax. Useful for vaginal discharge that occurs midway between menstrual periods. The discharge is white (similar to egg whites) and may be accompanied by the sensation that warm water is escaping from the vagina. The discharge is bland, non-irritating, and painless, and there is often great nervousness associated with this discharge.

Calcarea carb. Useful for vaginal discharge that is profuse (possibly gushing at times), itchy, milky, persistent, and burning. The discharge is sometimes seen in infants and young girls and is often experienced again before puberty. Vaginal discharge also occurs before and between menstrual periods. Useful for older women who experience heavy menstrual periods, chilliness, and cold, damp feet. There may be increased cravings for sweets. *Calcarea carb* is often used for women who are overweight.

Calcarea phos. Useful for vaginal discharge that is creamy or resembles egg whites. The discharge is often seen after the menstrual period and, as the flow diminishes, the vaginal discharge increases. The discharge is often worse in the morning and after bowel movements and urination. *Calcarea phos* is often associated with extreme weakness and may be used in girls and young women who experience disappointment in their love relationships.

Carbo veg. Useful for foul-smelling vaginal discharge that burns and causes the skin to become raw. The discharge tends to be thin and profuse, and seems worse in the morning when rising from bed. *Carbo veg* may be associated with post-menopausal women who are cold, experience shortness of breath, and like to fan themselves often to get more air. The person is generally weak and somewhat fragile. This remedy is also indicated in those who are bloated and experience belching and flatulence.

Caulophyllum. Useful for profuse, mucus-like vaginal discharge in young girls; the discharge may weaken them. *Caulophyllum* is also indicated in those whose periods are late because of anxiety and nervousness, especially young women. This remedy is also indicated in women weakened after childbirth and for those who have miscarried and developed a vaginal discharge, especially if there is a lot of anxiety and nervousness.

Causticum. Vaginal discharge that causes the vagina to become raw and sore can be helped by *Causticum.* The discharge tends to flow only at night and causes weakness.

Graphites. Useful for vaginal discharge that is pale, thin, profuse, and white. The discharge burns the vaginal tissue, and there is extreme weakness in the lower back. *Graphites* may also be associated with those who have eczema around the vaginal area, especially if it tends to crack and ooze an itchy, sticky discharge. Useful for those in the pre-menopausal period who are often overweight, pale, sensitive to cold, and constipated. Sometimes, a vaginal discharge replaces the menstrual period; periods generally are always late in this situation. An odd symptom with this remedy is the occurrence of hoarseness before the menstrual period. Vaginal discharge is profuse in the morning when rising from bed.

Helonias. Useful for vaginal discharge that causes vaginal tissue to become hot, red, swollen, burning, and itching. There is a sense of weight and soreness in the uterus, and the person is constantly aware of the uterus and its discomfort. Vaginal discharge is heavy and white and sometimes resembles sour, curdled milk. *Helonias* is often indicated in those who have heavy, long-lasting periods and who tend to become weak from their menstrual period. These people tend to get worse in cold weather and from exertion because of their anemia and fatigue. The person tends to be depressed, but seems better when busy and engaged in doing something.

Hydrastis. Useful for sticky, thick, ropy, and very itchy vaginal discharge. The discharge is bright yellow, often irritates the vaginal tissues, and tends to get worse after the menstrual period. General weakness, poor digestion, constipation, and depression are experienced.

Kali bich. Useful for vaginal discharge that is thick, sticky, greenish-yellow, and causes rawness in the vagina. This remedy is particularly indicated in those who are light-haired and overweight. The discharge is similar to the discharge of *Hydrastis,* except that it is not as hot as that of *Hydrastis* and tends to be more green (while discharge associated with *Hydrastis* is more yellow).

Kali mur. Useful for milky, white vaginal discharge that is thick, bland, and non-irritating. There are few mental symptoms associated with this remedy, and it is generally used in a lower potency (such as 6x).

Kreosote. This is an important remedy for extremely acrid, burning, irritating, odorous, and profuse vaginal discharge. The discharge tends to soil the person's underpants, staining them yellow. Vaginal discharge itches and burns excessively and is aggravated by urinating and relieved by washing with warm water or putting hot compresses on the vagina. The itching, which is very distressing, is located in the vulva, labia, and between the thighs. The discharge tends to be heaviest between menstrual periods. *Kreosote* is helpful for vaginitis during pregnancy, especially when there is excessive vaginal itching.

Mercurius sol. When irritating vaginal discharge causes the tissue in the vagina to become raw and swollen, *Mercurius sol* may be helpful. The discharge is greenish-yellow and gets worse at night and when in bed, especially when the person is overheated. Odor emanates from various parts of the body, including vaginal discharge, perspiration, and breath. This remedy is often indicated in infections that are more serious and bacterial in nature. Vaginal discharge tends to cause itching, and there is relief from scratching and from washing the affected area in cool water.

Natrum mur. Useful for thick, transparent or white vaginal discharge that may itch or irritate. *Natrum mur* is most useful for discharges associated with genital herpes. It may be associated with loss of pubic hair.

Natrum phos. Useful for vaginitis, especially after the use of antibiotics. It is helpful for yeast infections and may also be used for bacterial vaginosis (sometimes, or formerly, called hemophilus vaginitis). This remedy is helpful for vaginal discharge caused by eating too many acidic foods or sweets. Vaginal discharge tends to be yellow, and the tongue may have a characteristic yellow coating in the back that extends up to the roof of the mouth.

Nitric acid. Useful for corrosive vaginal discharge that causes the skin to become very sore around the vagina, sometimes causing ulcerations to form. The vaginal area is swollen and itchy. Vaginal discharge is odorous, reddish-brown, and tends to cause a sticking or stitching pain in the vaginal tissue. The hair on the genitals may fall out because the discharge is so corrosive. *Nitric acid* is especially indicated for warts on the vaginal tissues. Note that an infection with this degree of inflammation should be evaluated by a nurse practitioner or physician.

Pulsatilla. An important remedy for all kinds of vaginal infections that tend to get worse during menstrual periods and pregnancy. Vaginal discharge tends to be milky or watery and is generally not burning or painful, unless it is retained in the vagina too long. Generally, the discharge is mucus-like, thick, creamy, and white.

There is often chilliness, weepiness, a desire to walk in the cool air, and a desire to seek comfort when feeling sad. *Pulsatilla* is useful for yeast infections (along with *Natrum phos* and *Thuja*). Vaginal discharge sometimes occurs with sexual arousal.

Sepia. Useful for two types of vaginal discharge: yellow-green discharge that causes excessive itching, and milky discharge that gets worse before the menstrual period, with a bearing-down sensation as if the pelvic organs might fall out of the vagina. *Sepia* is indicated in young girls who have vaginal discharges, as well as in women who feel weak and depressed. The person may experience pain in the vagina that shoots up into the uterus, or may feel as though she is sitting on a ball. The discharge tends to make sexual intercourse painful, and may occur after sex. *Sepia* is also one of the most important remedies for genital herpes.

Staphysagria. Useful for vaginal discharge that is not irritating or corrosive. The genitals, however, are extremely sensitive, and the person cannot bear to be touched in this area. There is an increase in sexual thoughts, and vaginal itching and scratching tends to be somewhat erotic. Scratching tends to relieve the itching, but it starts up again in another area.

Sulphur. Useful for vaginal discharge that burns and causes soreness in the vaginal area. One of the most important symptoms with this remedy is a red and itchy vagina. *Sulphur* is indicated in those who have problems maintaining cleanliness and organization and in general are bothered by heat. Washing or bathing causes vaginal discomfort to get worse. Itching tends to become worse in the evening and from the warmth of bed, and it generally improves when it is cool outside or when the person feels cold.

Thuja. Vaginal discharge that is profuse, thick, and green can be relieved by *Thuja*. (Note that any discharge that is green or yellow should be evaluated by a nurse practitioner or physician.) This was an important remedy for gonorrhea before the days of antibiotics. The vagina is sensitive and vaginal warts, as well as warts on the anus and perineum, may appear. *Thuja* is also useful for helping cure yeast infections.

VARICOSE VEINS

Varicose veins are swollen veins in the legs that are blue and lumpy in appearance. Valves inside the veins and the support of the surrounding tissues around the veins generally help to prevent dilation or swelling of the veins. Because the superficial veins are not supported by muscles like the deeper veins are, the superficial veins tend to break down and the valves do not work properly.

Genetically, people may have fewer valves, or some important valves may be absent, which may result in varicose veins. Taller people have more problems because there is greater stress on the legs and a longer distance for the blood to travel back to the heart, creating more pressure in the lower extremities. Pregnancy, constipation, and long hours of standing are other factors that put downward pressure on the veins.

It is estimated that nearly 25 percent of American women and 10 percent of American men have some form of varicose veins. In severe cases, when fluid going out of the blood vessels into the tissues causes the skin to break down, an ulcer may develop.

Varicose veins are not life threatening and should not be confused with deep venous thrombosis or phlebitis. Treatment of varicose veins is difficult, because once they develop, there is not much a person can do to make veins healthy again. Sometimes surgery is necessary to remove painful or unsightly veins.

Weight control, regular exercise, and eating a high-fiber diet can prevent varicose veins from getting worse. The more weight supported by the circulatory system, the more the system is stressed. Excess body weight puts extra pressure on the veins and legs. Exercise not only reduces weight, but also stimulates the veins to push the blood back toward the heart. Elevating the legs as long as possible during the day is helpful to take some pressure off the veins. A high-fiber diet creates less straining when passing a bowel movement, which otherwise puts enormous pressure on the veins by closing off the flow of blood up the legs. A high fiber diet also helps prevent constipation, which puts pressure on the legs. Wearing support stockings can be helpful to squeeze the vein and help push blood back toward the heart. Lying with the legs above the hips can also be helpful. It is often recommended to lie on the ground and put the legs against the wall. Certain vitamins and supplements are known to help varicose veins.

The homeopathic remedies listed here can be useful for both treating the discomfort associated with varicose veins and helping strengthen the valves and tissues that are necessary for healthy vein function.

Apis. Useful for very swollen varicose veins that are accompanied by stinging pains. Cold applications provide relief, and warm applications aggravate the problem.

Arnica. Useful for varicose veins that are sore. *Arnica* is useful for the person who injures the veins or has sore veins. It is also helpful during pregnancy. The veins occasionally form into painful ulcers with crusts, and these ulcers sometimes discharge a watery fluid.

Arsenicum alb. Useful for inflamed varicose veins that burn like fire and become particularly worse at night. Warm applications relieve the burning; cold applications aggravate the burning. The person is restless and agitated. Varicose veins can occur anywhere on the legs and are sometimes worse during pregnancy.

Calcarea carb. Useful for inflamed, burning varicose veins. Sometimes networks of interlacing veins in the skin are formed. The veins are particularly numerous, painful, and discolored on the thighs and seem to be more sensitive during cold, damp weather. *Calcarea carb* is often useful for varicose veins in women who are overweight.

Carbo veg. Helps varicose veins of the lower legs, which sometimes form little networks of small blood vessels in the skin. The veins are distended and itch, especially in the evening and in bed. Varicose veins sometimes become black and blue and are slow to heal. The person is often chilly and suffers from indigestion (with flatulence or excessive belching). *Carbo veg* is particularly helpful during pregnancy when the veins are blue in color. Useful for varicose veins on the nose.

Graphites. Useful for varicose veins that itch and are accompanied by a cramping sensation and a drawing feeling in the veins. Sometimes the veins are actually covered with pimples. *Graphites* is usually associated with constipation.

Hamamelis. Helpful for inflamed, sore varicose veins of the lower legs that are very large, blue, and lumpy.

Pulsatilla. Useful for inflamed varicose veins of the lower legs. The veins become distended during the menstrual period. *Pulsatilla* is also useful during pregnancy. The veins sometimes bleed and are quite painful, often accompanied by stinging pain. This remedy is also useful for varicose veins under the tongue and on the thigh. The veins are blue and tend to bleed easily, especially when bumped. Sore, stinging black-and-blue spots form on the veins. The veins can become highly inflamed and extend down from the groin into the thighs. The pain is worse at night. The person is often weepy and chilly, yet wants to be in the open air. The person also may experience a lack of thirst and likes to have company.

Sepia. Useful for dark blue varicose veins that get worse during pregnancy. The person feels as if the pelvic organs are relaxed and have a sensation of heaviness. The person experiences the sensation that the entire pelvic region is engorged, which is when the varicose veins seem to be worse.

Sulphur. Helps burning, distended varicose veins. The veins itch, are painful, and become worse when warmth is applied. The veins sometimes break and form burning ulcers, which bleed easily, itch, and ooze an odorous discharge. The person has a difficult time standing because of aching and burning varicose veins and is often inclined to sit or slouch. When water contacts the legs, the veins itch and burn.

Zincum met. Useful for large varicose veins accompanied by perspiring legs and restless feet. *Zincum met* is particularly helpful during pregnancy for restless legs and achy varicose veins.

VERTIGO (ALSO CALLED DIZZINESS)

Vertigo can be described as feeling lightheaded or as though the person or room is spinning. It is a condition that can be simple, mild, and easily cured, or it can be a sign of a serious disease. It can be caused by a virus that gets into the inner ear, affecting the labyrinth system or semicircular canals. This causes swelling and leads to a feeling of being off-balance. Another common cause of vertigo is an ear or sinus infection, and if dizziness lasts more than a few days, is recurrent, or severe, a physician should be contacted. Conditions such as tumors, multiple sclerosis, Meniere's disease, anemia, or heart disease can also cause vertigo and may be long-lasting. A physician should also be contacted in these cases.

Aconite. Often associated with the early onset of an upper respiratory infection. Vertigo can occur after exposure to cold, dry wind. The person may experience ear pain and tends to fall to the right when dizzy. *Aconite* may help an associated headache and nausea. These symptoms may get worse during a woman's menstrual period. Vertigo is worse upon raising the head or rising from a prone position. There actually may be loss of vision during dizzy spells.

Argentum nit. Used for vertigo that is often associated with great weakness and trembling and may be associated with mental confusion. The person may experience the feeling that houses may fall while walking down the street, or that the walls may fall at the home. Dizziness gets worse upon closing the eyes, when in high places (such as in the mountains or in a tall building), and from walking and stooping. The person may also stagger while dizzy.

Arnica. Useful for dizziness or lightheadedness occurring after a head injury (such as being hit by a ball, being hit on the head with an object, or getting in an accident). The person may also experience ringing in the ears. Relief is found with rest. Report to a physician any of the following signs after a head injury: changes in consciousness, changes in emotions, confusion, dilation of pupils, nausea, vomiting, or seizure. The person should be watched for twenty-four hours and awakened at night to asses the level of consciousness.

Belladonna. Dizziness is often associated with upper respiratory infections from which the person is hot, red-faced, dry, thirsty, and agitated. *Belladonna* also helps high fevers. Vertigo usually worsens upon rising in the morning, and there is a tendency to fall to the left side or backward. The person experiences dizziness with headaches. Motion, moving the head, stooping, or rising from stooping aggravates, and the person feels as though objects are turning in a circle.

Borax. Vertigo occurs when the person is looking down or moving in a downward motion (such as descending in an airplane or walking down steep stairs).

Bromium. Useful for vertigo caused by looking at running water (such as a river) or watching anything moving rapidly. There is a tendency to fall backward. Vertigo is relieved by nosebleeds.

Bryonia. Typical symptoms of dizziness are that vertigo gets worse from any movement and gets better with rest. This remedy is often associated with stomach or gastric problems accompanied by thirst and pains that are relieved if the person remains absolutely still or if firm pressure is applied. This remedy is associated with nausea and vomiting. There is often a sensation of looseness in the brain when stooping. A sensation of sinking through the bed may occur while the person is lying down.

Calcarea carb. The person becomes dizzy when ascending or looking up (such as climbing stairs, tall mountains, or hills). Vertigo is worse in the open air and when turning the head. The condition worsens when the person has the chills. There may be a tendency to fall sideways when dizzy. A headache sometimes accompanies vertigo. Dizziness is worse when the head moves quickly.

Calcarea phos. Dizziness occurs with constipation. Vertigo is worse in windy weather.

China. For dizziness associated with weakness from excessive bleeding or diarrhea. The person feels weak and cannot move without feeling dizzy, fatigued, and lightheaded. A physician should be contacted in this situation.

Cocculus. This remedy is used when the person experiences vertigo while riding in a moving vehicle. Dizziness can also occur from staying up late at night and losing sleep and especially when caring for an ill or dying person. Dizziness is worse when the person sits up, and there is often a flushed face and hot head. Eating also makes the dizziness worse. The person is usually nauseated and vomits, and may feel intoxicated without drinking any alcohol. Vertigo is often associated with nervous people.

Conium maculatum. The person experiences vertigo when lying down and turning in bed. Vertigo is especially aggravated by turning the head sideways, whether in an upright or lying-down position. The person must lie perfectly still on the back because the smallest movement causes vertigo. Useful for the elderly, especially those who overuse tobacco. The person experiences vertigo upon rising or when going upstairs or downstairs. When the person looks steadily at an object, the sensation of turning in a circle is experienced.

Gelsemium. Dizziness can occur with influenza-like symptoms in which the person feels tired and weak. There may be aching muscles, and the person is lethargic and listless. Vertigo can occur with any movement. Vertigo is associated with heaviness of the head and seems to spread from the back of the head (occiput) and the nape of the neck. This remedy may be associated with dim or double vision. There can be staggering, trembling weakness when the person tries to move and a feeling of intoxication without drinking any alcohol. Urinating may actually help the dizziness. Vertigo can occur when a person is anxious about an upcoming event (such as giving a speech or flying in an airplane); dizziness may occur just thinking about the event.

Gratiola. The person feels worse after eating and being in a warm room. *Gratiola* is similar to *Nux vomica* in that it is often used by women who are excessively irritable and hypersensitive to noise, touch, and mental activity.

Ignatia. The person experiences dizziness during times of high anxiety; dizziness is especially brought on after hearing bad news (such as the death of a loved one). The person experiences vertigo that comes on with shock and grief.

Kali carb. Vertigo seems to start in the stomach area.

Lachesis. Dizziness may be experienced when closing the eyes; the person may stagger to the left side. Dizziness is aggravated upon waking in the morning or after a nap. Frequent short episodes of vertigo occur, especially when closing the eyes.

Natrum mur. Vertigo is associated with people who brood about past disappointments or feel sad about the loss of loved ones or broken relationships. They dislike words of comfort or sympathy. Dizziness occurs with headaches while the person is lying down. When reading or writing too much, dizziness may be associated with eye fatigue. Dizziness is worse upon rising in the morning and from drinking coffee. Dizziness occurs in high places and when looking steadily at one object for a long time (such as looking out a window). Objects seem to turn in a circle. Vertigo is better from applying cold to the head, such as ice packs or cold washcloths. Vertigo gets worse when tea is consumed. The person may experience vertigo during pregnancy. Note that while homeopathic remedies are safe during pregnancy, labor, and breastfeeding, a pregnant woman should confer with her obstetrician or midwife to coordinate treatment.

Natrum salicylicum. Useful for Meniere's disease, in which vertigo, deafness, and noises in the ear are experienced. Vertigo is worse upon raising the head, and all objects seem to move to the right. Vertigo often occurs after influenza.

Nux vomica. Useful for an irritable, oversensitive person who tends to overdo things (such as drinking too much alcohol or coffee or staying up too late partying or studying). *Nux vomica* may help nausea, vomiting, and general gastrointestinal upset. Any kind of mental activity can aggravate the dizziness. Noise, the smell of flowers, and the open air can cause dizziness in an oversensitive person. Dizziness is also worse when rising, especially in the morning. Dizziness becomes worse from stooping, and the person has a tendency to fall sideways. Dizziness becomes worse after eating. *Nux vomica* may help headaches accompanied by a sick feeling in the stomach, especially after drinking too much. The person feels intoxicated and staggers, trembles, and feels weak. Dizziness worsens when a fever is present, especially during the chills phase. The person may feel very lightheaded and experience dim vision during dizziness. The person feels that the room whirls in a circle.

Petroleum. Useful for seasickness when the person is dizzy and nauseated. The person feels worse when moving the eyes, especially while riding in a boat. The vertigo gets better when the person lies down and elevates the head. Vertigo is also associated with a feeling of heaviness at the back of the head, as if it were made of lead. Upon rising, the person experiences vertigo that is felt in the back of the head and nape of the neck. The person may feel intoxicated, even if no alcohol was consumed.

Phosphorus. This remedy is often associated with chronic and long-standing vertigo. *Phosphorus* can be useful for elderly people. A person who needs *Phosphorus* is hypersensitive to all sorts of internal impressions and becomes dizzy when smelling a strong odor (such as that of flowers). Vertigo tends to be worse when looking up or down. This remedy is associated with dizziness that accompanies anemia and loss of fluids and blood. Vertigo is worse upon rising from a seat or bed. Feelings of turning in a circle may be experienced. Emotionally, the person can be unfocused and overreact to normally minor setbacks. The person may feel faint and dizzy when things become overwhelming. Vertigo is worse when the person lies on the left side.

Pulsatilla. This remedy is associated with the particular *Pulsatilla* personality of a person who weeps, is easily discouraged, and wants to be consoled and pampered. When sick, the person may feel chilly, yet want cool air blowing, and is often thirstless. Dizziness compels the person to lie down and is worse when rising, especially in the morning. The vertigo is worse after eating and can be associated with nausea. A particular symptom with vertigo is that objects seem to be far away. The person sometimes feels as though being turned in a circle. Vertigo gets better when the person walks in the open air. Vertigo is worse during a woman's menstrual period, as well as when the period is late.

Rhus tox. Vertigo is accompanied by a tendency to fall, especially when rising from the bed. The person tends to fall backward or forward.

Sepia. Vertigo is accompanied by a sensation of something rolling around in the head. The person who needs *Sepia* feels better when blood circulation is increased (such as with strenuous exercise, dancing, or elevating the legs); this also helps the vertigo. Vertigo is worse when closing the eyes.

Silica. The person may experience vertigo when looking up. Conditions are worse when lying on the back and better when wrapped up warmly and lying on the left side. The person tends to fall forward, and has difficulty maintaining balance. Vertigo is associated with middle ear infections in which fluid causes the ear to be stuffed up.

Spigelia. For vertigo with very sensitive hearing. The person tends to fall when looking down, especially when looking steadily down for a long time. This remedy may help headaches and facial pains, especially on the left side.

Tabacum. For vertigo accompanied by a sick headache with severe nausea. The vertigo gets worse when the person opens the eyes. A tight feeling around the head, as if a band were wrapped around it, may be experienced. There may be vertigo from sea-sickness, accompanied by a sinking feeling in the pit of the stomach. The vertigo gets better when the person is in fresh, open air.

Theridion curassavicum. For vertigo accompanied by nausea and vomiting, and aggravated by the least movement, particularly closing the eyes. The person is very sensitive to noise, which seems to penetrate the body and cause vertigo.

WARTS

Warts are caused by a virus and can occur almost any place on the body, but the most common places for warts are the fingers, soles of the feet, genitalia, rectum, face, and forearms. They can be flat or raised, large or small, and look like a small blister or cauliflower. They are usually rough and have a pitted surface. They are very contagious. If a person has them, direct contact with other people's skin should be avoided, especially in moist environments. For example, a person who has plantar warts should not walk around barefoot in the shower where other people are showering. A person who has genital warts should not have sex without using a condom. Certain herbs and vitamins are known to help warts.

The homeopathic remedies listed here have been used effectively in treating warts. For many years, homeopaths have been called wart doctors because of their effectiveness in treating warts. Homeopathy is also useful for helping people decrease their susceptibility to the wart virus.

Antimonium crud. Useful for old, hard, horny warts located on any part of the body. This remedy is particularly helpful for plantar warts, those on the plantar surface of the foot (the sole), as well as warts on the palms of the hands. These warts tend to be fairly smooth and usually do not bleed easily.

Calcarea carb. Useful for warts that are either surrounded by a circle of ulcers or actually become ulcers. These warts often smell like old cheese and may pulsate. The warts are generally large, fleshy, and sometimes red. The warts can break down and ooze pus.

Causticum. Warts that are large and jagged and bleed easily can be helped with *Causticum.* These warts tend to be hard, dry, and horny. They commonly occur around the fingernails, the tips of the fingers, the nose, the eyebrows, and other parts of the face. Sometimes these warts are painful. The warts can have stalks and be scattered all over the body.

Dulcamara. Useful for flat, transparent warts (especially those located on the back of the hand). These warts are sometimes more visible in low, indirect light, rather than direct light. This remedy is also useful for large, soft, brownish warts that seem to be filled with water. These warts often occur on a person who lives in a very humid environment. Large, flat, fleshy warts can also occur on the face.

Graphites. Useful for warts located on the tip of the finger and around the nail. This type of wart often oozes a thin, sticky discharge.

Natrum mur. Watery, transparent warts that occur particularly on the soles of the feet and the palms of the hands can be treated with *Natrum mur.* These warts are dry and often have stalks.

Natrum sulph. Red warts that appear all over the body can be treated with *Natrum sulph.* This remedy is particularly helpful when the person develops warts due to continuous exposure to cold, damp weather.

Nitric acid. Useful for horny, golden-colored warts that tend to have bleeding, painful cracks. The pricking pain from these cracks feels like a thorn, stick, or needle. The warts may itch, are jagged, and sometimes form large, elevated, cauliflower-like masses.

Sabina. Useful for warty growths in the anus or genital region, especially when symptoms include intense burning and itching. These warts tend to bleed quite easily. *Sabina* is often useful when taken with or following *Thuja* and *Nitric acid.*

Staphysagria. Useful for large, fleshy moles and warts that are sensitive to touch.

Thuja. An excellent remedy for many different types of warts, but particularly helpful for warts on the hands, feet, and genitals. The warts often have little stalks and can appear on any part of the body. Sometimes the wart smells like old cheese. This remedy is particularly useful when the warts are brown or red and bleed easily. The characteristics of the warts vary: small or large, smooth or jagged, painful or painless, and flat and unnoticeable or extremely ugly. Genital warts can occur on the vagina, cervix, penis, or scrotum.

CHAPTER 3

Using *The Complete Homeopathic Resource* CD

While this book includes chapters on Basic Homeopathy and the Clinical Repertory, *The Complete Homeopathic Resource* CD contains a program that consists of four modules: Repertory, Clinical Repertory, Materia Medica, and Basic Homeopathy. The program is interactive with hyperlinks between sections and modules. In the CD, the Repertory, Clinical Repertory, and Materia Medica modules help you identify the best remedies for specific symptoms or illness. The Basic Homeopathy module provides a comprehensive overview on homeopathy and how this form of medicine can be used safely and effectively to treat a variety of illnesses; it is similar in content to Chapter 1 of this book.

The information in this chapter, along with additional facts and tips, can also be found in the Help section on the CD.

THE MODULES OF THE CD

The Repertory Module
A "repertory" is essentially an index to the materia medica. It contains a listing of symptoms (rubrics) and homeopathic remedies that are associated with and can treat the symptoms. The Repertory is especially useful when the sick person has many symptoms, when you, as the home prescriber, are unsure of the name of an illness, or when the total symptom set does not describe a single common illness.

The first module, the Repertory, can greatly assist in narrowing the choice of helpful homeopathic remedies. This program's repertory is a condensed version of Kent's *Repertory of the Homeopathic Materia Medica*.

More than one homeopathic repertory has been published, but Kent's is perhaps the most widely used. It was compiled by the American homeopathic physician, James Tyler Kent, M.D. (1849–1916), one of the most well-known homeopathic physicians. The first edition of Kent's Repertory was completed in 1877 and went through several revisions in the twentieth century. It is 1,423 pages long, includes more than 600 remedies, and has 65,000 rubrics.

The repertory in this program is a condensed version of Kent's Repertory. It includes approximately 9,000 rubrics. The following types of rubrics are included in this program:

- Rubrics that pertain to acute, self-limiting, or recurring conditions

- Rubrics with mental symptoms that are applicable to home use or basic clinical use

- Rubrics that correspond to the 105 remedies included in this program's Materia Medica

All repertories have their own logic and structure, and Kent's Repertory is no exception. Even though there may have been ways to reorganize Kent's Repertory to make it more immediately understandable, no major organizational changes have been made so as not to modify a very authoritative resource.

The Clinical Repertory Module

The second module, the Clinical Repertory, like the Repertory module, is very useful for narrowing the choice of helpful remedies. The Clinical Repertory is used when the name of an illness is known, or a complete set of symptoms describe a common affliction—an injury, a sore throat, an infection.

In the Clinical Repertory, you can choose to view illnesses alphabetically or by category. After you select an illness or illness category, the program displays a short list of candidate remedies, and then, upon your selection, a "remedy symptom picture" describing the symptoms commonly helped by that remedy. Or you can browse through the remedies, looking for the remedy symptom pictures that most closely match the symptoms you are confronting.

After reviewing the remedy symptom pictures in the Clinical Repertory, you can make a final remedy selection, or you can refer to the next module, Materia Medica, to get more specific information for making a final remedy selection.

The Materia Medica Module

"Materia medica" is Latin for "materials of medicine." Books (or CDs) that contain a materia medica provide detailed information on the symptoms that a substance is known to cause when given to healthy people and will initiate cure when given to sick people.

The third module, the Materia Medica, provides detailed descriptions of 105 commonly used remedies, and describes mental, emotional, and physical symptoms that can be helped by each remedy. In addition, the Materia Medica gives you guidelines on dosage and administering each remedy properly.

Often, review of a remedy in the Materia Medica is the last step in the remedy selection process. For a remedy to be most helpful, it is important that most of the symptoms appear in the materia medica of that remedy. However, all symptoms in the materia medica of a remedy need not be present for a remedy to be helpful.

There are many homeopathic materia medicas, one of the most well known being Boericke's *Homoeopathic Materia Medica and Repertory,* which was published in 1901. Basically, there are two kinds of materia medica: those that are compilations of raw proving data and those that interpret the data. In its most basic form, the materia medica is a collection of quotes from the people who proved the substance. Materia medicas come in many different sizes and styles. Some are contained in multi-volume sets, while others may be only a few pages. Some materia medicas are merely transcriptions of lectures given by homeopaths. Some contain only remedy constitutional type information, while others contain only specific physical symptoms. Some may contain modalities, remedy comparisons, dosages, and interactions, and others may not. Nearly all homeopathic books contain a materia medica of some sort.

The remedies in this program's Materia Medica were selected because they are very applicable to home prescribing for acute conditions. Many of them are useful for a wide variety of conditions, while some of them have been included because of their particular usefulness for conditions like allergies that a person often treats at home.

The Basic Homeopathy Module

The fourth module, Basic Homeopathy, provides a comprehensive overview of homeopathy. This section includes such varied information as the homeopathic approach to health and illness, and the laws and principles of homeopathy. It answers such questions as: "When is it safe and appropriate to use homeopathy?" and, "Where can I get the remedies?" It also instructs you on how to assemble your own home remedy kit.

THE REMEDY SELECTION PROCESS

Most of the time you will use the Repertory or the Clinical Repertory to analyze symptoms being experienced by you or a family member, and determine a short list of remedies to consider. You can then refer to the Materia Medica to make your final remedy choice. As you become more experienced in homeopathic prescribing, you may be able to select a remedy based on the Repertory, the Clinical Repertory, or the Materia Medica alone.

Using the Repertory

The Repertory is essentially an index to the Materia Medica. It contains a hierarchical listing of symptoms (rubrics) and homeopathic remedies that are associated with and can treat the symptoms.

The Repertory enables you to select one or more symptoms. The program then analyzes these symptoms to find the remedies that most closely match the symptoms and can therefore treat your condition. To find remedies that best match your condition, the program weighs, analyzes, and scores remedies based on the selected symptoms.

Kent's Repertory is divided into chapters organized by parts of the body and mind. In each chapter, the Repertory has a hierarchical listing of symptoms—the rubrics. Under each rubric is a listing of remedies and their grade. Grades are shown in three different typefaces: **bold,** *italicized,* and plain type. That formatting is followed in the CD program. The grade refers to the extent to which symptoms were brought out in the remedy provings. If the remedy is **bolded,** it brought out the symptoms in all or a majority of the provers. If the remedy is *italicized,* it brought out the symptoms in some of the provers. If a remedy is in plain type, it brought out the symptoms less often in the provers. Thus, the grade of the remedy is a measure of the probability that the remedy will produce similar symptoms in a healthy person, and hence help cure those symptoms in a sick individual.

Kent's Repertory relies upon complex indentation levels to demonstrate modifications to symptoms. This program maintains the hierarchy given by the indentation but presents it a bit differently on the computer screen to make it less confusing. Rather than formatting the Repertory as a series of indentations, the program separates the modifications by semicolons to keep the entire rubric on a line.

The program weighting calculations attempt to replicate what goes on in the mind of a professional homeopath as he or she analyzes a case. However, remember that this program is only a tool that may help you find an answer; it may not always provide the best answer or it may indicate several possible remedies. It is important for you to research the Materia Medica entries for the remedies that are indicated most prominently to find the best remedy for your symptoms.

Rubric

A rubric is a symptom in a repertory. A rubric is followed by a list of remedies that have either brought out the symptom during provings on healthy people or have cured the symptom when given to sick people for other problems. In this program, remedies associated with a rubric can be viewed by pressing the right mouse button. For more information, see Symptom Selection.

Opening the Repertory and Getting Started

Open the Repertory by clicking on the Repertory icon from any part of the program. The icon is highlighted when selected.

The Repertory consists of four screens that are used to select and analyze symptoms: Contents, Symptom Selection, Symptom Chart, and Symptom Analysis.

When the Repertory is first entered after beginning the program, a new session is automatically started and you may begin selecting symptoms. To open a previously saved session, select Open Session Open from the Repertory Tools menu. After symptoms have been selected, it is not necessary to save them (see Save Session) before using the other parts of the program. The selected symptoms remain in the Symptom Chart until Clear Session is selected or the program is closed.

Session

A repertory session is a record of all the information listed in the Symptom Chart: the session date, name, and the problem, with the selected symptoms. Each session is treated as a file that may be saved and reopened for further editing and analysis.

Contents

The Contents screen is seen upon first entering the Repertory. By clicking on the people or body part icon from any part of the Repertory, you can display condensed versions of the chapters in Kent's Repertory. The chapters (or symptom categories) are arranged around the people icon to make them easier to find.

Clicking on the appropriate selections of interest on the Contents screen results in a list of symptom characteristics for study and consideration. Symptom characteristics are selected from this list by dragging the pen to a symptom or condition, so the chosen symptom becomes highlighted with an underline.

When using homeopathy, it is important to consider symptoms of the mind, body part or function, and generalities, so that the entire illness is considered. As you choose categories from the Contents screen, it is important not to overlook the Generalities and Mind categories. Use the Generalities category to select symptoms that affect your (or the patient's) overall condition. For example, if all the symptoms are worse in the morning, you should select morning aggravation from Generalities. For further emphasis, you could also select morning aggravation under every symptom. Use the Mind category to select symptoms associated with your (or the person's) emotional and mental health. Symptoms that affect specific areas of the body should be selected under the other appropriate categories.

View a category by clicking on it. A list of symptoms for that category appears. From this list, select symptoms pertaining to the condition or illness. When you are satisfied with your selections, click on the clipboard at the top of the Repertory screen. The symptoms and associated remedies are now displayed on a Symptom Chart, which can be printed or saved for later reference and use. Next, click on the computer at the top of the Repertory screen. The symptoms and their remedies are analyzed by the *The Complete Homeopathic Resource* expert system, and the Symptom Analysis chart will display a list of remedies for consideration.

Several of the top-ranking remedies shown on the Symptom Analysis screen should be studied further to find the remedy that most closely matches the selected symptoms. You can study the remedies further in one, or both, of the next two modules: the Clinical Repertory or the Materia Medica.

Symptom Selection

Clicking on any category in the Contents accesses the Symptom Selection screen. This screen lists symptoms associated with the selected category. A general symptom often appears at the beginning of the list, followed by specific symptoms. As you move down the page within a general symptom, the symptoms get more and more specific. Below is an example of specific symptoms indented under the general symptom "Pain" in the "Female Genitals" category.

Female Genitals
Pain
    Ovaries
    Ovaries; right
    Ovaries; right; lying on right side amel
    Ovaries; left
    Ovaries; left; lying on left side agg
    Ovaries; left; extending to; right

The above symptoms are read in the following manner:

Female genital pain in general
Pain in the ovaries
Pain in the right ovary
Pain in the right ovary that is better (ameliorated) when lying on the right side
Pain in the left ovary
Pain in the left ovary that is worse (aggravated) when lying on the left side
Pain in the left ovary that extends to the right ovary

Under each general symptom that fits the condition, select the specific symptoms that best describe the condition. The more specific you can be with a symptom, the more appropriate the analysis will be for those symptoms. If none of the specific symptoms match the condition, select the general symptom.

Note: Gray-color (or "grayed out") symptoms are general symptoms that are not active because they have no remedies associated with them; these symptoms function only as headings for the symptoms that follow and are not selectable.

To view the remedies associated with any active (not gray) symptom, press the right mouse button on the symptom. The Symptom Remedies window appears.

Selecting Symptoms

1. Scroll through the list to find active (not gray) symptoms that match the condition.

2. Select matching symptoms by dragging the pen to each symptom. Selected symptoms appear underlined. If desired, drag the pen to any selected symptom to deselect it.

3. After you have selected all the matching symptoms from the current category, click on the people icon to return to the Contents screen and choose another category. Continue selecting symptoms until you have chosen the symptoms that describe the total symptomology of the case you're treating.

4. Click on the clipboard to view the Symptom Chart.

Symptom Remedies

The Symptom Remedies window appears after right-clicking on a symptom while in the Symptom Selection screen. The window lists the full text of the symptom, including the general symptom and category it came from and its associated remedies and weights. (For a description of how the program calculates the relative weights or matches of remedies, see Remedy Weighting Factors, below.)

Symptom Chart

The Symptom Chart screen is accessed by clicking on the clipboard from any part of the Repertory. This screen lists the set of symptoms that have been selected. You can verify that all of the symptoms were selected, and you can delete any symptoms that you no longer want to include. You may also emphasize a symptom that is very prominent in the condition. For example, you may want to emphasize a frontal headache if you feel it is the strongest symptom. The program then places more weight on the frontal headache when analyzing the symptoms. However, it is not necessary to emphasize any symptoms.

This screen also provides a place to enter the date, the name of the person with the symptoms, and the problem or condition. The date must be entered in the format "mm/dd/yy" (for example, 1/17/06). This session information is saved to give you a record of when and for whom the session was recorded. If the current session has a filename (that is, the session has been saved or opened), it is displayed in the Session field. See Save Session.

Tip: If you are editing a previously saved session and wish to include the current date instead of the old one, delete the existing text in the date field, click on the clipboard again, and then save the session.

Preparing the Symptoms for Analysis

Emphasize strong symptoms by dragging the exclamation point to the symptom. Emphasized symptoms appear in red. If desired, drag the exclamation point to any emphasized symptom to de-emphasize it.

If you no longer want to include a symptom, delete it by dragging the eraser to the symptom. The symptom disappears when the eraser is released.

When you have finished emphasizing and/or deleting symptoms, click on the computer icon to perform and view the Symptom Analysis.

Symptom Analysis

The Symptom Analysis screen is accessed by clicking on the computer icon from any part of the Repertory. This screen lists the remedies from the Symptom Chart in the order of their analyzed scores from highest to lowest. Each remedy's score is a percent of the top remedy's score displayed in bar graph form. The longer the remedy score bar, the higher the score is for that remedy. However, the first remedy on the Symptom Analysis is not necessarily the best remedy for your condition. High scores only indicate that the remedy may be helpful for the selected symptoms. It is important to refer to the Materia Medica before deciding which remedy to take.

To view a remedy's Materia Medica menu entry, click on the remedy name hypertext. Use the History tool or the footprints icon to return to the analysis when finished.

To speed up the analysis, raise the analysis cutoff value using the Preferences option on the Repertory Tools menu. Be careful not to raise the value too much, or remedies that should be considered may get cut off.

To print a copy of the session report, click on the printer icon. The option of including the chart, the analysis, or both in the report is available under the Preferences option on the Repertory Tools menu.

Remedy Weighting Factors

To find remedies that match the condition you're treating, the program weights, analyzes, and scores the remedies associated with the selected symptoms. The program weighting calculations attempt to replicate what goes on in the mind of a professional homeopath as he or she analyzes a case. The following factors are included in the weighting calculations and displayed on-screen.

Total remedy points. A remedy that appears bolded in the rubric receives maximum points, one that appears italicized is given two-thirds maximum points, and one that appears plain is given one-third maximum points. The points for each remedy are then collected from all the rubrics it appears under to give each remedy a total point score, which is then used in the analysis. The greater the points received, the heavier the emphasis.

The relative emphasis placed on a symptom. If a particular symptom is emphasized in the Symptom Chart, the remedies found under the emphasized symptom are given greater weight in the analysis.

The number of symptoms associated with a remedy. The more symptoms a remedy appears under, the greater weight it receives in the analysis.

The prominence of a remedy. The prominence or strength of a remedy under a symptom is taken into account in the analysis by considering the number of other remedies of equal or higher status under the same symptom. For example, an italicized remedy under a symptom, which has one other, italicized remedy and no bolded remedies receives greater emphasis than an italicized remedy under a symptom, which has two other, italicized remedies.

The number of remedies under the symptoms. The size of the symptom, or the number of remedies found under a symptom, is taken into consideration during the analysis. Remedies that are found under a symptom with fewer remedies are given greater emphasis than those found under a symptom with more remedies.

Whether the symptoms are related to the mind or are emotional in nature. Symptoms in the Mind category tend to be emotional in nature and the remedies found under Mind symptoms are given greater emphasis in the analysis.

Whether the symptoms are causal in nature. Some symptoms in the Repertory are considered causal in nature; that is, they could very well be the cause of the illness. When chosen, these particular symptoms and their remedies are given greater emphasis in the analysis.

The nature of the total symptom set chosen by the user. The nature of the chosen symptoms as a group is a very important consideration in the analysis. For example, if you have chosen a large group of symptoms with many remedies involved, the analysis may result in a large number of remedies of similar scores, making remedy selection more difficult. In this particular situation it is advantageous for the analysis to place a greater emphasis on the consideration of the size of the symptom and the prominence of certain remedies to help highlight certain remedies, thus making remedy selection easier.

Helpful Hints

Following are some tips that will make using the Repertory module more comprehensive and effective.

Look in more than one place. Sometimes material can appear in more than one place. Occasionally there are references to other sections, which make it easy to find the other locations. For example, if you are looking for a reference to a particular food, you can look in both the Generalities and Stomach sections—you will probably find something helpful in both sections.

Use the glossary. Though we did not change terms in order to avoid changing the meaning of symptoms, the glossary tool can help you understand some of the more old-fashioned words.

Remember that *amel* and *agg* mean made better and made worse. Throughout the Repertory the abbreviations amel and agg are used. Amel is an abbreviation for ameliorated (better from). Agg is an abbreviation for aggravated (worse from).

Study the Materia Medica. Once you have used the Repertory to narrow the field of remedies down to a few close matches, carefully study the Materia Medica entry for each identified remedy to determine which remedy picture most closely matches the condition.

Use the Clinical Repertory to verify your final remedy choice. While you can select a remedy using only the Repertory, you could verify your choice by checking appropriate conditions in the Clinical Repertory.

Spend some time browsing through the Repertory. To familiarize yourself with the format of the Repertory, it may be useful to spend some time browsing through the different sections of the Repertory.

Using the Clinical Repertory

The Clinical Repertory is a listing of specific illnesses or conditions and a description of the remedies that can be used to help the problems. Each remedy under the illness or condition headings has a brief description of its associated symptoms. From the remedy descriptions, you may be able to choose which remedy best matches the illness or symptoms you are treating.

The Clinical Repertory does not include chronic conditions or complicated conditions that are difficult to prescribe for. It also does not include serious diseases like heart disease, cancer, and multiple sclerosis, because they are not appropriate for home prescribing.

Some diseases, like chronic fatigue syndrome and mononucleosis, can be helped by homeopathy, but are not listed as separate conditions in this program. Because homeopathy emphasizes the symptoms rather than the disease, try reviewing more specific symptoms associated with this type of disease. For example, you could try reviewing the Clinical Repertory sections associated with sore throat or fever for help dealing with the symptoms of mononucleosis.

Opening the Clinical Repertory and Getting Started

Open the Clinical Repertory by clicking on the Clinical Repertory icon from any part of the program. The icon is highlighted when selected.

The Contents screen appears first. It lists clinical conditions either in alphabetical order or divided into categories, such as body areas or types of conditions. With either format, you can select a clinical condition and get a list of remedies that help the condition. You can then select a remedy and view its clinical description. After reading the clinical remedy descriptions and the associated Materia Medica entries, you can choose which remedy best fits the condition you are researching.

The Outline option is in the upper-right corner of every Clinical Repertory screen. It enables you to view the next level up in the topic hierarchy. If you are viewing a remedy description for a condition, clicking here brings you to the menu for that condition. Clicking again brings you to the category that the condition belongs to. Clicking again brings you back to the Contents.

Viewing Remedy Descriptions for a Condition

Select the format you prefer for listing the conditions: alphabetically or by category. If the conditions are listed alphabetically, click on a condition to see information. If the conditions are listed by category, click first on a category and then on a condition. The remedies for that condition then appear.

Click on a remedy to read its description or use the left arrow and right arrow to browse through the remedy descriptions.

To get an overall picture of a particular remedy, click on the remedy name at the top of the remedy description to jump to its Materia Medica topic menu. After reading the topic descriptions, use the History tool or Footprints option to return to the Clinical Repertory.

When finished reading the remedy descriptions, click on the Outline option to return to the remedy menu.

To view a different clinical condition, click on the Outline option again to return to the Contents screen.

Helpful Hints

Following are some tips that will make using the Clinical Repertory module more comprehensive and effective.

Use the browsing arrows to review remedies. If you need to read the descriptions of each remedy listed, you might find it easier to use the browsing arrows, rather than opening and closing each remedy.

You do not need a perfect match from the Clinical Repertory. Often a remedy description matches closely, but not perfectly. Your goal is to bring down the list of remedies to a manageable few by looking for the best matches among all the remedies. If you cannot make a remedy choice directly from the Clinical Repertory, you could consult Materia Medica to help make the final choice.

You do not always need to review the Materia Medica. Sometimes you can find the best remedy from the Clinical Repertory, without going to the Materia Medica for detailed study. For example, *Aconite* and *Arnica* are often the first remedies given for certain illnesses or conditions and you do not need to look any further. Or, you may find a remedy that seems to match the illness or condition perfectly and you may decide to look no further. More often than not, however, you need to finish your remedy search in the Materia Medica.

Using the Materia Medica

The Materia Medica includes descriptions of 105 commonly used homeopathic remedies. Each description provides an overall picture of a remedy, including the mental and physical symptoms associated with or helped by that remedy. These symptoms have been compiled as the result of provings on healthy people as well as symptoms observed to have been cured when the remedy was given to a sick person for other problems.

Remedies in the Materia Medica are listed by both their common name and Latin name. After selecting a remedy, you can click on the "Say It" bubble to hear the remedy pronunciation.

Opening the Materia Medica and Getting Started

Open the Materia Medica by clicking on the Materia Medica icon from any part of the program. The icon is highlighted when selected. The Contents screen appears first. It lists 105 homeopathic remedies by their common names (left column) and Latin names (right column). From this list, you can select a remedy and view its associated topics.

The Outline option is in the upper-right corner of every Materia Medica screen. It allows you to view the next level up in the topic hierarchy. If you are viewing a topic in a remedy, clicking here brings you to the menu for that remedy. Clicking again brings you back to the Contents.

Reading Remedy Descriptions

After choosing a remedy from the Contents, a listing of the sections for that remedy appears. Each Materia Medica entry may include any or all of the following sections:

- Quick Look
- Guiding Characteristics
- Deeper Pictures
- Major Symptoms
- Condition Better or Worse
- Dosage and Remedy Interactions
- Clinical Uses

Quick Look. This section provides a brief overview of the remedy, its uses, and the associated symptoms. The symptoms and uses are arranged from most prominent to least prominent. You could use this section to narrow down the field of remedies that you are considering, or in some cases the section might provide all the information you need to choose a remedy.

Guiding Characteristics. This section describes the overall remedy action. Each paragraph provides information on the symptoms and conditions associated with the remedy. This is a more philosophical and interpretive picture of the remedy, so it is useful for understanding the entire remedy picture. This section is especially useful when you are dealing with mental and emotional symptoms. Remember, as you read these symptoms, that these descriptions are meant to paint vivid verbal pictures using symptoms that provers experienced. In many cases, the mental symptoms reflect a certain type of person who is particularly sensitive to a remedy. Chances are that you won't recognize yourself or a family member totally in any of the remedies, but you may recognize some of the characteristics. Except where explicitly stated, you do not need to match all symptoms of a remedy to benefit from it. Simply look for the closest match.

Deeper Pictures. Here you will find more detailed information on a particular part of the remedy, such as its mental symptoms or uses for children. Not all remedies have a deeper picture associated with them.

Major Symptoms. This section summarizes the conditions that the remedy is useful for, categorized by body system. When you have a sore throat, for example, and want to see what sort of sore throat a remedy helps, you can use Major Symptoms to go directly to the throat section of the Materia Medica entry.

Condition Better or Worse. This section lists factors that relieve or aggravate a condition or symptom. These factors are also known as modalities. This section is *not* a listing of what you should and should not do to feel better. As with all of your or your family member's symptoms, you are trying to find the closest remedy match. Modalities are especially useful in differentiating between different remedies. If, for example, you are looking at two remedies with the symptom of throat pain, the modality "better by cool drinks" might be the clue you need to clarify which of the two remedies will help the condition.

There are three types of modalities included in this section: general modalities, specific modalities, and causations. For example, a general modality would be "generally feel worse when exposed to cold air"—the general modality describes when the person feels worse. A specific modality might state that "a person's headache is aggravated by exposure to cold air"—what aggravates, or makes worse, the symptom. A causation might state that a person "gets a sore throat or headache after exposure to cold air"—this is what causes the symptom to be aggravated. Causation modalities are the most important modalities, with general modalities second, and specific modalities of least importance.

Occasionally a modality lists a specific illness or problem in parentheses after a modality. For example, the modality "cold air" may have the condition "headache" in parentheses next to it. This means that the headache is aggravated or made worse by cold air. If there is nothing in parentheses after the modality, assume that the modality can be either specific, general, or causation. It is also useful to look at other parts of the Materia Medica or go to the Clinical Repertory to clarify the modalities. Under Condition Worse one might find "cold air," in this case.

Dosage and Remedy Interactions. This section provides instructions on how to take the remedy. It includes basic information such as the appropriate frequencies, amounts, and combinations of the remedy that will maximize its effect.

Clinical Uses. This is a cross-reference index to the Clinical Repertory. It lists all illnesses in the Clinical Repertory where the remedy is mentioned. Click on any of these conditions to jump to the Clinical Repertory entry for the condition.

Helpful Hints

Here are some tips for using the Materia Medica module more effectively.

You do not need to match all of the listed symptoms. Remember that the idea is to match your symptoms to those listed for a remedy. Your goal is to find the closest match, but it does not need to be 100 percent perfect. The majority of the symptoms you are treating should be seen in the picture of the remedy, but the condition does not need to match the majority of the symptoms listed under a remedy. There are sometimes thousands of symptoms associated with each remedy, and it is impossible for a person to match all of these symptoms.

Use the sections that are appropriate for the condition. Quick Look, Major Symptoms, and Guiding Characteristics are three different ways to look at the same information: Quick Look is a brief overview of the remedy; Guiding Characteristics is a narrative description of the remedy and tends to include more philosophical and interpretive information; and Major Symptoms categorizes the symptoms by body system. You could use Quick Look to narrow down the field of remedies that you are considering, or in some cases the section might provide all the information you need to choose a remedy. Guiding Characteristics helps especially when mental and emotional symptoms are present. Major Symptoms might be especially useful when, for example, you have a sore throat and you want to see what sort of sore throat a remedy helps. In this case, you could go directly to the throat section of the Materia Medica entry.

Keep the rank of your symptoms in mind. As you review the symptoms listed in the Materia Medica, keep in mind the rank of the symptoms present. All symptoms matter in the total picture. In general, however, mental, generalities, and modalities tend to be the most important categories when selecting a remedy. Strange, rare, and peculiar symptoms are listed under very few symptoms, so they are most useful in narrowing the field of remedies under consideration. Though they are helpful in describing the case, particular symptoms do not generally determine the final selection of a remedy.

Use the Notepad and Bookmark tools. As you study the remedies, use the Notepad to jot down notes. Or use the Bookmark tool to mark areas you may want to go back and review again.

Use the Materia Medica as an educational tool. Try browsing through the Materia Medica. There is a wealth of information to be found in this module, and you can learn a great deal about the individual remedies. The remedies offer a fascinating look at the interface between a person's body, mind, and emotions and the corresponding world of plants, animals, and minerals.

Using the Basic Homeopathy Module

Basic Homeopathy is an overview of the principles and practice of homeopathy. It describes how to practice homeopathy, how to get homeopathic remedies, what potencies to use, and how to choose a remedy.

Opening Basic Homeopathy and Getting Started

Open Basic Homeopathy by clicking on the Basic Homeopathy icon from any part of the program. The icon is highlighted when selected. The Contents screen appears first. It lists the available topics.

The Outline option is in the upper-right corner of every Basic Homeopathy screen. It allows you to view the next level up in the topic hierarchy. If you are viewing a subtopic, clicking here brings you to the topic menu. Clicking again brings you back to the Contents.

CHAPTER 4

Homeopathic Research and Clinical Studies

This chapter provides summary descriptions of research projects and clinical trials. The publications that contain detailed information on the research and resulting evidence are highlighted for each section.

EARLY RESEARCH

Clinical

A. M. Scofield, "Experimental Research in Homoeopathy: A Critical Review," *The British Homeopathic Journal*, vol. 73, no. 3 (July 1984), p. 162.

During World War II, the British military conducted a study on the prevention and treatment of mustard gas burns, using homeopathy, the primary medicine used in England before the widespread adoption of antibiotics.

The trial conducted by Paterson in 1944 in London used a selection of remedies, while one done in Glasgow used mustard gas in a 30c potency. In London, the results showed that *Rhus tox* produced a significant change in the frequency from deep to medium lesions with no change in the incidence of superficial lesions. In Glasgow, the results showed mustard gas, given before possible exposure, caused a significant shift in the frequency of both deep and medium lesions to medium and superficial lesions, therefore increasing the incidence of superficial lesions. A later analysis in 1982 showed statistical significance in favor of mustard gas, *Rhus tox*, and *Kali bich* over placebo. Other treatments did not show statistical significance.

Biochemical

H. L. Coulter, *Homeopathic Science and Modern Medicine* (Berkeley: North Atlantic Books, 1981), pp. 54–55.

A study by Boyd is considered by many to be a classic of homeopathic research because it used meticulous technique, control of variables, and extensive training for researchers. In 1954, Boyd tested the effect of high potencies of mercuric chloride on diastase activity, with the purpose of determining whether adding a small amount of mercuric chloride microdilution altered the speed of hydrolysis of starch with diastase. Five hundred comparisons were done between homeopathic dilution and control. The results were measured objectively and analyzed statistically. All tests gave significant results and various potencies stimulated the hydrolysis of starch when compared to distilled water controls. One independent statistician wrote that "significant difference is shown by every set of the series."

Botanical

H. L. Coulter, *Homeopathic Science and Modern Medicine* (Berkeley: North Atlantic Books, 1981), p. 56

Plants have long been considered a good medium for homeopathic research since it is difficult for critics of homeopathy to claim the placebo effect. In a controlled attempt to duplicate earlier studies, Pelikan and Unger in 1965 studied the effects of microdoses of *Argentum nit* on the growth of wheat seeds.

With the series repeated 240 times, the statistical analysis showed the varied effects of the different potencies. The effects on the growth of wheat seeds were dependent upon the potency. Some potencies were found to be more effective than others.

Bacteriological

H. L. Coulter, *Homeopathic Science and Modern Medicine* (Berkeley: North Atlantic Books, 1981), p. 57

In 1927, Junker investigated the effect of various microdilutions on paramecia cultures. He added microdilutions of various substances to the paramecia cultures and studied the daily growth changes related to the degree of dilution of the substance added. The effects on the daily growth changes of each paramecia culture were dependent upon the dilution of the substance. Some potencies were found to be more effective than others.

Zoological

H. L. Coulter, *Homeopathic Science and Modern Medicine* (Berkeley: North Atlantic Books, 1981), p. 58

In 1923, Krawkow first used microdilutions on animals. He studied the effect on the blood supply of the isolated rabbit ear. A biphasal effect resulted; a known principle of science states that while successive small doses of a substance have one effect, successive large doses of the same substance have the opposite effect. Microdilutions in strong concentrations relaxed the capillaries while microdilutions in weaker concentrations narrowed them.

META-ANALYSIS IN HOMEOPATHIC RESEARCH

Kleijnen's meta-analysis compiled all the efficacy studies in the field of homeopathy. This led the way to researchers improving the design quality of their studies. The early 1990s has given the field of homeopathy some of the best studies to date, with excellent design models.

J. Kleijnen, P. Knipschild, and G. ter Riet, "Clinical Trials of Homoeopathy," *British Medical Journal*, February 9, 1991, no. 302, pp. 316–323.

This is the best objective meta-analysis of clinical research prior to 1991. This meta-analysis reviewed 107 studies.

This extremely significant piece of research compiled, for the first time, all the efficacy studies in homeopathy in one place and assessed their methodological quality in an objective manner. This meta-analysis rigorously assessed the methodological quality of 107 controlled studies. Two trials were found to have uninterruptible results. Of the 105 trials assessed, 81 showed positive results (77%), and 24 did not show positive results (23%). Even when only the studies of high-quality design were included, 15 of 22 showed positive results (68%).

It has been stated that there are not a lot of controlled studies regarding homeopathy, but the number of studies that actually existed surprised the researchers. This level of scrutiny is infrequently applied to conventional studies. In fact, the editor of the *British Medical Journal* stated that "only about 15% of medical interventions are supported by solid scientific evidence ... partly because only 1% of the articles in medical journals are scientifically sound and partly because many treatments have not been assessed at all."[1]

While Kleijnen evaluated the clinical evidence for the efficacy of homeopathy, this included a variety of classical and modern homeopathy. Classical homeopathy relies heavily on the total symptom pattern of the patient (mental, emotional, and physical), rather than illness classifications, and uses only single remedies. The meta-analysis included 14 trials of classical homeopathy, 58 trials where a single remedy was given to patients with similar conventional diagnoses, 26 trials using combination homeopathic treatments, and 9 trials using isopathy.

Isopathy involves the use of the same substance (rather than a similar substance) as medicines for curing disease. For example, one trial used homeopathic doses of twelve common flowers that are known to aggravate the symptoms of people who suffer from hay fever. In the best trials methodologically, only one was classical and one was isopathic.

Individualized prescription was not a design criterion in this study, and the best methodological studies using this method were conducted after the time of Kleijnen's study. Kleijnen and fellow researchers would have been ready to accept that homeopathy is efficacious if the mechanism of action was understood.

D. Reilly, M. Taylor, C. McSharry, et al., "Is Homoeopathy a Placebo Response? Controlled Trial of Homoeopathic Potency, with Pollen in Hayfever as Model," *The Lancet*, 1986, pp. 881–885.

Reilly personally believed in the tenets of homeopathy, but not in microdilution, which is not an original tenet of homeopathic philosophy. As a skeptic, Reilly did not expect the results from his first study to be positive. He ran a pilot study that came out positive and was refused publication by *The Lancet,* a conventional medical journal.

He then incorporated all the criticisms and executed another study, five times larger. This second, well-designed, double-blind, placebo-controlled, randomized study tested the use of the 30c potency of twelve common flowers that create pollen to treat 144 hay fever patients. Subjects given this homeopathic medicine had six times fewer symptoms as those given a placebo and took antihistamines half as often.

Statisticians re-evaluated data considering patients' proximity to high-pollen-count areas and time of season; the significance of results was confirmed and strengthened. The study was positive with both clinical and statistical significance.

D. Reilly, M. Taylor, N. Beattie, et al., "Is Evidence for Homoeopathy Reproducible?" *The Lancet,* 1994, pp. 1601–1606.

This article reviews a study of the homeopathic treatment of asthma. This study was the third by these researchers on an allergic disorder. Patients given treatment were prescribed a 30c potency of the substance to which they were most allergic. This work represents some of the highest-caliber research in homeopathy, and it provides the strongest evidence of its efficacy.

This exceptionally well-designed study featured collaboration between homeopathic and conventional researchers and serves as a model for the future design of studies. The significance of this trial was that it reproduced statistically significant results using the same homeopathic immunotherapy model used in two previous studies. This study achieved the highest goals of scientific research: reproducibility, a clearly stated hypothesis, statistical significance, use of the double-blind method, use of conventional researchers and patients, and individualization of remedies. Reilly was awarded a research grant, which he used to design this study using conventional researchers and patients.

Twenty-eight patients with allergic asthma were involved in this study. Respiratory physicians using objective test measurements such as laboratory tests and histamine provocation rediagnosed the patients. The only involvement of homeopaths was in the design of the study and choosing the remedy. The medicines were made independently and homeopathically in France and sent double-blind to the pharmacists, who then recoded them and administered them to patients.

Patients were allowed to remain on their conventional therapy throughout the trial. The effect was measured on a daily visual analog scale of overall symptom intensity. This is an accepted objective tool used to measure subjective symptoms, such as pain. The difference in analog scores showing the active remedy to be more effective than placebo became apparent within one week and lasted for eight weeks. Patients taking homeopathic remedies showed a clinically statistically significant greater drop in symptoms.

With three positives in a row, Reilly questioned how much evidence is enough and concluded that "either homeopathy works or the clinical trial doesn't." All three of Reilly's studies (the pilot study, 1986, and 1994) used the same model of homeopathic immunotherapy in allergy. The first two trials used hay fever and the third used asthma. The comparison in all three trials was homeopathy as a system versus placebo.

When the data was pooled from all three trials, the average showed that improvement on homeopathy over placebo appeared by the second week and by the third week averaged a reduction of 33% in active remedy versus 10% in placebo. *The Lancet* published this as an editorial entitled "Reilly's Challenge" (1994, p. 1506).

J. Jacobs, W. B. Jonas, M. Jiménez-Pérez, and D. Crothers, "Homeopathy for Childhood Diarrhea: Combined Results and Meta-Analysis from Three Randomized-Controlled Clinical Trials," *Pediatric Infectious Disease Journal*, 2003, no. 22, pp. 229–234.

Three double-blind clinical trials of diarrhea in 242 children age 6 months to 5 years were analyzed as one group. Combined analysis shows a duration of diarrhea of 3.3 days in the homeopathy group compared with 4.1 days in the placebo group. The meta-analysis shows a consistent effect-size difference of approximately 0.66 days. Members of the same research team had done an earlier study in Nicaragua.

J. Jacobs, L. M. Jiménez, S. S. Gloyd, J. L. Gale, and D. Crothers, "Treatment of Acute Childhood Diarrhea with Homeopathic Medicine: A Randomized Clinical Trial in Nicaragua," *Pediatrics,* May 1994, pp. 719–725.

The design of this study was of such high quality that it was the first homeopathic research study to be published in a refereed medical journal in the United States. The purpose was to determine whether homeopathy is useful in treating childhood diarrhea. Jacobs and colleagues treated 81 children age 6 months to 5 years.

Individualized homeopathic medicine was prescribed and patients were put on oral rehydration therapy. This rehydration therapy treated dehydration but did not affect the duration of diarrhea. The group treated with homeopathy had a statistically significant decrease in the duration of diarrhea.

There was also a significant difference in the number of stools per day between the two groups after 72 hours of treatment. This may signify the usefulness of homeopathy in early stages of treatment. The decrease of 0.8 days per episode may decrease diarrhea and malnutrition and therefore decrease the burden to the mother. The 15% decrease in duration of diarrhea could reduce the morbidity rate.

W. B. Jonas, T. J. Kaptchuk, and K. Linde, "A Critical Overview of Homeopathy," *Annals in Internal Medicine,* March 4, 2003, no. 138, pp. 393–399.

Although this is not a meta-analysis, it is still a very good review of the clinical literature in homeopathy.

K. Linde, N. Clausius, G. Ramirez, et al., "Are the Clinical Effects of Homoeopathy Placebo Effects? A Meta-Analysis of Placebo-Controlled Trials," *The Lancet,* September 20, 1997, no. 350, pp. 834–843.

Even critics have called this meta-analysis "completely state of the art." It reviews 186 studies, 89 of which fit predefined criteria. Homeopathic medicines had a 2.45 times greater effect than placebo.

M. Wiesenauer and R. Ludtke, "A Meta-Analysis of the Homeopathic Treatment of Pollinosis with Galphimia Glauca," *Forsch Komplementarmed*, 3(1996), pp. 230–234.

This is a meta-analysis of seven randomized, double-blind, placebo-controlled trials and four non-placebo-controlled trials, representing a total of 1,038 patients. These studies found that patients given homeopathic doses of *Galphimia glauca* for hay fever experienced 1.25 times greater improvement in eye symptoms when compared with those given a placebo. This success rate is comparable with the success rate experienced with antihistamines, but the homeopathic medicine has no known side effects.

K. Linde, W. B. Jonas, D. Melchart, et al., "Critical Review and Meta-Analysis of Serial Agitated Dilutions in Experimental Toxicology," *Human and Experimental Toxicology*, 1994, no. 13, pp. 481–492.

This meta-analysis of more than 100 studies in toxicology showed that homeopathic medicines may be useful in treating toxic exposures. The researcher found that most of the studies were methodologically flawed. However, when reviewing only the higher-caliber studies, they found that animals given a homeopathic medicine excreted approximately 20% more of the toxic substance through their stools, urine, and sweat, when compared with animals given a placebo. The researchers also found that the best studies tended to test homeopathic medicines that were the most dilute.

DOUBLE-BLIND, PLACEBO-CONTROLLED CLINICAL TRIALS

I. R. Bell, D. A. Lewis II, A. J. Brooks, et al., "Improved Clinical Status in Fibromyalgia Patients Treated with Individualized Homeopathic Remedies Versus Placebo," *Rheumatology*, 2004, no. 43, pp. 1111–1115.

Participants on active treatment showed significantly greater improvements in tender-point count and tender-point pain, quality of life, and global health, along with a trend toward less depression, compared with those on placebo. People on homeopathic treatment also experienced changes in EEG readings. "Helpfulness from treatment" in homeopathic patients was very significant.

M. Oberbaum, I. Yaniv, Y. Ben-Gal, et al., "A Randomized, Controlled Clinical Trial of the Homeopathic Medication Traumeel S⁻ in the Treatment of Chemotherapy-Induced Stomatitis in Children Undergoing Stem Cell Transplantation," *Cancer*, 2001, 92(3), pp. 684–690.

The homeopathic medication Traumeel S⁻ may significantly reduce the severity and duration of chemotherapy-induced stomatitis in patients undergoing bone marrow transplantation. Thirty patients age 3 to 25 years who had undergone allogeneic (n=15) or autologous (n=15) stem cell transplantation were randomly assigned to either a Traumeel S⁻ group or a placebo group. Patients in the homeopathy group were instructed to rinse their mouths with Traumeel S⁻ five times daily for a minimum of fourteen days or until all signs of stomatitis were absent for at least two days.

At treatment conclusion, mean stomatitis scores were significantly lower in the homeopathy group than for those in the placebo group. Five patients (33%) in the Traumeel S⁻ group did not develop stomatitis, compared to 1 patient (7%) in the placebo group. Stomatitis worsened in only 7 patients (47%) in the Traumeel S⁻ group, compared with 14 patients (93%) in the placebo group.

J. Jacobs, D. A. Springer, and D. Crothers, "Homeopathic Treatment of Acute Otitis Media in Children: A Preliminary Randomized Placebo-Controlled Trial, *Pediatric Infectious Disease Journal*, 20(2), February 2001, pp. 177–183.

This randomized, double-blind, placebo-controlled study prescribed individualized homeopathic medicine or placebo to 75 children. There were 19.9% more treatment failures in children given a placebo. Diary scores showed a significant decrease in symptoms at 24 and 64 hours after treatment in favor of those given a homeopathic medicine.

M. A. Taylor, D. Reilly, R. H. Llewellyn-Jones, et al., "Randomised Controlled Trial of Homoeopathy Versus Placebo in Perennial Allergic Rhinitis with Overview of Four Trial Series," *British Medical Journal,* August 19, 2000, no. 321, pp. 471–476.

This trial of 51 patients with perennial allergic rhinitis showed a substantially significant difference in the objective measure of nasal airflow in patients given a 30c potency of the specific substance to which they were most allergic, as compared to those patients given a placebo. There was, however, no statistically significant difference in visual analog scales. In reviewing the four trials with allergy patients (n=253), the researchers found a 28% improvement in visual analog scores in those given a homeopathic medicine, compared to a 3% improvement in patients given a placebo.

E. Chapman, R. Weintraub, M. Milburn, et al., "Homeopathic Treatment of Mild Traumatic Brain Injury: A Randomized, Double-Blind, Placebo-Controlled Trial," *Journal of Head Trauma Rehabilitation,* 14(6), Dec. 1999, pp. 521–542.

Sixty patients were prescribed an individualized remedy (1 of 18 different ones) at Spaulding Rehabilitation Hospital (affiliated with Harvard). Compared with placebo recipients, patients given a homeopathic medicine experienced improvement in a subject-rated Function Assessment composed of three scales: a difficulty with situations scale, a symptom rating scale, and a participation in daily activities scale.

R. A. van Haselen and P. A. Fisher, "A Randomized Controlled Trial Comparing Topical Piroxicam Gel with a Homeopathic Gel in Osteoarthritis of the Knee, *Rheumatology,* 2000, no. 39, pp. 714–719.

This randomized, double-blind trial found that a homeopathic topical gel was as effective and as tolerated as Piroxicam gel, a non-steroidal anti-inflammatory drug. This trial evaluated the care of 172 osteoarthritic patients over four weeks as they applied either a homeopathic gel or Piroxicam gel three times daily. The homeopathic gel contained *Symphytum, Rhus toxicodendron,* and *Ledum palustre.*

M. Weiser, W. Strosser, and P. Klein, "Homeopathic vs. Conventional Treatment of Vertigo: A Randomized Double-Blind Controlled Clinical Trial," *Archives of Otolaryngology—Head and Neck Surgery,* August 1998, no. 124, pp. 879–885.

This was a comparative trial of a homeopathic combination medicine versus betahistine hydrocholoride, a leading vertigo drug in Europe.

R. Papp, G. Schuback, E. Beck, et al., "Oscillococcinum in Patients with Influenza-Like Syndromes: A Placebo-Controlled Double-Blind Evaluation," *The British Homeopathic Journal,* 87 (April 1998), pp. 69–76.

This study of 372 patients replicated an earlier trial of 487 patients. Both trials found statistically significant results with Oscillococcinum in the treatment of patients with influenza-like syndromes. The earlier trial: J. P. Ferley, et al., "A Controlled Evaluation of a Homeopathic Preparation in the Treatment of Influenza-Like Syndrome," *British Journal of Clinical Pharmacology,* March 1989, no. 27, pp. 329–335.

R. G. Gibson, et al., "Homeopathic Therapy in Rheumatoid Arthritis: Evaluation by Double-Blind Clinical Therapeutic Trial," *British Journal of Clinical Pharmacology,* 9 (May 1980), pp. 453–459.

This was an attempt to improve on the design of Gibson's earlier study and was a double-blind trial in the treatment of rheumatoid arthritis. This was the first homeopathic-allopathic collaborative trial since the mid-nineteenth century, and was the first reported in an allopathic journal overseas.

This study used individualized prescribing. It compared 23

patients receiving orthodox anti-inflammatory therapy and homeopathy with a similar group of 23 patients receiving orthodox anti-inflammatory therapy and placebo.

Results showed significant improvement in subjective pain, articular index, stiffness, and grip strength in those patients using homeopathy, while there was no statistical difference in patients receiving placebo. What might the results have been if patients had taken homeopathy alone?

Fisher, et al., "Effect of Homeopathic Treatment on Fibrositis (Primary Fibromyalgia)," *British Medical Journal*, no. 299 (1989), pp. 365–366.

This was a crossover study; patients received active and placebo treatment for one month each in random order. Patients did better in all variables when using *Rhus tox*. The number of patients on active treatment showing improved pain level or sleep (according to visual analog scores) was virtually double. The number of tender spots was reduced by 25% in patients on active treatment. Tender spots are the best indicator for fibrositis.

Ferley, et al., "A Controlled Evaluation of a Homeopathic Preparation in the Treatment of Influenza-Like Syndromes," *British Journal of Clinical Pharmacology*, no. 27 (1989), pp. 329–335.

This well-designed trial found positive results in studying the effectiveness of a combination remedy in the treatment of influenza-like syndromes. The study used mostly general practitioners who were not homeopathic physicians. The remedy was a combination drug consisting of *Anas barbariae hepatis* and *Cordis extractum* 200c (commercial name: Oscillococcinum).

Two hundred thirty-seven patients received the remedy and 241 patients received a placebo. Parameters measured included rectal temperature and presence or absence of five symptoms: headache, stiffness, lumbar pain, articular pain, and shivers. All symptoms were recorded twice a day in diaries. Recovery was defined as a rectal temperature less than 37.5°C (99.5°F) and complete resolution of the five symptoms. Seven percent more of the homeopathy patients recovered within 48 hours than placebo patients.

Results showed that patients under age 30 had a higher percentage of recovery and patients on the active remedy had a higher percent of recovery if the flu syndrome was mild or moderate. This may indicate that for severe flu, a single remedy may be a better choice.

de Lange de Klerk, et al., "Effect of Homeopathic Medicines on Daily Burden of Symptoms in Children with Recurrent Upper Respiratory Tract Infections," *British Medical Journal,* no. 309 (November 19, 1994), pp. 1329–1332.

This was a well-designed study with results that did not find statistical significance. Discussion at a Homeopathic Research Network meeting suggested that, had the number of participants increased by a small number, the study would have yielded statistically significant positive results. This brings up the debate regarding the importance of sample size (the number in the group studied). While many researchers believe a large number is necessary to cancel out the effects of randomization, some statisticians will argue that even one result must be taken as fact if it is found to be statistically significant.

The object was to the determine the effect of individually prescribed homeopathic medicine in children with recurrent respiratory tract infections. Outcome measures included the mean score for daily symptoms, the number of antibiotic courses, and the number of adenoidectomies and tonsillectomies over one year of follow-up.

The results found a small numerical difference in daily symptom scores in favor of homeopathy, but the difference was not statistically significant. The use of antibiotics was reduced by 54.8% in those receiving homeopathy, while those receiving placebo had a 37.7% reduction; a difference of 17.1% was not statistically significant.

All the children in the study had had at least two courses of antibiotics, which may have changed the symptom pattern that is fundamental to homeopathic prescribing. While the *British Medical Journal* presented results as an either-or alternative, the decreased use of antibiotics should be viewed as a significant benefit, even if not statistically significant.

M. Wiesenauer and R. Ludtke, "The Treatment of Pollinosis with Galphimia Glauca D4: A Randomized Placebo Controlled Double-Blind Clinical Trial," *Alternative Therapies in Health and Medicine*, vol. 1, no. 5 (November 1995), pp. 101–102, Abstract.

The goal of this study was to duplicate an earlier trial and confirm that using a homeopathic preparation of *Galphimia glauca* in the treatment of pollinosis was effective. This was a randomized, placebo-controlled, double-blind clinical trial. The researchers used the general medical practices of 27 practitioners in Germany; 132 patients suffering from pollinosis were followed for 1 month.

The participants were randomized to active remedy or placebo but physicians were allowed to individualize the prescription. The measurements were collected by rating ocular and nasal symptoms on a scale of 1 to 4: 1—symptom free; 2—obvious relief; 3—slight improvement; and 4—no improvement.

The difference between those on active medication who were symptom free and those on placebo who received obvious relief was statistically significant. The improvement of the nasal symptoms in the group receiving active remedy was significant after two weeks and improvement of the eye symptoms was significant after four weeks. The researchers concluded that the efficacy of *Galphimia glauca* for the treatment of pollinosis was confirmed.

"Influence of Potassium Dichromate on Tracheal Secretions in Critically Ill Patients, *Chest,* vol. 127, no. 3 (March 2005), pp. 936–941.

A prospective, randomized, double-blind, placebo-controlled study with parallel assignment was performed to assess the influence of sublingually administered *Kali bichromicum* (potassium dichromate) 30c on critically ill patients with a history of tobacco use and COPD (chronic obstructive pulmonary disease). Fifty patients received either *Kali bichromicum* 30c globules (group 1) or placebo (group 2). The amount of tracheal secretions was reduced significantly in group 1. Extubation (the removal of obstructive mucus from the lung with a tube) could be performed significantly earlier in group 1. Similarly, length of stay was significantly shorter in group 1 (4.20 ± 1.61 days versus 7.68 ± 3.60 days). This data suggest that potentized (diluted and vigorously shaken) *Kali bichromicum* may help to decrease the amount of stringy tracheal secretions in COPD patients.

M. Frass, M. Linkesch, S. Banjya, et al., "Adjunctive Homeopathic Treatment in Patients with Severe Sepsis: A Randomized, Double-Blind, Placebo-Controlled Trial in an Intensive Care Unit," *Homeopathy,* 2005, no. 94, pp. 75–80.

At a University of Vienna hospital, seventy patients with severe sepsis were enrolled in a randomized double-blind, placebo-controlled clinical trial, measuring survival rates at 30 days and at 180 days. Those patients given a homeopathic medicine were prescribed it in the 200c potency only (in 12-hour intervals during their hospital stay). The survival rate at day 30 was 81.8% for homeopathic patients and 67.7% for those given a placebo. At day 180, 75.8% of homeopathic patients survived and only 50.0% of the placebo patients survived. One patient was saved for every four who were treated.

CLINICAL OUTCOMES STUDIES

F. Sharples and R. van Haselen, "Patients' Perspective on Using a Complementary Medicine Approach to Their Health: A Survey at the Royal London Homoeopathic Hospital," *NHS Trust Report,* 1998.

The researchers gave 541 questionnaires to adult outpatients who had at least three visits; 506 were returned, and 499 analyzed. Of these, 63% had had their main problem for more than 5 years; 80% reported that their main problem had very much, moderately, or slightly improved, and 90% were satisfied or very satisfied with their care. Of the 262 patients who were using a conventional drug, 76 (29%) had stopped and 84 (32%) had decreased their usage since receiving homeopathic care.

D. Riley, M. Fischer, B. Singh, et al., "Homeopathy and Conventional Medicine: An Outcomes Study Comparing Effectiveness in a Primary Care Setting," *Journal of Alternative and Complementary Medicine,* April, 2001, pp. 149–160.

Thirty clinicians in 6 clinics in 4 countries enrolled 500 patients with upper respiratory tract complaints, lower respiratory tract complaints, or ear complaints. Half the patients received homeopathic medicines alone, while the other half received conventional drugs alone. Of patients receiving homeopathic care, 82.6% experienced improvement, while only 68% of those receiving a conventional medication experienced a similar degree of improvement. Rapidity of improvement was also notable: 67.3% of homeopathic patients experienced improvement within 3 days, while only 56.6% of patients given conventional medicines experienced improvement (16.4% of homeopathic patients improved within 24 hours, and 5.7% in the conventional-medicine group). In both treatment groups, 60% of patient visits lasted 5 to 15 minutes. In the homeopathic treatment group, 84% received no conventional drugs, suggesting that homeopathy is usually a substitute for conventional drugs, not an adjunctive treatment.

LABORATORY STUDIES

J. Cazin, M. Cazin, J. L. Gaborit, et al., "A Study of the Effect of Decimal and Centesimal Dilutions of Arsenic on the Retention and Mobilization of Arsenic in the Rat," *Human Toxicology,* 1987, no. 6, pp. 315–320.

This study showed the usefulness of homeopathy in the elimination of toxins and brings up two questions: Can homeopathy be used in humans to eliminate environmental toxins? And can this be proven through research studies?

Here, the researchers studied the retention of arsenic in rats and its mobilization under the influence of infinitesimal doses. Previous studies determined that a rat is the best animal in which to study the retention and mobilization of arsenic. Both decimal and centesimal dilutions were studied. All active dilutions showed increased arsenic excretion in comparison to potentized water.

P. Belon, J. Cumps, M. Ennis, P. F. Mannaioni, M. Roberfroid, J. Ste-Laudy, and F. A. C. Wiegant, "Histamine Dilutions Modulate Basophil Activity," *Inflammation Research*, 2004, no. 53, pp. 181–188. (An earlier, less detailed review was published as Belon, Cumps, Ennis, et al., "Inhibition of Human Basophil Degranulation by Successive Histamine Dilutions: Results of a European Multi-Centre Trial, *Inflammation Research*, 1999, pp. S17–S18.

Four independent laboratories, each associated with a university, conducted a series of experiments using dilutions of histamine beyond Avogadro's number (the 15th through 19th centesimal dilution, that is, 10^{-15} to 10^{-19}. The researchers found inhibitory effects of histamine dilutions on basophil degranulation triggered by anti-IgE, a type of antibody (immunoglobulin) produced by cells of the lining of the respiratory and intestinal tracts, considered to be responsible for allergic reactions. A total of 3,674 data points were collected from the four laboratories. The overall effects were highly significant. The test solutions were made in independent laboratories, the participants were blinded to the content of the test solutions, and the data analysis was performed by a biostatistician who was not involved in any other part of the trial.

L. Rey, "Thermoluminescence of Ultra-High Dilutions of Lithium Chloride and Sodium Chloride," *Physica A*, no. 323, 2003, pp. 67–74.

Homeopathic doses (15c) of lithium chloride and sodium chloride had a substantially different effect on thermoluninescence in water with deuterium oxide. Lithium chloride was chosen because it is known to suppress hydrogen bonds, and the researchers theorized that thermoluminescence is dependent upon the hydrogen-bond network. (This research was featured in *New Scientist*, June 11, 2003.)

W. Jonas, Y. Lin, and F. Tortella, "Neuroprotection from Glutamate Toxicity with Ultra-Low Dose Glutamate," *Neuroreports*, 12(2), Feb. 12, 2001, pp. 335–339.

From the abstract:

The protective effects of ultra-low doses (ULD) of glutamate against glutamate toxicity were studied in primary rat spinal, cortical, and cerebellar neurons. Neurons were exposed to four subtoxic, ultra-low concentrations of glutamate (10[-18] M, 10[-20] M, 10[-22] M and 10[-30] M) for 72 h[ours] and then subsequently challenged with toxic concentrations (25 [micro] M) of glutamate. Neuron viability was consistently 10% higher in spinal and cortical neurons pre-exposed to glutamate concentrations of 10[-18] M and 10[-22] M, and in cerebellar neurons pre-exposed to 10[-20] M and 10(-30) M. Using laser scanning confocal microscopy and the fluorescent calcium probe fluo-3, [the researchers] found no alterations in intracellular calcium dynamics in the protected cells.

This protective effect is consistent with a growing body of evidence for tolerance induced by low-dose toxin exposure but it is the first time that such tolerance has been demonstrated with ultra-low glutamate exposure. [The] data show that pre-exposure of neuronal cells to ULD glutamate can protect against subsequent exposure to toxic levels of glutamate.

S. Samal and K. Geckeler, "Unexpected Solute Aggregation in Water on Dilution," *Chemical Communications*, Oct. 2001, pp. 2224–2225.

This study made a surprising discovery that molecules form clusters that increase in size with dilution, and that the size occurs nonlinearly with dilution. (This important study by two chemists in South Korea was featured in *New Scientist*, Nov. 10, 2001, pp. 4–5.)

W. Jonas, Y. Lin, A. Williams, et al., "Treatment of Experimental Stroke with Low-Dose Glutamate and Homeopathic Arnica montana," *Perfusion*, November 1999, vol. 12, no. 11, pp. 452–456, 460–462.

This study evaluated the ability of *Arnica* to reduce long-term damage and mortality from brain injury in rats that were experimentally induced into a stroke. After seven days, *Arnica* 200c reduced by 50% (!) the long-term damage (infarct volume) and mortality (40% died, compared to 66% in the control group) from brain injury, but may exacerbate the immediate effects of the stroke, though this was not statistically significant.

Resources

BIBLIOGRAPHY FOR THIS BOOK AND THE CD MODULES

Allen, H. C. *Allen's Key Notes.* New Delhi: B. Jain Publishers; 1988.

Allen, T. F. *Handbook of Materia Medica and Homoeopathic Therapeutics.* New Delhi: B. Jain Publishers, 1979.

Allen, T. F. *Encyclopedia of the Materia Medica,* New Delhi: B. Jain Publishers, 1979.

Bellavite, P., and Signorini, A. *The Emerging Science of Homeopathy.* Berkeley: North Atlantic Books, 2002.

Bhanja, K. C. *The Homeopathic Prescriber.* Calcutta: National Homeopathic Laboratory, 1978.

Boericke, W. *Homoeopathic Materia Medica and Repertory.* New Delhi: Homeopathic Publications, 1927.

Boericke, W. *Organon of Medicine of Samual Hahnemann.* New Delhi: B. Jain Publishers, 1974.

Boericke, W., and Dewey, W. *The Twelve Tissue Salts of Schussler.* Philadelphia: Boericke and Tafel, 1914.

Boger, C. M. *A Synoptic Key to Materia Medica.* New Delhi: B. Jain Publishers, 1931.

Bridgman, P. W. *The Physics of High Pressure.* London: G. Bell, 1949.

Chernin, D., Buegel, D., and Lewis, B. *Homeopathic Remedies for Health Professionals and Laypeople.* Honesdale, Pa.: Himalayan Institute Press, 1992.

Clark, J. *A Dictionary of Practical Materia Medica.* New Delhi: B. Jain Publlishers, 1978.

Coulter, H. L. *Divided Legacy: A History of the Schism in Medical Thought.* Berkeley: North Atlantic Books, 1975.

Coulter, H. L. *Homeopathic Science and Modern Medicine.* Berkeley: North Atlantic Books, 1981.

Cummings, S., Ullman, D. *Everybody's Guide to Homeopathic Medicines.* New York: Jeremy P. Tarcher/Putnam, 2004.

Dewey, W. A. *Practical Homoeopathic Therapeutics.* New Delhi: B. Jain Publishers, 1976.

Dossey, L. "How Should Alternative Therapies Be Evaluated?" *Alternative Therapies in Health and Medicine,* vol. 1, no. 2 (May 1995).

Dubos, R. *Drugs in Our Society* (Baltimore: John Hopkins, 1964).

Farrington, E. A. *Clinical Materia Medica.* New Delhi: B. Jain Publishers, 1976.

Gibson, D. *Studies of Homoeopathic Remedies.* Bucks, England: Beaconsfield Publishers Limited, 1987.

Grossinger, R. *Planet Medicine.* Boulder, Colo.: Shambhala, 1982.

Hahnemann, S. *The Organon of Medicine.* New Delhi: B. Jain Publishers, 1974.

Hering, C. *The Guiding Symptoms of the Materia Medica.* New Delhi: B. Jain Publishers, 1974.

Hering, C. *The Homeopathic Domestic Physician.* New Delhi: B. Jain Publishers, 1974.

Jouanny, J. *The Essentials of Homeopathic Materia Medica.* France: Laboratoires, 1985.

Kent, J. T. *Lectures on Homeopathic Philosophy,* 1919. Reprint, Berkeley: North Atlantic Books, 1979.

Kent, J. T. *Repertory of the Homeopathic Materia Medica.* New Delhi: B. Jain Publishers, 1988.

Lilienthal, S. Homeopathic Therapeutics. New Delhi: B. Jain Publishers, 1925.

Murphy, R. *Homeopathic Remedy* Guide. Blacksburg, Va.: Hahnemann Academy of North America, 2000.

Nash, E. B. *Leaders in Homeopathic Therapeutics.* Philadelphia: Boericke and Tafel, 1926.

Pierce, W.I. *Plain Talks on Materia Medica.* Calcutta: Haren & Brother, 1970.

Tyler, M. L. *Homoeopathic Drug Pictures.* Devon, England: Health Sciences Press, 1975.

Ullman, D. *Homeopathic Medicine for Children and Infants.* New York: Jeremy P. Tarcher/Putnam, 1992.

Ullman, D. *The Consumer's Guide to Homeopathy.* New York: Jeremy P. Tarcher/Putnam, 1995.

Ullman, D. "Principles of Homeopathy," *Co-evolution Quarterly,* Spring 1981.

Ullman, D., Cummings, S. *Everybody's Guide to Homeopathic Medicines.* New York: Jeremy P. Tarcher/Putnam, 2004.

Vithoulkas, G. *Homeopathy, Medicine of the New Man.* Wellingborough: Thorsons, 1979.

Vithoulkas, G. *The Science of Homeopathy.* New York: Grove Press, 1981.

RESEARCH

Bellavite, P., and Signorini, A. *The Emerging Science of Homeopathy: Complexity, Biodynamics, and Nanopharmacology* (Berkeley: North Atlantic Books, 2002). The original 1995 edition was entitled *Homeopathy: A Frontier in Medical Science.* This is the best book on homeopathic research to date. Some chapters present compelling theories on how homeopathic medicines may work, in the light of new physics, biophysics, fractals, chaos, and complexity theory. Some chapters are technical.

Dana Ullman, *Homeopathic Family Medicine* (an ebook). This is the best and most up-to-date review and description of clinical research in homeopathy. Available as a one-time download or as a subscription from www.homeopathic.com.

Homeopathy. This publication is an excellent academic journal in homeopathy. To subscribe, go to www.elsevier.com.

Three Internet sites have information on homeopathic research:

- Homeopathic Educational Services (www.homeopathic.com)
- Samueli Institute for Information Biology (www.samueli-institute.org)
- National Center for Homeopathy (www.homeopathic.org)

MAGAZINES

Homeopathy Today (published by the National Center for Homeopathy)

American Journal of Homeopathic Medicine (published by the American Institute of Homeopathy)

Simillimum (published by the Homeopathic Academy of Naturopathic Physicians)

ORGANIZATIONS

American Institute of Homeopathy

The American Institute of Homeopathy (AIH) is an organization of medical doctors, osteopathic doctors, and dentists. They publish the *Journal of the American Institute of Homeopathy*.

- The oldest medical professional organization in this country, AIH was founded in 1844 (the AMA was founded in 1847).

- The organization's purpose is to promote homeopathy and disseminate homeopathic medical knowledge.

- The AIH helps establish standards of medical practice.

Contact: American Institute of Homeopathy, 539 Harkle Road, Suite A, Sante Fe, NM 87505; 505-989-1457.

National Center for Homeopathy

The National Center for Homeopathy, a nonprofit membership organization dedicated to promoting health through homeopathy, is the largest homeopathic organization in the United States. Some of the benefits of membership include:

- NCH annual directory of practitioners, study groups, pharmacies, resources—updated every year

- NCH-affiliated study groups (more than 165 study groups nationwide)—a unique opportunity to learn homeopathic self-care with others

- Summer school—annual weekend and week-long courses taught by experienced clinicians

- Annual conference—held in a different location around the country every year

- A strong voice in the health care reform and media debate for increased access to homeopathic health care

- *Homeopathy Today,* the monthly magazine full of practical information on using homeopathy, along with news updates, events listings, and seminar announcements

Contact: National Center for Homeopathy, 801 North Fairfax Street, Suite 306, Alexandria, VA 22314; 703-548-7790, 703-548-7792 fax; e-mail info@homeopathic.org.

NATUROPATHIC MEDICAL SCHOOLS

Five naturopathic medical schools teach homeopathy to their students. All are four-year programs.

Bastyr University, 14500 Juanita Dr. NE, Bothell, WA 98011; 425-823-1300; www.bastyr.edu

Canadian College of Naturopathic Medicine, 1255 Sheppard Ave. E., Toronto, Ont., M2K 1E2 Canada; 416-498-1255; www.ccnm.edu

National College of Naturopathic Medicine, 049 SW Porter, Portland, OR 97201; 503-255-4860; www.ncnm.edu

Southwest College of Naturopathic Medicine, 2140 E. Broadway, Tempe, AZ 85282; 480-858-9100; www.scnm.edu

University of Bridgeport, College of Naturopathic Medicine, 60 Lafayette., Bridgeport, CT 06601; 800-392-3582

INTENSIVE HOMEOPATHIC TRAINING PROGRAMS (U.S.)

American Medical College of Homeopathy (2001 W. Camelback #150, Phoenix, AZ 85015; 602-347-7950; www.chiaz.com). Todd Rowe, M.D., who also teaches at the Hahnemann College of Homeopathy, has developed his own school, which also includes clinical supervision.

American University of Complementary Medicine (formerly Curentur University) offers a state-approved course leading to a Master's degree (11543 Olympic Blvd., Los Angeles, CA 90064; 310-914-1446; www.aucm.org).

Evolution of the Self School of Homeopathy (2700 Woodlands Village, #300-250, Flagstaff, AZ 86001; 520-525-2228) offers four- and six-year programs (primary teacher is the highly respected Vega Rozenberg, R.S.Hom).

Homeopathic Academy of Southern California (2236 Rutherford Rd. #115, Carlsbad, CA 92008; 760-494-0542; www.homeopathic-academy.com) has a three-year course with excellent teachers (Allison Maslan, R.S.Hom, and William Mann, LAc).

Homeopathy School of Colorado (P.O. Box 20340, Boulder, CO 80308; 303-440-3717; www.homeopathyschool.org) has a two-year program.

Institute of Classical Homeopathy (2325 Third St. #426, San Francisco, CA 94107; 415-551-1020; www.classichomeopathy.org) offers a four-year program in Napa County, taught by Nikki Henriques.

Luminos Homeopathic Courses (E-31, Bowen Island, BC V0N 1G0, Canada; 604-947-0757; www.homeopathycourses.com) has courses in select cities in the U.S. and Canada.

National Center for Homeopathy (801 N. Fairfax St. #306, Alexandria, VA 22314; 703-548-7790; www. homeopathic.org) offers summer courses for health professionals, including dentists and veterinarians, and laypeople.

New England School of Homeopathy was founded by famed homeopath-naturopath Paul Herscu, N.D., and offers training programs in Massachusetts, Washington, D.C., and occasionally other locations. For information: 356 Middle St., Amherst, MA 01002; 413-256-5949; postgrad@nesh.com.

Northwestern Academy of Homeopathy (5201 Eden Ave. #245, Edina, MN 55436; 612-794-6445; www.homeopathicschool.org) offers a three-year program.

Pacific Academy of Homeopathy (1199 Sanchez St., San Francisco, CA 94114; 415-695-2710; www.Homeopathy-academy.org) sponsors a three-year course for both laypeople and professionals.

Renaissance Institute of Classical Homeopathy (P.O. Box 31025, Santa Fe, NM 87594; www.drluc.com) offers courses in Las Vegas, Nevada and Boston.

South Texas Center for Classical Homeopathy (13526 George Rd. #101, San Antonio, TX 78230; 210-733-0990).

Teleosis School of Homeopathy (5A Lancaster St., Cambridge, MA 02140; 617-547-8500; info@teleosis.com) offers a two-year program plus two years of clinical training. Founder: Joel Kreisberg, DC, CCH. Open only to licensed professionals. Held at Massachusetts College of Pharmacy.

Texas Institute for Homeopathy (1406 Brookstone, San Antonio, TX 78258; 210-492-3162; www.texashomeopathy.com).

INTENSIVE HOMEOPATHIC TRAINING PROGRAMS (CANADA)

Canadian Academy of Homeopathy (1173 Blvd. Du Mont-Royal, Outremont, Quebec H2V 2H6, Canada; 514-279-6629; www.homeopathy.ca).

Canadian College of Naturopathic Medicine (1255 Sheppard Ave. E., N. York, Ont., M2K 1E2 Canada; 416-498-1255; www.ccnm.edu).

Hahnemann Center for Homeopathy and Heilkunst (1445 St. Joseph Blvd., Ottawa, Ontario K1C 7K9; 613-830-2556; www.homeopathy.com).

Toronto School of Homeopathic Medicine (17 Yorkville Ave., #200, Toronto, Ontario M4W 1L1, Canada; 416-966-2350; www.homeopathycanada.com).

Vancouver Homeopathic Academy (P.O. Box 34095, Station D, Vancouver, BC, V6J 4M1 Canada; 604-708-9387).

TRAINING IN HOMEOPATHY
FOR DENTISTS AND VETERINARIANS

Special trainings for dentists are available from **National Dental Seminars** (P.O. Box 123, Marengo, IL 60152).

Training in veterinary homeopathy is available through **Richard Pitcairn**, D.V.M, Ph.D. (1283 Lincoln St., Eugene, OR 97401; 541-342-7665).

CORRESPONDENCE COURSES

Caduceus Institute of Classical Homeopathy (516 Caledonia, Santa Cruz, CA 95012; 800-396-9778 or 831-466-0516). Instructor: Willa Esterson Keizer, C.CH.

Homeopathic Educational Services represents the British Institute of Homeopathy that was developed by pharmacist Trevor Cook, former pharmacist to the Queen of England. One- or two-year courses are available and feature books, tapes, and written material. Various specialty courses in case taking, repertorization, women's health, veterinary care, herbs and nutrition, homeopathic pharmacy, anatomy and physiology, and pathology and the nature of disease are also offered. Contact 800-359-9051 or 510-649-0294; www.homeopathic.com.

CERTIFICATION ORGANIZATIONS

American Board of Homeotherapeutics (617 W. Main St. 4th floor, Charlottesville, VA 22903; 703-548-7790), for certified M.D.s and D.O.s.

Council on Homeopathic Certification (PMB 187, 16915 SE 272nd St. #100, Covington, WA 98042; 866-242-3399; www.homeopathicdirectory.com).

Homeopathic Academy of Naturopathic Physicians (www.hanp. net) is the certifying organization for naturopathic physicians.

North American Society of Homeopaths (P.O. Box 450039, Sunrise, FL 33345; 206-720-7000; www.homeopathy.org).

FOREIGN PROGRAMS OF STUDY

Foundation for Homeopathic Research, founded by one of Rajan Sankaran's leading students, offers a month-long course specifically designed for American and European students and practitioners. Write: FHR, 8-5-Giriraj, Neelkanth Valley, Ghatkopar, Bombay 400 077, India.

Royal London Homoeopathic Hospital (Great Ormond St., London WC1N 3HR, England) offers training programs for M.D.s, D.O.s, and pharmacists.

Also in England are numerous four-year training programs for anyone interested. Contact the **Society of Homoeopaths** for a list of these schools: 11 Brookfield, Duncan Close, Moulton Park, Northampton NN3 6WL, England; 01604-817890; www.homeopathy-soh.org.

A training program for physicians is available at the **University of Oxford's Dept of Continuing Education.** Write: HPTG, 22 Farndon Road, Oxford OX2 6RT, England.

In addition to these various courses, one excellent way to augment one's study of homeopathy is through courses on audiotape and videotape. By reviewing Homeopathic Educational Services' comprehensive catalog, you will find numerous courses of immense value.

MAIN SOURCES FOR HOMEOPATHIC MEDICINES IN THE U.S.

Single remedies and select combination remedies are available at most health food stores. Many pharmacies also sell homeopathic remedies to the public.

Boiron (6 Campus Blvd., Newtown Square, PA 19073; 800-258-8823)

Hahnemann Laboratories (1940 Fourth St., San Rafael, CA 94901; 888-427-6422; www.hahnemannlabs.com)

Homeopathic Educational Services (2124 Kittredge St., Berkeley, CA 94704; 800-359-9051; www.homeopathic.com) (This company sells all products from Boiron, Hahnemann Labs, and Standard.)

Standard Homeopathic (210 West 131st St., Los Angeles, CA 90061; 800-624-9659)

Washington Homeopathic (33 Fairfax St., Berkeley Springs, WV 25411; 800-336-1695; www.homeopathyworks.com)

Notes

Chapter 1: What Is Homeopathy?
1. H. L. Coulter, *Divided Legacy: A History of the Schism in Medical Thought,* p. 432.
2. S. Hahnemann, *The Organon of Medicine,* p. 189.
3. R. Dubos, *Drugs in Our Society,* pp. 38–39.
4. P. W. Bridgman, *The Physics of High Pressure.*
5. D. Ullman, "Principles of Homeopathy," *Co-evolution Quarterly,* Spring, 1981, p. 66.
6. D. Ullman, *The Consumer's Guide to Homeopathy,* p. 14.
7. R. Grossinger, *Planet Medicine,* Chapter 10.

Chapter 4: Homeopathic Research and Clinical Studies
1. R. Smith, "Where Is the Wisdom?" quoted in L. Dossey, "How Should Alternative Therapies Be Evaluated?" *Alternative Therapies in Health and Medicine,* vol. 1, no. 2 (May 1995), p. 83.

About the Author

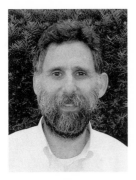

Dennis K. Chernin, MD, MPH, is a medical doctor, a homeopath, and the medical director of two county public health departments in Michigan. He has practiced homeopathic medicine since 1976. Currently, Dr. Chernin practices holistic and family medicine in Ann Arbor, Michigan, where he uses homeopathy as well as nutritional and meditational approaches to health care. He often lectures at the University of Michigan Medical School.

Dr. Chernin received his BA and the Phi Beta Kappa honorary from Northwestern University and his MD and MPH from the University of Michigan. He did residencies in psychiatry and preventive medicine and is board certified in preventive medicine. His three other published books include *Health: A Holistic Approach; Homeopathic Remedies for Health Professionals and Laypeople;* and *How to Meditate Using Chakras, Mantras, and Breath* (with audio CDs).

INSTALLATION INSTRUCTIONS

For Windows operating systems 2000, ME, and XP.

1. Insert the CD.
2. Double-click on My Computer to browse to the CD (on the D: or E: drive).
3. Double-click on the CD drive.
4. Double-click on "setup.exe" (the computer icon), or "setup" if file extensions are hidden on your computer, to run the installation program.

RUNNING THE PROGRAM AFTER INITIAL INSTALLATION

CD must be in drive

Click "Start, Programs, Homeopathy Resource, Homeopathy Resource." To exit, click Main, then Exit.

TO ACCESS THE HR CD TUTORIAL

CD must be in drive

Double-click on My Computer, drive D or E (with HR CD), Tutorial, Chw 16.

To exit the tutorial, click on screen and click Exit, or press the escape key.